ENDOCRINOLOGY RESEARCH AND CLINICAL DEVELOPMENTS

NEW DEVELOPMENTS IN MELATONIN RESEARCH

ENDOCRINOLOGY RESEARCH AND CLINICAL DEVELOPMENTS

Additional books in this series can be found on Nova's website under the Series tab.

Additional e-books in this series can be found on Nova's website under the e-book tab.

BIOCHEMISTRY RESEARCH TRENDS

Additional books in this series can be found on Nova's website under the Series tab.

Additional e-books in this series can be found on Nova's website under the e-book tab.

ENDOCRINOLOGY RESEARCH AND CLINICAL DEVELOPMENTS

NEW DEVELOPMENTS IN MELATONIN RESEARCH

DARIO ACUÑA-CASTROVIEJO
IRYNA RUSANOVA
AND
GERMAINE ESCAMES
EDITORS

New York

For permission to use material from this book please contact us:
Telephone 631-231-7269; Fax 631-231-8175
Web Site: http://www.novapublishers.com

Library of Congress Cataloging-in-Publication Data

ISBN: 978-1-62618-843-3

Library of Congress Control Number: 2013938555

Published by Nova Science Publishers, Inc. † New York

Contents

Preface

From the discovery of melatonin in 1958 by Lerner, it has been a long road of worldwide studies on the physiology, characteristics and medical applications of this molecule. The present book provides updated knowledge on melatonin as versatile non-toxic and beneficial molecule, which begins to have important clinical applications in the treatment of on some disease.

Melatonin is a highly conserved neurohormone present in nearly all studied species. Melatonin is nearly exclusively synthesized during the night in the pineal gland, and mediates information concerning the temporal position and the duration of darkness. Many biological and functional characteristics of this indole hormone, including its chronobiotic, antioxidant and anti-inflammatory properties, have been established to date. These properties account for some interesting applications of the indoleamine, and they can be summarized as follows:

- Circulating melatonin is a main synchronizer of the sleep/wake cycle control and human mood and behavior. Melatonin, as regulator of circadian and seasonal rhythms, can be a useful co-treatment in bipolar patients with sleep alterations. Furthermore, melatonin may have an important role in migraines therapy and other types of headache, particularly those related to sleep phase syndrome disruption.
- Melatonin is a very potent free radical scavenger, especially against the highly toxic hydroxyl radical, and stimulates the endogenous antioxidative system. Melatonin also has anti-inflammatory and immunomodulatory properties and, together with its antioxidant activity, can be useful in counteracting and/or preventing a number of sequels in diseases coursing with oxidative stress and inflammation, including metabolic syndrome, cardiovascular diseases, glaucoma, and neurodegenerative disorders.
- Administration of melatonin has shown not only a promising role on the inhibition of numerous cancer pathways by its oncostatic properties, but also improvements in the quality of life and functional status of patients suffering from aggressive cancers, such as breast, prostate, colorectal, liver, and pancreatic cancer.
- Melatonin acts on the ovary via the hypothalamus-pituitary pathway and directly through its ovarian receptors, influencing the reproductive physiology. Melatonin seems a promising safe putative fertility medication and might open new horizons in infertile management, as it improves oocyte quality, increases fertilization rates and reduces follicular fluid oxidative damage.

- Besides animal species, it is now known that melatonin has a primary function in plants as an antioxidant, yielding protection against environmental insults. Regulation of mitosis, delay of flower induction, stimulation of root growth, adventitious and lateral root regeneration, protection against cold-induced apoptosis, and protection from oxidative damage, are some of the physiological roles of melatonin in plants. These actions are now being evaluated due to their importance in the agro-food field.
- Melatonin has a high safety profile and it reduces the toxicity of many pharmaceutical agents. Thus, besides its direct actions above mentioned, melatonin has additional importance when used in combination with other drugs, reducing their side effects.

The present review provides new information on the molecular pathways of melatonin actions, and on new pharmaceutical formulations of the indoleamine. Due to the studies reporting the safety of melatonin in humans, melatonin is widely employed as a prescription drug and/or nutritional supplement mainly claiming for its effectiveness in sleep-wake cycle regularization. Considering melatonin's high efficacy in reducing oxidative and inflammatory damage, there is increasing interest in its potential use for improving human health, either as a single molecule and/or in a combinatory therapy with other drugs.

We hope that the abundant information presented in this book helps to encourage the better understanding the importance of melatonin in biomedicine, and provide the necessary tools for the clinical use of this molecule.

In: New Developments in Melatonin Research ISBN: 978-1-62618-843-3
Editors: D.Acuña-Castroviejo, I.Rusanova, G.Escames © 2013 Nova Science Publishers, Inc.

Chapter 1

Roles of Melatonin in Humans and Plants

Virginia Sarropoulou*, Kortessa Dimassi-Theriou and Ioannis Therios
Laboratory of Pomology, Department of Horticulture,
School of Agriculture, Aristotle University of Thessaloniki, Greece

Abstract

In this chapter, the important physiological roles of melatonin in humans and in plants are analysed. Melatonin has shown promise in treating sleep onset insomnia in children with autism spectrum disorders (ASD). Furthermore, melatonin due to its antioxidant activity has protective effect in the aging processes. Moreover, melatonin could be involved in the etiology of the breast tumor supporting the hypothesis of a possible oncostatic role of melatonin on hormone-dependent tumors. A number of studies have shown that melatonin levels are lower in Alzheimer's disease (AD) patients compared with aged matched controls. Furthermore, melatonin may play an important role for the treatment of migraines and other types of headache, particularly those related to sleep phase syndrome. As a potent free radical scavenger and antioxidant melatonin scavenges especially highly toxic hydroxyl radicals, and additionally stimulates a number of antioxidative enzymes. Decrease in melatonin concentrations has been observed following stimulation of growth hormone (GH) in children. Melatonin may have a direct effect on bone and act as a bone protector, may impair osteoclast activity, through its free radical scavengering and antioxidant properties. Human studies have shown melatonin to be potentially radioprotective, it has important protective actions in the central nervous system and it is especially beneficial in preserving brain morphology, biochemistry and neurobehavior that are disrupted by ischemia/reperfusion (I/R) or a stroke. Furthermore,

* Corresponding author: Virginia Sarropoulou, Laboratory of Pomology, Department of Horticulture, School of Agriculture. Aristotle University of Thessaloniki, 54124, Thessaloniki, Greece, Emails: vsarropo@agro.auth.gr, vsarrop@gmail.com, Tel: +30 2310 908377, +30 6942037688.

it plays a role in the regulation of biological rhythms. The body temperature presents circadian variations with lower levels during nighttime, when melatonin levels are very high, and thyroid hormones influence shiver independent thermogenesis. A primary function of melatonin in plants is to serve as an antioxidant and plant protector agaist environmental insults. Preservation of the functional chlorophyll is of importance for survival, growth and finally production of plants. Another area in which melatonin promotes plant growth seems to emerge in seeds, seedlings, and in the root system. Regulation of mitosis, delay of flower induction, stimulation of hypocotyls, coleoptile, and root growth, adventitious and lateral root regeneration, protection against cold-induced apoptosis, protection from toxic copper ions, chlorophyll degradation and oxidative damage are some of the physiological roles of melatonin in plants. In higher plants, melatonin affects circadian rhythms and photoperiodic reactions and increases the activities of several antioxidant enzymes. Melatonin's actions via Ca^{2+}-calmodulin may be a potential mechanism of signaling in plants. Melatonin also plays a significant role in the regulation of the reproductive physiology and flower development of *Hypericum perforatum* (St John's wort).

Keywords: Antioxidant, circadian rhythm, flowering, growth, IAA, melatonin synthesis, therapeutic involvement

Introduction

The pineal gland has been known for more than 2000 years. However, there was a common belief that this organ is insignificant and functionless and only after the isolation in 1958 of the active substance of this gland named melatonin (N-acetyl-5-methoxytryptamine) the situation changed. After the discovery of melatonin many scientists including human doctors and plant physiologists become interested in this gland. The last years, a significant progress resulted in the research concerning the roles of this hormone in humans and in plants.

Melatonin is not only produced by the pineal gland but also it was found in varying concentrations in a variety of plants. Its presence was verified by gas chromatography/mass spectrometry. Consumption of plant materials that contain high levels of melatonin could alter blood melatonin levels as well as provide protection of macromolecules against oxidative damage.

Melatonin in Humans – Physiology and Pathology

Melatonin Synthesis in Humans

Melatonin is an indolic hormone mainly secreted by the pineal gland. One of the most striking characteristics of this hormone is that it is secreted only during the night, or more exactly, in darkness. Consequently, the melatonin concentration in plasma is low during the day (in light) and reaches a peak value of about 1 nM during the night (in darkness). The nocturnal secretion of melatonin is very sensitive to the inhibitory effects of light, and the exposure to light at night, even if it is a short-time exposure to light of low intensity, can cause the nocturnal melatonin peak to become either decreased or fully suppressed [1].

Insomnia

Supplemental melatonin has shown promise in treating sleep onset insomnia in children with autism spectrum disorders (ASD). Twenty-four children, free of psychotropic medications, completed an open-label doseescalation study to assess dose–response, tolerability, safety, feasibility of collecting actigraphy data, and ability of outcome measures to detect change during a 14-week intervention. Supplemental melatonin improved sleep latency, as measured by actigraphy, in most children at 1 or 3 mg doses. It was effective the first week of treatment, maintained effects over several months, was well tolerated and safe, and showed improvement in sleep, behavior, and parenting stress. These findings contribute to the growing literature on supplemental melatonin for insomnia in ASD and inform planning for a large randomized trial in this population [2].

Melatonin as an Antioxidant

Melatonin's potential role in aging lies in its non-receptor mediated interactions as a potent oxygen radical scavenger. Studies have shown that endogenous levels of melatonin have oxidative protective effects, with a greater reduction in DNA damage at night, reflecting melatonin's phasic secretion pattern [3]. It scavenges both the superoxide anion and the hydroxyl radical, protecting nuclear DNA, proteins, and membrane lipids against free radical damage, as well as stimulating the activity of glutathione peroxidase, putatively the most important antioxidant in the brain. The indole's lipo- and hydrophilicity are properties unique to antioxidants and allow for rapid diffusion and accessibility to all subcellular components as well as freely crossing the blood-brain barrier. Other antioxidants are confined to particular cellular compartments, such as lipid cell membranes for vitamin E and the cytosol for vitamin C.

It has been discovered, recently, that melatonin is involved in antioxidative defense system of the organism, designed to protect molecules from damage by toxic oxygen radicals [4;5]. Melatonin is a potent free radical scavenger and antioxidant that scavenges especially highly toxic hydroxyl radicals, and additionally stimulates a number of antioxidative enzymes. Because it is both lipophilic and hydrophilic, easily passes all morphophysiological barriers; enters all cells and may carry out its antioxidant function with equal efficiency in multiple cellular compartments, i.e. in the nucleus, cytosol and membranes [6]. Moreover, it is the only antioxidant known to decrease substantially after middle age, and this decrease closely correlates with a decrease in total antioxidant capacity of human serum with age [7]. Question is still open, whether melatonin is efficient free radical scavenger also in physiological concentration or whether the observations made to date are of pharmacological importance only.

However, it should be stressed that compared to two well-known scavengers, glutathione and mannitol, melatonin is 4x and 14x more effective, respectively [8]. Free radical scavenging ability of melatonin has implications for a variety of diseases, including age-associated neurodegenerative diseases and cancer initiation.

Melatonin seems to function *via* a number of means to reduce oxidative stress. Thus, the experimental evidence supports its actions as a direct free radical scavenger [9-11], as an indirect antioxidant when stimulating antioxidant enzymes [12;13], its stimulation of the synthesis of glutathione (an essential intracellular antioxidant) [14], its ability to augment the activities of other antioxidants (or *vice versa*) [15], its protection of antioxidative enzymes from oxidative damage [16;17], and its ability to increase the efficiency of mitochondrial electron transport chain (ETC) thereby lowering electron leakage and reducing free radical generation [18;19].

Melatonin and Aging Process

As the result of the aging process, non-regenerative neuroendocrine cells of the pineal gland, the pinealocytes, degenerate and may have reduced sympathetic innervation as well.

This leads to a concomitant decrease in melatonin production, although studies have shown that caloric restriction helps maintain age-related decline of melatonin production. A reduction in circulating melatonin deprives the brain's capacity for antioxidative defense, furthering the rate of cellular damage with advancing age. It is interesting to note however, that melatonin synthesis is lowest during the light cycle, when oxidative stress reaches maximum values [4;20].

Clinical interests in melatonin reside in its potential as a therapeutic, as the possibility of delaying the aging process sparks great interest among clinicians, scientists, and the general populace alike, along with other clinical uses, such as its potential to resynchronize circadian rhythms for treatment of jet lag after eastward travel [21]. In one study, therapeutic doses of melatonin have shown to increase life-span of an animal model by roughly 20% [22]. Although this and other studies have yet to provide conclusive evidence of melatonin's efficacy as a therapeutic, its pharmacological characteristics at least do not prohibit its use. Melatonin is non-toxic, readily absorbed gastrointestinally, and has low-protein binding and rapid and extensive distribution after oral ingestion. It also readily crosses the blood-brain barrier [3].

Notwithstanding proven efficacy, melatonin can be bought over-the-counter and has already been used as a dietary supplement in hopes of slowing the aging process.

Does Melatonin Play a Role in Aging Processes?

Although there is not clear evidence indicating that melatonin may delay aging there are some reasons to postulate a role for this compound in the aging process: (i) melatonin participates in many vital life processes, and its secretion falls gradually over the life-span; (ii) diminished melatonin secretion in advanced age may be related to deterioration of many circadian rhythms, as a consequence of a reduced function of suprachiasmatic nucleus; (iii) Melatonin acts as endogenous sleep-inducing agent, and its reduced concentrations may result in lowered sleep efficacy very often associated with advancing age; (iv) melatonin exhibits immunoenhancing properties, and suppressed immunocompetence has been implicated in the acceleration of aging processes; (v) melatonin is a potent free radical scavenger, and free radicals cause damage to vital cellular constituents, accumulating with age which has significance not only for aging per se but also for many age-related diseases [23-25]. It has been proposed that melatonin may be of some therapeutic significance.

Moreover, in some countries (e.g. Argentina, China, Poland, USA) melatonin has become recently available as either an over the counter (OTC) drug or food supplement.

There are some widely accepted indications for therapeutic use of melatonin but also perspectives for its broader use. It should be stressed that toxicity of melatonin is remarkably low, and no serious negative side effects of melatonin have been reported, so far [26].

Melatonin and Reproductive System

A relationship exists between melatonin of the pineal gland and reproductive system of animals. This relationship indicates that melatonin regulates the reproduction in seasonally breeding animals by acting at various levels of hypothalamic-pituitary-gonadal axis.

Such relationship between melatonin and reproductive system has been suggested for humans. Hence, melatonin plays a significant role in the normal development of puberty. Abnormal melatonin levels cause precocious or delayed puberty. Furthermore, melatonin may affect the seasonal fluctuation in human reproductive function.

Oncostatic Roles of Melatonin

Animal and human studies, point to immunomodulatory role of melatonin. Such parameters of immune reactivity as number of immune cells and their subpopulations, lymphocyte proliferation and blood level of different cytokines exhibit circadian rhythmicity and these diurnal changes seem to be controlled by the pineal melatonin synthesis. It appeard that melatonin may exert a direct effect on the immune system because melatonin receptors have been discovered in immune organs and cells of humans. Cultured human lymphocytes synthesize and release large amount of melatonin which could act, in addition to its endocrine effect, as an intacrine, autocrine, and/or paracrine substance for the local coordination of the immune response. Hence, endogenous melatonin is an essential part for an accurate response of human lymphocytes through the modulation on interleukin-2/interleukin-2 receptor system. Anyway, the relationship between melatonin and immune system seems to be complex and needs further study.

Among the proposed actions of melatonin [27;28], those supporting the hypothesis of a possible oncostatic role of melatonin on hormone-dependent tumors are: (a) the down-regulation of the hormones of the neuroendocrine reproductive axis, leading to a decrease in the circulating levels of gonadal steroids, and (b) the ability of melatonin to counteract the effects of estrogens at the level of the estrogen targets, that is to say, to behave as a naturally occurring antiestrogen. Both the enhancement of immune function induced by melatonin [29] as well as the antioxidant properties of this indolamine [4] has also been considered among those mechanisms involved in its oncostatic actions. In 1978 an article published in *The Lancet* [30] proposed, for the first time, the theory of the possible role of the pineal gland on the etiology of breast cancer. These authors suggested that a decrease in pineal function, whatever its cause, and the consequent reduction in melatonin secretion, could induce a state of relative hyperestrogenism, and the early and prolonged exposure of the breast tissue to the estrogens could be involved in etiology of the breast tumor. A few years later, Tamarkin et al. [31], in an article in *Science*, described a relationship between plasma melatonin concentration and breast cancer. Women with estrogen receptor (ER)-positive breast adenocarcinomas had nocturnal plasmatic concentrations of melatonin significantly lower than healthy women or women suffering ER-negative breast tumors. Whether these changes in melatonin secretion were the origin or the consequence of the tumoral process was not, however, clarified.

From that promising article until now, the data supporting a possible role of melatonin on human breast cancer have, unfortunately, been very scarce and most of them consist of indirect evidence resulting from epidemiological studies. These studies suggest a relationship between pineal function and the risk of breast cancer, based on the low incidence of breast cancer among blind women [32-34] as well as on the inverse association between breast cancer incidence and degree of visual impairment [35]. In these cases, the total or partial suppression of the light input could mediate an increase in melatonin circulating levels that could explain the low incidence of tumors. On the other hand, the high incidence of breast cancer among women exposed to light during the night (such as shift workers) [36] or exposed to low frequency electromagnetic fields [37;38] could be explained by the decreased melatonin synthesis under these environmental conditions.

In conclusion, (1) Melatonin, through its antigonadotropic and antiestrogenic actions, behaves as an antitumoral agent on hormonedependent mammary tumors. (2) These oncostatic properties of melatonin have consistently been demonstrated on *in vivo* models of chemically induced rat mammary tumors as well as *in vitro* on MCF-7 human breast cancer cells. (3) The possible role of melatonin on human breast tumors is only supported by indirect data. (4) The characteristics of melatonin's oncostatic actions, comprising different aspects of tumor biology such as initiation, proliferation, and metastasis as well as the physiological doses at which the effect is accomplished, give special value to these findings and encourage clinical studies on the possible therapeutic value of melatonin in breast cancer [39].

Alzheimer's Disease (AD)

In Alzheimer's disease (AD) patients with disturbed sleep-wake rhythms there is also a higher degree of irregularities in melatonin secretion [40]. An impairment of melatonin secretion is present that is related to both age and severity of mental impairment. The nocturnal growth hormone secretion and both the mean levels and nadir values of plasma cortisol are also related to mental impairments [41].

Pineal Changes

A number of studies have shown that melatonin levels are lower in AD patients compared with aged matched controls [40;42-45]. The daily variations in pineal melatonin and 5-methoxytryptophol content disappeared in AD patients [45;46] maybe linked with the clinical observations of sleep disorders and sundowning in these patients. Others have reported that there is a selective impairment of the nocturnal melatonin peak in dementia [42] or that the melatonin levels are increased in AD patients during daytime and that these patients do not react to bright light [44].

SCN Changes

The neurodegenerative process in AD affects the hypothalamic suprachiasmatic nuclei (SCN) pacemaker which, in turn, affects melatonin rhythmicity [47].

Retina

Not only the retina but also the optic nerve, which provides direct and indirect light input to the SCN, show degenerative changes in AD [48-51]. In the macula of AD patients retinal cell degeneration has been observed without neurofibrillary tangles, neuritic plaques or amyloid angiopathy being present in the retina or optic nerves [48;49;52]. Extensive neuronal loss (36%) was reported throughout the entire retina of AD patients, but being most pronounced in the superior and inferior quadrants. The ratio of astrocytes to neurons is significantly higher in AD [48;49;52], indicating that a process of neurodegeneration takes place.

On the other hand, there are also a number of observations suggesting that visual deficits in AD do not stem from neuroretinal dysfunction. Although earlier work showed a higher proportion of abnormalities in the retinal nerve fiber layer of AD patients than in controls [53] by scanning laser polarimetry the retinal nerve fiber layer thickness was not altered in the earlier stages of AD [54].

Effect of Melatonin on Sundowning in AD Patients

Melatonin decreases sundowning in AD patients [55]. A significant decrease in agitated behaviors and confusion in the evening hours, or 'sundowning' has been seen following melatonin administration [56]. In addition to melatonin's ability to phase shift circadian rhythms [57], in in vitro experiments melatonin was found to function as an antioxidant and neuroprotector in rat and primate brain tissue [12;58;59]. Melatonin has also been reported to protect neurones against b-amyloid toxicity [60;61], to prevent b-amyloid-induced lipid peroxidation [62] and to alter the metabolism of the b-amyloid precursor protein [63]. The decreased levels of melatonin in AD may thus be involved in the pathogenesis of AD. However, this remains to be proven [47].

Role of Melatonin in the Regulation of Human Circadian Rhythms and Sleep

The circadian rhythm of pineal melatonin is the best marker of internal time under low ambient light levels. The endogenous melatonin rhythm exhibits a close association with the endogenous circadian component of the sleep propensity rhythm. This has led to the idea that melatonin is an internal sleep 'facilitator' in humans, and therefore useful in the treatment of insomnia and the readjustment of circadian rhythms. There is evidence that administration of melatonin is able: (i) to induce sleep when the homeostatic drive to sleep is insufficient; (ii) to inhibit the drive for wakefulness emanating from the circadian pacemaker; and (iii) induce phase shifts in the circadian clock such that the circadian phase of increased sleep propensity occurs at a new, desired time. Therefore, exogenous melatonin can act as soporific agent, a chronohypnotic, and/or a chronobiotic [64].

Therapeutic Potential of Melatonin in Migraines and Other Headache Types

Melatonin may play an important therapeutic role for the treatment of migraines and other types of headaches, particularly those related to delayed sleep phase syndrome. Current research supports the hypothesis that migraines are a response to a pineal gland circadian irregularity in which the administration of melatonin normalizes this circadian cycle; i.e., melatonin may play a role in resynchronizing biological rhythms to lifestyle and subsequently relieve migraines and other forms of headaches. In addition, research testing the administration of melatonin found that it is safe in migraine sufferers, with few or no side effects [65].

The Pineal Gland, Melatonin and the Migraine Connection

The pineal gland is considered a photoneuroendocrine transducer that translates environmental information into neuroendocrine molecules [66-68] explain that melatonin, an indole compound, is the net result of this transduction. Melatonin is synthesized from serotonin via the enzyme N-acetyltransferase, which is emitted in a circadian cycle from the suprachiasmatic nucleus [66]. Also, the suprachiasmatic nucleus receives light stimuli via the retinohypothalamic tract. Of interest is Jacobsen's description of an oculocephalic sympathetic abnormality associated with migraine sufferers, the neural pathway of which regulates the secretion of melatonin by the pineal gland [68].

Biochemical Studies of Melatonin and Migraines

Migraine sufferers without depression had lower nocturnal plasma melatonin levels than controls, and migraine patients with superimposed depression exhibited the greatest deficiency of melatonin compared to the control group [65]. In another study, Brun and colleagues (1995) collected urine samples (between 7 p.m. and 7 a.m.) throughout an entire menstrual cycle, and measured melatonin levels in 10 female patients suffering menstrually associated migraines without aura. Controls consisted of nine females matched for age, body surface area, length of cycle, and fertility [66]. Compared to controls, the migraine patients had lower mean nocturnal melatonin throughout the entire menstrual cycle with no differences between luteal and follicular phases, whereas controls displayed only lower follicular phase melatonin. No correlation was found between time of headache or intensity of pain and nocturnal melatonin excretion. The highest levels of melatonin in migraine patients were during menses; the authors note this could reflect rhythmic changes due to pain and/or dyssomnia. However, since lower levels of melatonin were noted outside attacks, the authors speculated that decreases of melatonin might serve as a marker of impending migraine. The authors conclude that the abnormality of melatonin secretion in migraine patients over the entire cycle could be a sympathetic hypofunction and represents a "vulnerability of the rhythmic organization of the central nervous system." Murialdo et al. [69] state that, "Sympathetic dysfunction in migraine, enhanced during the acute pain attack, could explain the decreased urinary levels of melatonin in our patients and the further fall in indole excretion during headache episodes." Although only three studies could be found that directly test melatonin in migraine patients, together they suggest female migraine sufferers have decreased nocturnal plasma melatonin levels both overall and during migraine attacks.

Melatonin and Growth Hormone (GH)

The relationship between melatonin and growth hormone (GH) is poorly understood. Decrease in melatonin concentrations has been observed following stimulation of GH (due to insulin-induced hypoglycemia, arginine infusion, clonidine administration, or growth hormone releasing hormone stimulation) in children. Moreover, our recent results showed that melatonin levels were significantly higher in children with GH deficiency in comparison with children with idiopathic short stature, and there was negative correlation between GH peak after stimulation test and nocturnal melatonin concentrations [70]. Administration of melatonin caused either enhancement of spontaneous and exercise-induced GH secretion [71;72], or did not exert any effect [73]. However, the role of melatonin in mechanisms of regulation of growth hormone secretion seems to be secondary and not important.

Melatonin and Neurodegenerative Diseases

A role for melatonin in neurodegenerative diseases (such as Alzheimer's and Parkinson's diseases) has been recently suggested. The experimental findings indicate that melatonin may act in a variety of ways to reduce neuronal loss in Alzheimer's disease by altering the process of generation and action of amyloid-b leading to increased cellular survival. Melatonin concentrations decrease in some, but not all, patients suffering from Alzheimer's disease. Decreased nocturnal melatonin levels were found both in preclinical and definite Alzheimer's patients. Many reports demonstrated that melatonin treatment seems to constitute a selection therapy to improve sleep, to ameliorate sundowning, and to slow evolution of cognitive impairment in Alzheimer's patients [74;75]. There are also experimental data suggesting a role of melatonin in another neurodegenerative disorder, Parkinson's disease which is characterized by the progressive deterioration of dopamine-containing neurons in the pars compact of the substantia nigra in the brain stem due to the oxidation of dopamine [76]. There is evidence that melatonin may reduce dopamine auto-oxidation under experimental conditions [77] although its administration did not slow progression of the Parkinson disease [74].

Melatonin as a Bone Protector

Melatonin may have a direct effect on bone health and acts as a bone protector. Suppression of melatonin secretion lowered serum calcium concentration, an effect prevented by melatonin administration. Treatment of ovariectomized rats with melatonin prevents bone loss by an effect partly dependent on residual estradiol levels. Melatonin presumably acts as an autacoid in bone cells since it is present in high quantities in bone marrow, where bone cell precursors are located. Melatonin dose-dependently augments proteins that are incorporated into the bone matrix, like procollagen type I c-peptide.

Osteoprotegerin, an osteoblastic protein that inhibits the differentiation of osteoclasts is also augmented by melatonin in vitro. Melatonin through its free radical scavenging and antioxidant properties may impair osteoclast activity [78].

Radioprotective Effect of Melatonin

Human studies have shown melatonin to be potentially radioprotective [79;80]. Moreover, it is a more efficient protector than amifostine, a commonly used agent for this purpose [81]. The mechanism of melatonin in protection against ionizing radiation is thought to involve scavenging of free radicals [82].

It is estimated that nearly 70% of biological damage caused by ionizing radiation is attributable to the free radical, especially the hydroxyl radical that attacks DNA, proteins, and cellular membranes. Melatonin has been suggested as a radioprotective agent, with the proposed advantages of being broadly protective, readily available, orally self-administered, and without major known side effects [83].

Melatonin Protects Against Ischemia/Reperfusion (I/R) Injury

The multifaceted functions of melatonin have proven that this molecule has important protective actions in the central nervous system and it has been shown to be especially beneficial in preserving brain morphology, biochemistry and neurobehavior that are disrupted by ischemia/reperfusion (I/R) or a stroke. Unfortunately, many methods that have been found to be effective in protecting the brain in experimental I/R models, have failed to be useful in the clinical situation. With regard to melatonin, it has never been examined as to its potential protective actions during ischemia and reperfusion of the brain of humans. It has, however, been widely tested in humans where it possesses potent antioxidant activity (as in animals) [84-86] and, furthermore, it has never been found to be toxic or to have significant side effects. In view of this, it should be given consideration not only for protection of the brain from I/R injury but other organs as well where the consequences of hypoxia and reoxygenation are highly detrimental.

The Hypothalamic-Pituitary Axis and Melatonin in Humans: Possible Interactions in the Control of Body Temperature

Melatonin plays a role in the regulation of biological rhythms, such as in body temperature which presents circadian variations with lower levels during nighttime, when melatonin levels are very high, and thyroid hormones influence shiver independent thermogenesis [87]. Melatonin has been demonstrated to play an important role in the regulation of biological rhythms [88]. The secretion of melatonin by the pineal gland is regulated by a neural pathway including the retina, a specific retino-hypothalamic tract leading to the suprachiasmatic nucleus, which projects fibers to the superior cervical ganglion, that innervates the pineal with sympathetic fibers [89]. Activity of the retino-hypothalamic-pineal system is influenced by environmental lighting conditions, with an inhibitory effect of light on melatonin secretion, whose variations are able to convey within the organism information about photoperiodic changes [90]. The melatonin mediated photoperiodic message is a fundamental cue for the circadian and seasonal coordination of biological functions [28]. The body temperature in humans presents a circadian rhythm, influenced but dissociable from the sleep/wake cycle, with a minimum during nighttime, when melatonin levels are at their maximum [91;92]. Thyroid hormones increase thermogenesis by enhancement of mitochondrial oxidative metabolism [93]. In the pineal gland a type II thyroxine 5'-deiodinating activity (5'–D II) with nighttime increase has been found, melatonin stimulates this 5'–D II activity in the brown adipose tissue (BAT) and a complex interaction among light, pineal, fat body mass and serum thyroxine has been demonstrated in experimental animals [94;95].

Thyroid secretion is positively correlated with thyrotropin-releasing hormone (TRH) serum levels during the day and negatively correlated with thyroid-stimulating hormone (TSH) and melatonin serum levels at night, while TRH and TSH serum levels are positively correlated late at night and in the morning. Body temperature is positively correlated with free-thyroxine (FT4) serum levels in the morning and negatively correlated with melatonin serum levels at night [87]. Melatonin may infuence thermoregulation increasing vasodilation and peripheral heat loss and may also regulate thermogenesis [96-98]. Thyroid hormones are photoperiod-dependent in animals [99] and an inhibitory action of the pineal gland on hypothalamic-pituitary-thyroid axis (with reduced thyroid response to TSH in the presence of elevated melatonin levels) has been evidenced in hamsters and rats and in vitro (100). The response of anterior pituitary to hypothalamic TRH and of thyroid to hypophyseal TSH may be influenced by melatonin levels, so that melatonin may modulate the function of the hypothalamic-pituitary-thyroid axis and influence the circadian variability of body temperature [87].

Physiological Functions of Melatonin in Plants

Several early studies have shown that melatonin exhibits effects similar to those of the plant growth hormone, auxin, which stimulates plant growth [101]. Other studies have pointed out that melatonin may promote or inhibit plant flowering as well as the maturation of plants [102-106].

Rather, progressively more data support the idea that a primary function of melatonin in plants is to serve as an antioxidant and a plant protector against environmental stresses. This suggestion is initiated by the observations that cold stress significantly elevates melatonin production in plants [107]. This observation was followed by the identification of high levels of melatonin in a pollutant resistant plant, the water hyacinth Eichhornia crassipes [82]. This species tolerates extremely polluted environments and, therefore, it is used in phytoremediation [108]. The high levels of melatonin in this plant are believed to play a pivotal role in preparing it against the environmental insults that generate ROS. Numerous studies have, in fact, mentioned the protective effects of exogenously applied melatonin to plants against a variety of oxidative stresses and harsh environments. These stressors include extremely cold or hot environments [109-111], UV irradiation [112;113], copper [82], cadmium, salted soil and hydrogen peroxide toxicity [114]. The protective effects of melatonin against these stressors were attributed to its free radical scavenging and antioxidant capacity [114;115].

Plants lack mobility like that of animals, except for leaf movements, and the high levels of antioxidants including melatonin in plants may be a compensatory mechanism for them to tolerate and survive in hostile environments. Oxidative stress, such as UV irradiation, probably consumes large quantities of melatonin in plants. This is supported by a recent field of study which showed that when grapes are in the shade of leaves and branches (passive avoidance of UV irradiation compared with active avoidance by animals), melatonin concentrations in these grapes are 10-fold higher than those that are directly exposed to sunlight [114;116]. It is documented that melatonin directly scavenges ROS in plants and decreases the levels of malonldiadehyde (MDA) in leaves of mung bean plant (*Vigna radiata*) exposed to UV-B [117] and dose-dependently protects against oxidative DNA damage as well as promoting DNA repair in plant protoplasts of *Gentiana macrophylla* after irradiation with different doses of UV-B [113]. In seedlings of cucumbers subjected to heat stress, melatonin sprayed on the leaves significantly reduced the concentration of MDA, superoxide anion, and hydrogen peroxide in these tissues [111].

In addition to the direct interactions of melatonin with ROS, melatonin application also elevates the endogenous antioxidant enzymes in plants. These include peroxidase, superoxide anion dismutase (SOD), catalase (CAT), ascorbate peroxidase, monodehydroascorbate reductase (MDHAR), and glutathione reductase [111]. As a result, the content of other antioxidants, namely ascorbic acid, vitamin E, and glutathione, are protected from oxidative damage [101].

Studies also have shown that not only exogenously applied but also endogenously produced melatonin in the plants possesses the same antioxidant capacity. Transgenic plants rich in endogenous melatonin have a higher total antioxidative capacity and lower oxidatively damaged or damaging products (reduced MDA, O^-_2, and H_2O_2) compared with their non-transgenic wild-type counterparts which have lower endogenous melatonin levels [111;117]. Outcomes of high melatonin levels in plants are elevated rates of germination of seeds under unfavourable conditions [118], an enhanced survival rate [119], and improved quality of the plant products. The quality of the plant products can be judged from the contents of the nutritional ingredients they contain. Studies document that elevated levels of melatonin in plants essentially completely preserve the content of b-carotenoids, double the levels of vitamin E, and significantly increase the quantities of vitamin C and glutathione [111;117]. The preservation of other antioxidants by melatonin strongly suggests that melatonin is the first line of defence against the oxidative stress occurring in plants. Other antioxidants preserved by melatonin may be used for other purposes, for example to intensify the colour of the flowers or function as back-up protection after melatonin is consumed [115].

Another important feature of melatonin as the first-line defence against oxidative stress is its stress-inducible characteristic in plants. A broad spectrum of stresses including cold temperature, UV exposure, H_2O_2, copper, and other environmental toxic chemicals significantly up-regulate endogenous melatonin production [101;112;120]. An obvious advantage of a stress-inducible antioxidant such as melatonin is to upgrade the antioxidant capacity of the organisms when they experience low intensity insults and to pre-condition them to cope with upcoming stronger stressors. This increases their chance of survival; without pre-conditioning, a given species would be damaged or even destroyed by a rapid onset intensive stress. Whether the antioxidant capacity of melatonin in plants is exclusively dependent on its direct interaction with ROS or whether this is mediated by melatonin receptors is currently unknown. Melatonin receptors have not been reported in plants [101].

Several investigators have studied the physiological roles of melatonin in plants [106;121]. Studies suggest that melatonin is involved in many functions in plants, including regulation of mitosis [122;123] delaying flower induction [106], the stimulation of hypocotyl, coleoptile, and root growth [124;125], adventitious and lateral root regeneration [120;124] and protection against cold-induced apoptosis (109), toxic copper ions [126], chlorophyll degradation [127], and oxidative damage [112].

Chlorophyll Preservation, Photosynthetic Stimulation, and the Potential for Improving Crop Production

In green plants or other organisms such as green algae, chlorophyll is the major molecule responsible for photosynthesis. Via this process, energy contained in photons is captured by chlorophyll and used for the synthesis of carbohydrates. Chlorophyll is fragile and easily injured by ROS which are generated either during the photosynthetic process or by the environmental variations including cold or hot temperatures and extensive visible or UV irradiation [128;129]. Preservation of the functional chlorophyll is of importance for the survival, growth, and finally the production of plants.

As an antioxidant, melatonin certainly has the capability of protecting against the degradation of chlorophyll. Arnao and Hernandez-Ruiz incubated barley leaves with a solution containing 1 mM melatonin for 48 h and found that the chlorophyll content in the melatonin-treated leaves was 2-fold higher than that in untreated leaves [127]. This was the first report to show that melatonin protected chlorophyll against oxidative stress. Thereafter, the chlorophyll-preserving effects of melatonin were confirmed in cucumber seedling subjected to heat stress [110] and also in a photosynthetic green macroalga (Ulva sp.) [130]. In Ulva, both endogenously produced and exogenously applied melatonin preserved the chlorophylls when the algae were subjected to hostile weather or metals which are toxic for this organism, namely zinc, lead, and cadmium. The chlorophyll protective effects of melatonin in the green macroalga relate to the radical scavenging activity of this indoleamine. Accordingly, melatonin levels in the green macroalga under these environmental stresses were found to be significantly up-regulated, which indicates an inducible characteristic of melatonin responsive to stressors also in this organism [130].

The findings on chlorophyll preservation may be in accordance with earlier findings on melatonin's capacity to delay leaf senescence under conditions of abiotic stress, in both monocots (corn) and dicots (cucumber and tobacco). In addition to preserving the integrity of chlorophyll, melatonin also increases the photosynthetic efficiency of chlorophyll in plants. When melatonin was sprayed on cucumber seedlings at a concentration of 25–100 μM, the net photosynthetic rate was increased both under normal temperature conditions and when the seedlings were subjected to heat stress. Accordingly, the intercellular CO_2 concentrations were reduced [110]. This indicates that more CO_2 contained in the leaves is being converted to carbohydrates with the accelerated photosynthesis as a consequence of melatonin treatment. Melatonin treatment also preserves the chlorophyll content of apple leaves which are subjected to oxidative stress following exposure to H_2O_2; the indoleamine also maximizes their photosysten II efficiency as well as elevates their ascorbic acid levels [131].

Another area in which melatonin apparently promotes plant growth seems to emerge in seeds, seedlings, and in the root system [101]. Melatonin promotes seed germination as reported in cucumber and in red cabbage [118;126]. A currently ongoing study, conducted at cold temperatures, in which pea seeds were hydroprimed with or without melatonin (5 μM), showed that the germination rate of melatonin-treated seeds was 73.2%, whereas 53.7% of the non-melatonin-treated seeds germinated (RJ Reiter et al., unpublished observations). In another preliminary study, Posmyk hydroprimed corn seeds with or without melatonin. After germination, the seedlings were planted in the field without further treatment and allowed to grow naturally. At harvesting, the melatonin-treated corn plants had a larger root system compared with non-melatonin-treated corn plants. This interesting observation implies that during the seed germination stage, melatonin initiated the irreversible gene expression for root development and this effect had consequences for, or even persisted throughout, the rest of the growing season. The one time melatonin treated corn seeds also developed plants with notably larger corn cobs than those of non-melatonin-treated plants. It was estimated that the production of the corn from the melatonin-treated plants was 20% greater than that from the non-melatonin-treated plants.

One well-designed study has reported that in plants (barley and lupin) the highest melatonin levels are in the roots with an obvious gradient between different root parts. The order from high to low melatonin levels is apical, central, and basal portions of the root system [132]. The root-promoting action has also been observed in high level melatonin transgenic rice plants. In these plants, the chlorophyll content and root system are elevated above those in wild-type plants [133]. In addition to promoting root growth, melatonin stimulates root regeneration [114]. Sarropoulou et al. recently observed that melatonin, at the concentration of 1 μM, dramatically enhanced adventitious root regeneration in in vitro shoot tip explants of the commercial sweet cherry rootstocks CAB-6P (*Prunus cerasus*), however, at a concentration of 10 μM, melatonin had an inhibitory effect on root generation. This is the first report to show that melatonin influences root development in a fruit tree [134].

Recently, it has been reported that *Hordeum vulgare* L. leaves treated with melatonin solutions clearly slowed the senescence process, as estimated from the chrorophyll loss in leaves; this protective effect against senescence was melatonin concentration-dependent. These authors suggest that melatonin may have a specific action on the chrorophyll-degrading enzymeschlorophyllase, pheophorbide a oxygenase or red-chlorophyll catabolite reductase. They also did not preclude the possibility that the indole may prevent the generation of free radicals and thereby delay the senescence process [127].

Discoveries to date indicate that the beneficial effects of melatonin in plants may be multifaceted: (i) melatonin increases the plant germination rate; (ii) enhances the capacities of plants to resist a variety of environmental insults, especially cold and hot temperatures which are important factors in determining crop production; (iii) preserves the chlorophyll content and promotes its photosynthetic rate; as a result, plants synthesize more carbohydrates and increase their biomass; and (iv) promotes the development of the root system, which could lead to a greater absorptive capacity of nutrients from the soil [101].

Melatonin as a Growth Promoter in Plants

The protective role of melatonin against apoptosis during cold-treatment in cell suspensions of Daucus carota has been described [109]. Other actions ascribed to melatonin include a possible role as plant growth regulator, for example in the dicot Lupinus albus L. and in several monocots (wheat, barley, oat and canary grass). Indeed, growth-promotion activity in hypocotyls and coleoptiles and a growth-inhibition in roots by melatonin has been described [103;125]. Also, the generation capacity of de novo roots (rhizogenesis) by melatonin has been studied in primary and adventitious roots of lupin seedlings [114], and the expansion of cotyledons through cellular expansion in lupin has been added to its specific roles in plants [132]. Recently, it has been reported that barley leaves treated with melatonin clearly delay the dark-induced senescence process [127]. Lei et al. demonstrated that melatonin treatment (at different concentrations) of Daucus carota L. cultured root cells attenuated cold-induced cell apoptosis [109]. Also, the incubation of Brassica oleracea L. seeds with exogenous melatonin solutions (hydropriming) had a protective effect against copper, a highly toxic metal [126]. Tan et al. demonstrated that melatonin added to the soil enhanced the tolerance and survival of pea plants against copper contamination, proposing that the presence of melatonin in plants can be used for phytoremediation applications [82].

Additional evidence indicating the involvement of melatonin in root formation was obtained in a study of the etiolated hypocotyls of Lupinus albus [114]. Exogenously applied melatonin stimulated adventitious root generation in amounts proportional to concentrations from 0.001 to 10 μM. In the same concentration range of melatonin, lateral root induction was optimal at 1 μM.

Melatonin affects the cytoskeleton, causing either microtubule enlargement or depolymerization. It was proposed that at physiological concentrations (10^{-9} M) melatonin antagonizes the inhibition of tubulin polymerization caused by calmodulin and thus stimulates microtubule growth. At pharmacological levels (10^{-7}–10^{-5} M), melatonin binds to tubulin and prevents its polymerization [135]. These effects were observed in both animals and plants. In higher plants, 10^{-4} M melatonin increases birefringence of the mitotic spindle (i.e. stimulates microtubule assembly) in Haemanthus katherinae [123]. In contrast, $8x10^{-4}$ M melatonin causes microtubule depolymerization and therefore disrupts the mitotic apparatus in onion root tips [122].

Melatonin's action in plants via Ca^{2+}-calmodulin may be a potential mechanism of signalling in plants in view of the Ca^{2+}-dependent activity of auxin in several physiological responses. Melatonin is known to have a high affinity for calmodulin and, moreover, it has remarkable effects on the cytoskeleton in plants [136]. Melatonin causes protein-kinase Ca^{2+}-dependent inhibition, with the interaction of calmodulin-kinase being relevant to rearrangements of the cytoskeleton, which represents some of the earliest effects described for melatonin, including plants [137]. In fact, melatonin was reported to stimulate the microtubule assembly in Haemanthus katharinae Baker while, in contrast, it caused microtubule depolymerization, disrupting the mitotic apparatus in the onion root tip [106]. On the other hand, the activation of calcium channels that change cell polarity resulted in an increase in melatonin (and the related indoles auxin and serotonin) in Echinacea purpurea (L.) Moench explants, together with an inhibition in thidiazuron-induced callus induction [104]. Since, at physiological concentrations, melatonin has been proposed to antagonize the inhibition of tubulin polymerization caused by calmodulin, thereby stimulating microtubule growth, and at pharmacological levels the indole binds to tubulin preventing its polymerization [135], these observations may possibly be related to the growth-promoting effects with low concentrations of melatonin and the inhibition provoked by high concentrations of melatonin reviewed in this section.

Melatonin has also been proposed to play a significant role in the regulation of the reproductive physiology and flower development of Hypericum perforatum L. (St John's wort) because the highest concentrations of the indole are detected during uninucleate microsporogenesis and the enhanced regenerative potential of isolated anthers at the stage of elevated melatonin contents [138]. Melatonin might also contribute to the maintenance of dormancy germs or to a differentiated state in fruit tissue [139]. Elevated levels in some juicy fruits may indicate a role in fruit ripening and/or a function in the maintenance of developmental stages that may extend to the persistence of dormancy.

Cell elongation is a key process in root growth. Reactive oxygen species (ROS), including the hydroxyl radical, reportedly activate Ca^{2+} channels allowing Ca^{2+} influx, which enhances cell elongation [140]. Another study indicated that the hydroxyl radical makes cell membranes more permeable, also leading to enhanced cell elongation [141]. Moreover, one of the metabolites formed when melatonin scavenges radicals is N^1-acetyl-N^2-formyl-5-methoxykynuramine (AFMK) [82], which likely fuctions as an antioxidant [142]. Thus, high concentrations of melatonin and AFMK might reduce ROS in root cells and thereby inhibit ROS-induced cell growth [112]. Melatonin has a high affinity to Ca^{2+}/calmodulin (CaM), which inhibits intercellular Ca^{2+}/CaM-dependent functions [137;143]. It has been shown that CaM inhibitors reduce root growth and that this inhibitory action can be counteracted by the addition of exogenous CaM. Thus, the negative effect of high concentrations of melatonin on root elongation may be a result of melatonin-related changes in CaM antagonism [124].

Growth Regulation and Plant Development

Auxin inhibits the elongation of preexisting roots in contrast that it stimulates root formation. Exogenously applied melatonin inhibited root growth in mustard in a manner similar to auxin [124] (However, it is still unclear whether melatonin induces auxin biosynthesis or if melatonin itself can be metabolized and converted to IAA. According to Park (2011), the effects of exogenously applied melatonin on vegetative development are: increase of germination rate, stimulation of coleoptile elongation, promotion of lateral leaflet generation, inhibition of root elongation and, adventitious and lateral root formation in regeneration system. Regarding reproductive development, the effects or characteristic changes of melatonin are: influence on flowering, stage-specific accumulation during fruit development, and high accumulation in maturating seeds. As concerns senescence, preservation of chlorophyll during senescence and attenuation of apoptosis are the characteristic effects of melatonin while as regards stress resistance, protective effects against oxidative stress, resistance against cold stress and tolerance to photodamage and UV-B are the physiological roles of melatonin in plants.

Regulation of Circadian Rhythms and Photoperiodic Reactions in Higher Plants

Several authors therefore tested whether melatonin affects circadian rhythms and/or photoperiodic reactions also in higher plants. This possibility is indirectly supported by the finding that melatonin levels in the dicot plant *Chenopodium rubrum* exhibit a diurnal rhythm with a night maximum [105]. Because melatonin application in long days causes short-day responses in some vertebrates, effects of melatonin administration were investigated in several species of plants with photoperiodically controlled flowering [105;144]. Similarly, melatonin treatment 1, 2, or 4 hr before lights off does not induce flowering of the water plants *Spirodela polyrhiza, Lemna minor*, and *Lemna trisulca* in non-inductive photoperiods [105;139]. Melatonin at concentrations 10^{-4} or $5x10^{-4}$ M also does not significantly influence flowering of the long-day plant *Chenopodium murale*. The most convincing effect of melatonin on a photoperiodic response in a higher plant was found in the short-day plant *C. rubrum* [106].

Melatonin as an Antioxidant in Plants

Leaves of different varieties of Nicotiana tabacum L. (tobacco) were differentially sensitive to ozone damage, with the sensitivity being reduced in leaves with the highest melatonin concentrations [145]. Therefore, sufficiently high melatonin levels seem to protect plants against damage from ozone, a free radical generator, which in high concentrations decreases plant height, results in visible foliar injury at all growth stages, and progressively reduces the fresh weight of fruits when applied at flowering [145;146].

The high amounts of melatonin detected in seeds have been hypothesized to be essential for protecting germ and reproductive tissues from oxidative damage due to UV light, drought, extremes in temperature, and environmental toxins [147;148]. As an example, its presence in Juglans regia L. (walnut) may be to protect the highly oxidizable lipids from oxidation, thereby preserving the viability of the nut (seed) so it will subsequently germinate successfully [13]. It has also been suggested that the amphiphility of melatonin may favour its accumulation especially in oily seeds, presumably providing antioxidative protection within a dormant and more or less dry system, in which enzymes are poorly effective and cannot be upregulated. Melatonin increases activities of several antioxidant enzymes: superoxide dismutase (SOD, both MnSOD and CuSOD), catalase, glutathione peroxidase (GPx), glutathione reductase (GRd) and glucose-6-phosphate dehydrogenase [12;16]. Melatonin stimulates the rate-limiting enzyme of glutathione (GSH) synthesis, c-glutamylcysteine synthase, and thus increases intracellular concentration of GSH [14]. Melatonin also increases the expression of genes coding for antioxidative enzymes, especially SOD [149].

Conclusion

In conclusion, melatonin plays very important roles in humans and plants both by its endogenous levels and by exogenous application.

References

[1] Brainard GC, Rollag MD, Hanifin JP. Photic regulation of melatonin in humans: ocular and neural signal transduction. *J. Biol. Rhythms* 1997 Dec;12(6):537-46.

[2] Malow B, Adkins KW, McGrew SG, Wang L, Goldman SE, Fawkes D, et al. Melatonin for sleep in children with autism: a controlled trial examining dose, tolerability, and outcomes. *J. Autism Dev. Disord.* 2012 Aug;42(8):1729-37.

[3] Arendt J, Broadway J. Light and melatonin as zeitgebers in man. *Chronobiol. Int.* 1987;4(2):273-82.

[4] Reiter RJ. Oxygen radical detoxification processes during aging: the functional importance of melatonin. *Aging* (Milano) 1995 Oct;7(5):340-51.

[5] Reiter RJ. Functional diversity of the pineal hormone melatonin: its role as an antioxidant. *Exp. Clin. Endocrinol. Diabetes* 1996;104(1):10-6.

[6] Reiter RJ. Oxidative damage in the central nervous system: protection by melatonin. *Prog. Neurobiol.* 1998 Oct;56(3):359-84.

[7] Benot S, Goberna R, Reiter RJ, Garcia-Maurino S, Osuna C, Guerrero JM. Physiological levels of melatonin contribute to the antioxidant capacity of human serum. *J. Pineal. Res.* 1999 Aug;27(1):59-64.

[8] Tan DX, Poeggeler B, Reiter RJ, Chen LD, Chen S, Manchester LC, et al. The pineal hormone melatonin inhibits DNA-adduct formation induced by the chemical carcinogen safrole in vivo. *Cancer Lett.* 1993 Jun 15;70(1-2):65-71.

[9] Allegra M, Reiter RJ, Tan DX, Gentile C, Tesoriere L, Livrea MA. The chemistry of melatonin's interaction with reactive species. *J. Pineal. Res.* 2003 Jan;34(1):1-10.

[10] Hardeland R, Reiter RJ, Poeggeler B, Tan DX. The significance of the metabolism of the neurohormone melatonin: antioxidative protection and formation of bioactive substances. *Neurosci. Biobehav. Rev.* 1993;17(3):347-57.

[11] Hardeland R, Balzer I, Poeggeler B, Fuhrberg B, Uria H, Behrmann G, et al. On the primary functions of melatonin in evolution: mediation of photoperiodic signals in a unicell, photooxidation, and scavenging of free radicals. *J. Pineal. Res.* 1995 Mar;18(2):104-11.

[12] Reiter RJ, Tan DX, Osuna C, Gitto E. Actions of melatonin in the reduction of oxidative stress. A review. *J. Biomed. Sci.* 2000 Nov;7(6):444-58.

[13] Reiter RJ, Manchester LC, Tan DX. Melatonin in walnuts: influence on levels of melatonin and total antioxidant capacity of blood. *Nutrition* 2005 Sep;21(9):920-4.

[14] Urata Y, Honma S, Goto S, Todoroki S, Iida T, Cho S, et al. Melatonin induces gamma-glutamylcysteine synthetase mediated by activator protein-1 in human vascular endothelial cells. *Free Radic. Biol. Med.* 1999 Oct;27(7-8):838-47.

[15] Gitto E, Tan DX, Reiter RJ, Karbownik M, Manchester LC, Cuzzocrea S, et al. Individual and synergistic antioxidative actions of melatonin: studies with vitamin E,

vitamin C, glutathione and desferrioxamine (desferoxamine) in rat liver homogenates. *J. Pharm. Pharmacol.* 2001 Oct;53(10):1393-401.

[16] Mayo JC, Sainz RM, Antoli I, Herrera F, Martin V, Rodriguez C. Melatonin regulation of antioxidant enzyme gene expression. *Cell Mol. Life Sci.* 2002 Oct;59(10):1706-13.

[17] Mayo JC, Tan DX, Sainz RM, Lopez-Burillo S, Reiter RJ. Oxidative damage to catalase induced by peroxyl radicals: functional protection by melatonin and other antioxidants. *Free Radic. Res.* 2003 May;37(5):543-53.

[18] Acuna CD, Escames G, Carazo A, Leon J, Khaldy H, Reiter RJ. Melatonin, mitochondrial homeostasis and mitochondrial-related diseases. *Curr. Top Med. Chem.* 2002 Feb;2(2):133-51.

[19] Okatani Y, Wakatsuki A, Reiter RJ, Miyahara Y. Acutely administered melatonin restores hepatic mitochondrial physiology in old mice. *Int. J. Biochem. Cell Biol.* 2003 Mar;35(3):367-75.

[20] Reiter RJ, Melchiorri D, Sewerynek E, Poeggeler B, Barlow-Walden L, Chuang J, et al. A review of the evidence supporting melatonin's role as an antioxidant. *J. Pineal. Res.* 1995 Jan;18(1):1-11.

[21] Pierpaoli W. The pineal gland as ontogenetic scanner of reproduction, immunity, and aging. The aging clock. *Ann. NY Acad. Sci.* 1994 Nov 25;741:46-9.

[22] Lissoni P, Barni S, Meregalli S, Fossati V, Cazzaniga M, Esposti D, et al. Modulation of cancer endocrine therapy by melatonin: a phase II study of tamoxifen plus melatonin in metastatic breast cancer patients progressing under tamoxifen alone. *Br. J. Cancer* 1995 Apr;71(4):854-6.

[23] Karasek M, Reiter RJ. Melatonin and aging. *Neuro Endocrinol. Lett* 2002 Apr;23 Suppl 1:14-6.

[24] Karasek M. Melatonin, human aging, and age-related diseases. *Exp. Gerontol.* 2004 Nov;39(11-12):1723-9.

[25] Pandi-Perumal SR, Srinivasan V, Maestroni GJ, Cardinali DP, Poeggeler B, Hardeland R. Melatonin: Nature's most versatile biological signal?. *FEBS J.* 2006 Jul;273(13):2813-38.

[26] Karasek M, Reiter RJ, Cardinali DP, Pawlikowski M. Future of melatonin as a therapeutic agent. *Neuro Endocrinol. Lett.* 2002 Apr;23 Suppl 1:118-21.

[27] Brzezinski A. Melatonin in humans. *N. Engl. J. Med.* 1997 Jan 16;336(3):186-95.

[28] Reiter RJ. The pineal and its hormones in the control of reproduction in mammals. *Endocr. Rev.* 1980;1(2):109-31.

[29] Maestroni GJ. The immunoneuroendocrine role of melatonin. *J. Pineal. Res.* 1993 Jan;14(1):1-10.

[30] Cohen M, Lippman M, Chabner B. Role of pineal gland in aetiology and treatment of breast cancer. *Lancet* 1978 Oct 14;2(8094):814-6.

[31] Tamarkin L, Danforth D, Lichter A, DeMoss E, Cohen M, Chabner B, et al. Decreased nocturnal plasma melatonin peak in patients with estrogen receptor positive breast cancer. *Science* 1982 May 28;216(4549):1003-5.

[32] Coleman MP, Reiter RJ. Breast cancer, blindness and melatonin. *Eur. J. Cancer* 1992;28(2-3):501-3.

[33] Feychting M, Osterlund B, Ahlbom A. Reduced cancer incidence among the blind. *Epidemiology* 1998 Sep;9(5):490-4.

[34] Kliukiene J, Tynes T, Andersen A. Risk of breast cancer among Norwegian women with visual impairment. *Br. J. Cancer* 2001 Feb 2;84(3):397-9.

[35] Verkasalo PK, Pukkala E, Stevens RG, Ojamo M, Rudanko SL. Inverse association between breast cancer incidence and degree of visual impairment in Finland. *Br. J. Cancer* 1999 Jul;80(9):1459-60.

[36] Kheifets LI, Matkin CC. Industrialization, electromagnetic fields, and breast cancer risk. *Environ. Health Perspect.* 1999 Feb;107 Suppl 1:145-54.

[37] Brainard GC, Kavet R, Kheifets LI. The relationship between electromagnetic field and light exposures to melatonin and breast cancer risk: a review of the relevant literature. *J. Pineal. Res.* 1999 Mar;26(2):65-100.

[38] Caplan LS, Schoenfeld ER, O'Leary ES, Leske MC. Breast cancer and electromagnetic fields--a review. *Ann. Epidemiol.* 2000 Jan;10(1):31-44.

[39] Sanchez-Barcelo EJ, Cos S, Fernandez R, Mediavilla MD. Melatonin and mammary cancer: a short review. *Endocr. Relat. Cancer* 2003 Jun;10(2):153-9.

[40] Mishima K, Tozawa T, Satoh K, Matsumoto Y, Hishikawa Y, Okawa M. Melatonin secretion rhythm disorders in patients with senile dementia of Alzheimer's type with disturbed sleep-waking. *Biol. Psychiatry 1999* Feb 15;45(4):417-21.

[41] Magri F, Locatelli M, Balza G, Molla G, Cuzzoni G, Fioravanti M, et al. Changes in endocrine circadian rhythms as markers of physiological and pathological brain aging. *Chronobiol. Int.* 1997 Jul;14(4):385-96.

[42] Ferrari E, Arcaini A, Gornati R, Pelanconi L, Cravello L, Fioravanti M, et al. Pineal and pituitary-adrenocortical function in physiological aging and in senile dementia. *Exp. Gerontol.* 2000 Dec;35(9-10):1239-50.

[43] Liu RY, Zhou JN, van HJ, Hofman MA, Swaab DF. Decreased melatonin levels in postmortem cerebrospinal fluid in relation to aging, Alzheimer's disease, and apolipoprotein E-epsilon4/4 genotype. *J. Clin. Endocrinol. Metab.* 1999 Jan;84(1): 323-7.

[44] Ohashi Y, Okamoto N, Uchida K, Iyo M, Mori N, Morita Y. Daily rhythm of serum melatonin levels and effect of light exposure in patients with dementia of the Alzheimer's type. *Biol. Psychiatry* 1999 Jun 15;45(12):1646-52.

[45] Skene DJ, Vivien-Roels B, Sparks DL, Hunsaker JC, Pevet P, Ravid D, et al. Daily variation in the concentration of melatonin and 5-methoxytryptophol in the human pineal gland: effect of age and Alzheimer's disease. *Brain Res.* 1990 Sep 24;528(1):170-4.

[46] Skene DJ, Bojkowski CJ, Currie JE, Wright J, Boulter PS, Arendt J. 6-sulphatoxymelatonin production in breast cancer patients. *J. Pineal Res.* 1990;8(3):269-76.

[47] Skene DJ, Swaab DF. Melatonin rhythmicity: effect of age and Alzheimer's disease. *Exp. Gerontol.* 2003 Jan;38(1-2):199-206.

[48] Blanks JC, Torigoe Y, Hinton DR, Blanks RH. Retinal pathology in Alzheimer's disease. I. Ganglion cell loss in foveal/parafoveal retina. *Neurobiol. Aging* 1996 May;17(3):377-84.

[49] Blanks JC, Schmidt SY, Torigoe Y, Porrello KV, Hinton DR, Blanks RH. Retinal pathology in Alzheimer's disease. II. Regional neuron loss and glial changes in GCL. *Neurobiol. Aging* 1996 May;17(3):385-95.

[50] Hinton DR, Sadun AA, Blanks JC, Miller CA. Optic-nerve degeneration in Alzheimer's disease. *N. Engl. J. Med.* 1986 Aug 21;315(8):485-7.

[51] Katz B, Rimmer S, Iragui V, Katzman R. Abnormal pattern electroretinogram in Alzheimer's disease: evidence for retinal ganglion cell degeneration? *Ann. Neurol.* 1989 Aug;26(2):221-5.

[52] Blanks JC, Hinton DR, Sadun AA, Miller CA. Retinal ganglion cell degeneration in Alzheimer's disease. *Brain Res.* 1989 Nov 6;501(2):364-72.

[53] Hedges TR, III, Perez GR, Speigelman D, Barbas NR, Peli E, Yardley CJ. Retinal nerve fiber layer abnormalities in Alzheimer's disease. *Acta Ophthalmol. Scand.* 1996 Jun;74(3):271-5.

[54] Kergoat H, Kergoat MJ, Justino L, Chertkow H, Robillard A, Bergman H. An evaluation of the retinal nerve fiber layer thickness by scanning laser polarimetry in individuals with dementia of the Alzheimer type. *Acta Ophthalmol. Scand.* 2001 Apr;79(2):187-91.

[55] Brusco LI, Fainstein I, Marquez M, Cardinali DP. Effect of melatonin in selected populations of sleep-disturbed patients. *Biol. Signals Recept.* 1999 Jan;8(1-2):126-31.

[56] Cohen-Mansfield J, Garfinkel D, Lipson S. Melatonin for treatment of sundowning in elderly persons with dementia - a preliminary study. *Arch. Gerontol. Geriatr.* 2000 Aug 1;31(1):65-76.

[57] Deacon S, English J, Arendt J. Acute phase-shifting effects of melatonin associated with suppression of core body temperature in humans. *Neurosci. Lett.* 1994 Aug 29;178(1):32-4.

[58] Pappolla MA, Chyan YJ, Poeggeler B, Frangione B, Wilson G, Ghiso J, et al. An assessment of the antioxidant and the antiamyloidogenic properties of melatonin: implications for Alzheimer's disease. *J. Neural. Transm.* 2000;107(2):203-31.

[59] Tan DX, Manchester LC, Reiter RJ, Plummer BF, Limson J, Weintraub ST, et al. Melatonin directly scavenges hydrogen peroxide: a potentially new metabolic pathway of melatonin biotransformation. *Free Radic. Biol. Med.* 2000 Dec;29(11):1177-85.

[60] Pappolla M, Bozner P, Soto C, Shao H, Robakis NK, Zagorski M, et al. Inhibition of Alzheimer beta-fibrillogenesis by melatonin. *J. Biol. Chem.* 1998 Mar 27;273(13):7185-8.

[61] Pappolla MA, Sos M, Omar RA, Bick RJ, Hickson-Bick DL, Reiter RJ, et al. Melatonin prevents death of neuroblastoma cells exposed to the Alzheimer amyloid peptide. *J. Neurosci.* 1997 Mar 1;17(5):1683-90.

[62] Daniels WM, van Rensburg SJ, van Zyl JM, Taljaard JJ. Melatonin prevents beta-amyloid-induced lipid peroxidation. *J. Pineal. Res.* 1998 Mar;24(2):78-82.

[63] Song W, Lahiri DK. Melatonin alters the metabolism of the beta-amyloid precursor protein in the neuroendocrine cell line PC12. *J. Mol. Neurosci.* 1997 Oct;9(2):75-92.

[64] Cajochen C, Krauchi K, Wirz-Justice A. Role of melatonin in the regulation of human circadian rhythms and sleep. *J. Neuroendocrinol.* 2003 Apr;15(4):432-7.

[65] Gagnier JJ. The therapeutic potential of melatonin in migraines and other headache types. *Altern. Med. Rev.* 2001 Aug;6(4):383-9.

[66] Brun J, Claustrat B, Saddier P, Chazot G. Nocturnal melatonin excretion is decreased in patients with migraine without aura attacks associated with menses. *Cephalalgia* 1995 Apr;15(2):136-9.

[67] Sandyk R. The influence of the pineal gland on migraine and cluster headaches and effects of treatment with picoTesla magnetic fields. *Int. J. Neurosci.* 1992 Nov;67(1-4):145-71.

[68] Toglia JU. Is migraine due to a deficiency of pineal melatonin?. *Ital. J. Neurol. Sci.* 1986 Jun;7(3):319-23.

[69] Murialdo G, Fonzi S, Costelli P, Solinas GP, Parodi C, Marabini S, et al. Urinary melatonin excretion throughout the ovarian cycle in menstrually related migraine. *Cephalalgia* 1994 Jun;14(3):205-9.

[70] Karasek M, Stawerska R, Smyczynska J, Lewinski A. Increased melatonin concentrations in children with growth hormone deficiency. *J. Pineal. Res.* 2007 Mar;42(2):119-24.

[71] Meeking DR, Wallace JD, Cuneo RC, Forsling M, Russell-Jones DL. Exercise-induced GH secretion is enhanced by the oral ingestion of melatonin in healthy adult male subjects. *Eur. J. Endocrinol.* 1999 Jul;141(1):22-6.

[72] Valcavi R, Dieguez C, Azzarito C, Edwards CA, Dotti C, Page MD, et al. Effect of oral administration of melatonin on GH responses to GRF 1-44 in normal subjects. *Clin. Endocrinol.* (Oxf) 1987 Apr;26(4):453-8.

[73] Waldhauser F, Lieberman HR, Lynch HJ, Waldhauser M, Herkner K, Frisch H, et al. A pharmacological dose of melatonin increases PRL levels in males without altering those of GH, LH, FSH, TSH, testosterone or cortisol. *Neuroendocrinology* 1987 Aug;46(2):125-30.

[74] Srinivasan V, Pandi-Perumal SR, Cardinali DP, Poeggeler B, Hardeland R. Melatonin in Alzheimer's disease and other neurodegenerative disorders. *Behav. Brain. Funct.* 2006;2:15.

[75] Wu YH, Swaab DF. The human pineal gland and melatonin in aging and Alzheimer's disease. *J. Pineal. Res.* 2005 Apr;38(3):145-52.

[76] Fahn S, Cohen G. The oxidant stress hypothesis in Parkinson's disease: evidence supporting it. *Ann. Neurol.* 1992 Dec;32(6):804-12.

[77] Miller JW, Selhub J, Joseph JA. Oxidative damage caused by free radicals produced during catecholamine autoxidation: protective effects of O-methylation and melatonin. *Free Radic. Biol. Med.* 1996;21(2):241-9.

[78] Cardinali DP, Garcia AP, Cano P, Esquifino AI. Melatonin role in experimental arthritis. C*urr. Drug Targets Immune Endocr. Metabol. Disord.* 2004 Mar;4(1):1-10.

[79] Vijayalaxmi, Reiter RJ, Herman TS, Meltz ML. Melatonin and radioprotection from genetic damage: in vivo/in vitro studies with human volunteers. *Mutat. Res.* 1996 Dec 20;371(3-4):221-8.

[80] Vijayalaxmi, Reiter RJ, Herman TS, Meltz ML. Melatonin reduces gamma radiation-induced primary DNA damage in human blood lymphocytes. *Mutat. Res.* 1998 Feb 2;397(2):203-8.

[81] Topkan E, Tufan H, Yavuz AA, Bacanli D, Onal C, Kosdak S, et al. Comparison of the protective effects of melatonin and amifostine on radiation-induced epiphyseal injury. *Int. J. Radiat. Biol.* 2008 Oct;84(10):796-802.

[82] Tan DX, Manchester LC, Helton P, Reiter RJ. Phytoremediative capacity of plants enriched with melatonin. *Plant Signal Behav.* 2007 Nov;2(6):514-6.

[83] Shirazi A, Ghobadi G, Ghazi-Khansari M. A radiobiological review on melatonin: a novel radioprotector. *J. Radiat. Res.* 2007 Jul;48(4):263-72.

[84] Gitto E, Pellegrino S, D'Arrigo S, Barberi I, Reiter RJ. Oxidative stress in resuscitation and in ventilation of newborns. *Eur. Respir. J.* 2009 Dec;34(6):1461-9.
[85] Jan JE, Wasdell MB, Freeman RD, Bax M. Evidence supporting the use of melatonin in short gestation infants. *J. Pineal. Res.* 2007 Jan;42(1):22-7.
[86] Kedziora-Kornatowska K, Szewczyk-Golec K, Czuczejko J, Pawluk H, van Marke de LK, Kozakiewicz M, et al. Antioxidative effects of melatonin administration in elderly primary essential hypertension patients. *J. Pineal. Res.* 2008 Oct;45(3):312-7.
[87] Mazzoccoli G, Giuliani A, Carughi S, De CA, Puzzolante F, La VM, et al. The hypothalamic-pituitary-thyroid axis and melatonin in humans: possible interactions in the control of body temperature. *Neuro Endocrinol. Lett.* 2004 Oct;25(5):368-72.
[88] Petterborg LJ, Thalen BE, Kjellman BF, Wetterberg L. Effect of melatonin replacement on serum hormone rhythms in a patient lacking endogenous melatonin. *Brain Res. Bull.* 1991 Aug;27(2):181-5.
[89] Moore RY. Neural control of pineal function in mammals and birds. *J. Neural Transm. Suppl.* 1978;(13):47-58.
[90] Cardinali DP. Pineal and melatonin actions in reproductive endocrinology. *Arch. Biol. Med. Exp.* (Santiago) 1984 Dec;17(3-4):239-47.
[91] Cagnacci A, Elliott JA, Yen SS. Melatonin: a major regulator of the circadian rhythm of core temperature in humans. *J. Clin. Endocrinol. Metab.* 1992 Aug;75(2):447-52.
[92] Williams G, Pirmohamed J, Minors D, Waterhouse J, Buchan I, Arendt J, et al. Dissociation of body-temperature and melatonin secretion circadian rhythms in patients with chronic fatigue syndrome. *Clin. Physiol.* 1996 Jul;16(4):327-37.
[93] Sterling K. Thyroid hormone action at the cell level (first of two parts). *N. Engl. J. Med.* 1979 Jan 18;300(3):117-23.
[94] Guerrero JM, Puig-Domingo M, Reiter RJ. Thyroxine 5'-deiodinase activity in pineal gland and frontal cortex: nighttime increase and the effect of either continuous light exposure or superior cervical ganglionectomy. *Endocrinology* 1988 Jan;122(1):236-41.
[95] Guerrero JM, Reiter RJ. Iodothyronine 5'-deiodinating activity in the pineal gland. *Int. J. Biochem.* 1992 Oct;24(10):1513-23.
[96] Cagnacci A, Krauchi K, Wirz-Justice A, Volpe A. Homeostatic versus circadian effects of melatonin on core body temperature in humans. *J. Biol. Rhythms* 1997 Dec;12(6):509-17.
[97] Gilbert SS, van den Heuvel CJ, Kennaway DJ, Dawson D. Peripheral heat loss: a predictor of the hypothermic response to melatonin administration in young and older women. *Physiol. Behav.* 1999 Apr;66(2):365-70.
[98] Gilbert SS, van den Heuvel CJ, Dawson D. Daytime melatonin and temazepam in young adult humans: equivalent effects on sleep latency and body temperatures. *J. Physiol.* 1999 Feb 1;514 (Pt 3):905-14.
[99] Vriend J. Evidence for pineal gland modulation of the neuroendocrine-thyroid axis. *Neuroendocrinology* 1983;36(1):68-78.
[100] Wright ML, Pikula A, Babski AM, Labieniec KE, Wolan RB. Effect of melatonin on the response of the thyroid to thyrotropin stimulation in vitro. *Gen. Comp. Endocrinol.* 1997 Nov;108(2):298-305.
[101] Tan DX, Hardeland R, Manchester LC, Korkmaz A, Ma S, Rosales-Corral S, et al. Functional roles of melatonin in plants, and perspectives in nutritional and agricultural science. *J. Exp. Bot.* 2012 Jan;63(2):577-97.

[102] Arnao MB, Hernandez-Ruiz J. Melatonin promotes adventitious- and lateral root regeneration in etiolated hypocotyls of Lupinus albus L. *J. Pineal. Res.* 2007 Mar;42(2):147-52.

[103] Hernandez-Ruiz J, Cano A, Arnao MB. Melatonin acts as a growth-stimulating compound in some monocot species. *J. Pineal. Res.* 2005 Sep;39(2):137-42.

[104] Jones MP, Cao J, O'Brien R, Murch SJ, Saxena PK. The mode of action of thidiazuron: auxins, indoleamines, and ion channels in the regeneration of Echinacea purpurea L. *Plant Cell Rep.* 2007 Sep;26(9):1481-90.

[105] Kolar J, Johnson CH, Machackova I. Presence and possible role of melatonin in a short-day flowering plant, Chenopodium rubrum. *Adv. Exp. Med. Biol.* 1999;460:391-3.

[106] Kolar J, Machackova I. Melatonin in higher plants: occurrence and possible functions. *J. Pineal. Res.* 2005 Nov;39(4):333-41.

[107] Tan DX, Manchester LC, Terron MP, Flores LJ, Reiter RJ. One molecule, many derivatives: a never-ending interaction of melatonin with reactive oxygen and nitrogen species?. *J. Pineal. Res.* 2007 Jan;42(1):28-42.

[108] Agunbiade FO, Olu-Owolabi BI, Adebowale KO. Phytoremediation potential of Eichornia crassipes in metal-contaminated coastal water. *Bioresour. Technol.* 2009 Oct;100(19):4521-6.

[109] Lei XY, Zhu RY, Zhang GY, Dai YR. Attenuation of cold-induced apoptosis by exogenous melatonin in carrot suspension cells: the possible involvement of polyamines. *J. Pineal. Res.* 2004 Mar;36(2):126-31.

[110] Xu XD, Sun Y, Sun B, Zhang J, Guo XQ. [Effects of exogenous melatonin on active oxygen metabolism of cucumber seedlings under high temperature stress]. Ying Yong Sheng Tai Xue Bao 2010 May;21(5):1295-300.

[111] Xu XD, Sun Y, Guo XQ, Sun B, Zhang J. [Effects of exogenous melatonin on ascorbate metabolism system in cucumber seedlings under high temperature stress]. Ying Yong Sheng Tai Xue Bao 2010 Oct;21(10):2580-6.

[112] Afreen F, Zobayed SM, Kozai T. Melatonin in Glycyrrhiza uralensis: response of plant roots to spectral quality of light and UV-B radiation. *J. Pineal. Res. 2006* Sep;41(2):108-15.

[113] Zhang LJ, Jia JF, Hao JG, Cen JR, Li TK. A modified protocol for the comet assay allowing the processing of multiple samples. *Mutat. Res.* 2011 Apr 3;721(2):153-6.

[114] Arnao MB, Hernandez-Ruiz J. Melatonin promotes adventitious- and lateral root regeneration in etiolated hypocotyls of Lupinus albus L. *J. Pineal. Res.* 2007 Mar;42(2):147-52.

[115] Tan DX, Hardeland R, Manchester LC, Paredes SD, Korkmaz A, Sainz RM, et al. The changing biological roles of melatonin during evolution: from an antioxidant to signals of darkness, sexual selection and fitness. *Biol. Rev. Camb. Philos. Soc.* 2010 Aug;85(3):607-23.

[116] Boccalandro HE, Gonzalez CV, Wunderlin DA, Silva MF. Melatonin levels, determined by LC-ESI-MS/MS, fluctuate during the day/night cycle in Vitis vinifera cv Malbec: evidence of its antioxidant role in fruits. *J. Pineal. Res.* 2011 Sep;51(2):226-32.

[117] Wang Y, Ji J, Bu H, Zhao Y, Xu Y, Johnson CH, et al. [Genetic transformation of Nicotiana tabacum L. by Agrobacterium tumefaciens carrying genes in the melatonin

biosynthesis pathway and the enhancement of antioxidative capability in transgenic plants]. Sheng Wu Gong Cheng Xue Bao 2009 Jul;25(7):1014-21.

[118] Posmyk MM, Balabusta M, Wieczorek M, Sliwinska E, Janas KM. Melatonin applied to cucumber (Cucumis sativus L.) seeds improves germination during chilling stress. *J. Pineal. Res.* 2009 Mar;46(2):214-23.

[119] Zhao Y, Qi LW, Wang WM, Saxena PK, Liu CZ. Melatonin improves the survival of cryopreserved callus of Rhodiola crenulata. J. Pineal. Res. 2011 Jan;50(1):83-8.

[120] Arnao MB, Hernandez-Ruiz J. Chemical stress by different agents affects the melatonin content of barley roots. *J. Pineal. Res.* 2009 Apr;46(3):295-9.

[121] Paredes SD, Korkmaz A, Manchester LC, Tan DX, Reiter RJ. Phytomelatonin: a review. *J. Exp. Bot.* 2009;60(1):57-69.

[122] Banerjee S, Margulis L. Mitotic arrest by melatonin. *Exp. Cell Res.* 1973 Apr;78(2):314-8.

[123] Jackson WT. Regulation of mitosis. II. Interaction of isopropyl N-phenylcarbamate and melatonin. *J. Cell Sci.* 1969 Nov;5(3):745-55.

[124] Chen Q, Qi WB, Reiter RJ, Wei W, Wang BM. Exogenously applied melatonin stimulates root growth and raises endogenous indoleacetic acid in roots of etiolated seedlings of Brassica juncea. *J. Plant. Physiol.* 2009 Feb 15;166(3):324-8.

[125] Hernandez-Ruiz J, Cano A, Arnao MB. Melatonin: a growth-stimulating compound present in lupin tissues. *Planta* 2004 Nov;220(1):140-4.

[126] Posmyk MM, Kuran H, Marciniak K, Janas KM. Presowing seed treatment with melatonin protects red cabbage seedlings against toxic copper ion concentrations. *J. Pineal. Res.* 2008 Aug;45(1):24-31.

[127] Arnao MB, Hernandez-Ruiz J. Protective effect of melatonin against chlorophyll degradation during the senescence of barley leaves. *J. Pineal. Res.* 2009 Jan;46(1):58-63.

[128] Triantaphylides C, Havaux M. Singlet oxygen in plants: production, detoxification and signaling. *Trends Plant. Sci.* 2009 Apr;14(4):219-28.

[129] Yamano HO, Matsushita HO, Yanagiwara S. Plasma concentration of rabeprazole after 8-week administration in gastroesophageal reflux disease patients and intragastric pH elevation. *J. Gastroenterol. Hepatol.* 2008 Apr;23(4):534-40.

[130] Tal O, Haim A, Harel O, Gerchman Y. Melatonin as an antioxidant and its semi-lunar rhythm in green macroalga Ulva sp. *J. Exp. Bot.* 2011 Mar;62(6):1903-10.

[131] Wang YM, Jin BZ, Ai F, Duan CH, Lu YZ, Dong TF, et al. The efficacy and safety of melatonin in concurrent chemotherapy or radiotherapy for solid tumors: a meta-analysis of randomized controlled trials. *Cancer Chemother. Pharmacol.* 2012 May;69(5):1213-20.

[132] Hernandez-Ruiz J, Arnao MB. Distribution of melatonin in different zones of lupin and barley plants at different ages in the presence and absence of light. *J. Agric. Food Chem.* 2008 Nov 26;56(22):10567-73.

[133] Kang K, Lee K, Park S, Kim YS, Back K. Enhanced production of melatonin by ectopic overexpression of human serotonin N-acetyltransferase plays a role in cold resistance in transgenic rice seedlings. *J. Pineal. Res.* 2010 Sep;49(2):176-82.

[134] Sarropoulou V, Dimassi-Theriou K, Therios I, Koukourikou-Petridou M. Melatonin enhances root regeneration, photosynthetic pigments, biomass, total carbohydrates and

proline content in the cherry rootstock PHL-C (Prunus avium x Prunus cerasus). *Plant. Physiol. Biochem.* 2012 Dec;61:162-8.

[135] Benitez-King G, Anton-Tay F. Calmodulin mediates melatonin cytoskeletal effects. *Experientia* 1993 Aug 15;49(8):635-41.

[136] Hardeland R. New actions of melatonin and their relevance to biometeorology. *Int. J. Biometeorol.* 1997 Nov;41(2):47-57.

[137] Hardeland R. Melatonin, hormone of darkness and more: occurrence, control mechanisms, actions and bioactive metabolites. *Cell Mol. Life Sci.* 2008 Jul;65(13):2001-18.

[138] Murch SJ, Saxena PK. Mammalian neurohormones: potential significance in reproductive physiology of St. John's wort (Hypericum perforatum L.)?. *Naturwissenschaften* 2002 Dec;89(12):555-60.

[139] Hardeland R, Poeggeler B. Non-vertebrate melatonin. *J. Pineal. Res.* 2003 May;34(4):233-41.

[140] Foreman J, Demidchik V, Bothwell JH, Mylona P, Miedema H, Torres MA, et al. Reactive oxygen species produced by NADPH oxidase regulate plant cell growth. *Nature* 2003 Mar 27;422(6930):442-6.

[141] Schopfer P. Hydroxyl radical-induced cell-wall loosening in vitro and in vivo: implications for the control of elongation growth. *Plant J.* 2001 Dec;28(6):679-88.

[142] Tan DX, Manchester LC, Di MP, Martinez GR, Prado FM, Reiter RJ. Novel rhythms of N1-acetyl-N2-formyl-5-methoxykynuramine and its precursor melatonin in water hyacinth: importance for phytoremediation. *FASEB J.* 2007 Jun;21(8):1724-9.

[143] Hardeland R. New actions of melatonin and their relevance to biometeorology. Int J Biometeorol 1997 Nov;41(2):47-57.

[144] Van Tassel DL, Roberts N, Lewy A, O'Neill SD. Melatonin in plant organs. *J. Pineal. Res.* 2001 Aug;31(1):8-15.

[145] Dubbels R, Reiter RJ, Klenke E, Goebel A, Schnakenberg E, Ehlers C, et al. Melatonin in edible plants identified by radioimmunoassay and by high performance liquid chromatography-mass spectrometry. *J. Pineal. Res.* 1995 Jan;18(1):28-31.

[146] Badria FA. Melatonin, serotonin, and tryptamine in some egyptian food and medicinal plants. *J. Med. Food.* 2002;5(3):153-7.

[147] Burkhardt S, Tan DX, Manchester LC, Hardeland R, Reiter RJ. Detection and quantification of the antioxidant melatonin in Montmorency and Balaton tart cherries (Prunus cerasus). *J. Agric. Food. Chem.* 2001 Oct;49(10):4898-902.

[148] Manchester LC, Tan DX, Reiter RJ, Park W, Monis K, Qi W. High levels of melatonin in the seeds of edible plants: possible function in germ tissue protection. *Life Sci.* 2000 Nov 10;67(25):3023-9.

[149] Antolin I, Rodriguez C, Sainz RM, Mayo JC, Uria H, Kotler ML, et al. Neurohormone melatonin prevents cell damage: effect on gene expression for antioxidant enzymes. *FASEB J.* 1996 Jun;10(8):882-90.

Reviewed by Christos Chatzissavvidis, Assistant Professor, Democritus University of Thrace, Department of Agriculture and Development, Pantazidou 193, Orestiada 68200, Fax: +30 2552041191, email: cchatz@agro.duth.gr

In: New Developments in Melatonin Research ISBN: 978-1-62618-843-3
Editors: D.Acuña-Castroviejo, I.Rusanova, G.Escames © 2013 Nova Science Publishers, Inc.

Chapter 2

Melatonin as a Circadian Hormone in Invertebrates

Beatriz Fuentes-Pardo*, Carolina Barriga-Montoya and Araceli de la O-Martínez
Laboratorio de Cronobiología, Departamento de Fisiología, Facultad de Medicina, Universidad Nacional Autónoma de México (UNAM). Circuito Interior S/N, Ciudad Universitaria, México, D. F. México

Abstract

Melatonin is a highly conserved molecule present in nearly all studied species. In mammals and birds, it is well accepted that the circulating levels of this hormone function during daytime, allowing the synchronization of many circadian rhythms. The cellular mechanisms of melatonin action are produced through the activation of specialized membrane and nuclear receptors. However, the mechanism of their actions, from signaling pathways to the integrative level, is far from being understood.

Comparative studies provide important contributions toward understanding the action of melatonin. Studies in invertebrates, notably in crustaceans and insects, can greatly help to elucidate various aspects of melatonin action: the common challenge of organisms to face their temporal organization has apparently been achieved by a phylogenetically conserved strategy. In this chapter we will compile information about the following: 1) the presence of melatonin in invertebrates 2) their biological effects, and 3) their mechanisms of action.

* Corresponding author: Beatriz Fuentes-Pardo, Universidad Nacional Autónoma de México (UNAM). Circuito Interior S/N, Ciudad Universitaria, 04510, México, D. F. México, bfpardo@unam.mx.

Introduction

To date, it is well accepted that under constant environmental conditions, the majority of the physiological variables of living organisms display endogenous, sustained oscillations with a period close to but different from 24 h, known as circadian rhythms. These rhythms allow organisms to predict, instead of merely react to, cyclic changes in the environment; also, they provide the different species with the possibility of temporal organization. Because these circadian cycles can be synchronized with external signals, organisms are also able to adjust themselves to exogenous rhythms such as the day/night cycles [1].

It is common to say that circadian rhythms evolved as an adaptation to environmental changes deriving from the Earth's rotation. The most important property in relation to this adaptative argument is ubiquity: all tested living organisms have exhibited circadian activity. Even, more so, the way that these rhythms have behaved in the laboratory under several experimental treatments is surprisingly similar among all species. Namely, if a physiological mechanism is found in each living organism and in all studied species, it appears to work in the same manner, thus, the mechanism must have originated early in the species' phylogeny due to natural selection. The importance of comparative studies for understanding the underlying mechanisms cannot be dennied. There are several key biological questions that have been understood when the phenomenon has been situated within an adaptative and evolutionary context.

At present, it is accepted that daily rhythms are controlled by a network of circadian clocks that are able to reset themselves into a new phase when appropriate input signals arrive, in order to impose the corresponding circadian signal on effector organs, mainly peripheral tissues. In mammals, organization of the circadian network appeared to be hierarchical, with the master clock localized in the suprachiasmatic nuclei at the top of the hierarchy [2]. However, recent findings have challenged the dominant role of these structures in physiological regulation, and it has become increasingly evident that close interaction between different central and peripheral clocks is necessary to maintain robust circadian rhythms in functions and metabolism [3]. In the circadian pacemaking system of birds, a hypothalamic region has also been detected that is possibly equivalent to the mammalian suprachiasmatic nuclei [4]. On the other hand, circadian biology of invertebrates has led to a different hypothesis: circadian system of pacemakers is distributed in which no master clock has been identified. The model of distributed clockwork involves oscillators such as retinular cells, neurosecretory systems in the optic lobes, and putative brain pacemakers [5-7].

Melatonin (5-Methoxy-N-acetyltryptamine) is an evolutionary, highly conserved molecule occurring in organisms as different as algae and humans. This widespread process indicates a high evolutionary age for this indolamine. In vertebrates, melatonin plays a well established role as a chemical mediator of darkness and is perhaps the most important signal carrying information about circadian cyclicities. At present, it is known that photoperiodic messages are encoded through melatonin secretion. Photoperiodic changes, which act via nervous system, alter the synthesis of a release of melatonin mainly from the pineal gland. Changes in melatonin concentration drive the rhythms of many physiological variables. That is because it is known as the circadian hormone [8-11].

In invertebrates as well as vertebrates, light is the main temporal cue to indicate the time of day: light is the most powerful synchronizer. The mechanisms underlying this process, as in vertebrates, are not completely understood, but it is sufficiently well accepted that, as in vertebrates, hormone melatonin is involved.

Studies in invertebrates, notably in crustaceans and insects, can greatly help to elucidate various aspects of melatonin action in animals: the common challenge of organisms in confronying their temporal organization has apparently been achieved by a phylogenetically conserved strategy. In consequence, in this chapter we will review in the context of circadian rhythms in invertebrates: as follows 1) the presence of melatonin 2) their biological effects, and 3) their mechanisms of action.

Presence of Melatonin in Invertebrates

Because of the number of species alive, we are able to recognize the following eight particularly important phyla in invertebrates: Porifera (approximately 5,500 species); Cnidaria (approximately 10,000 species); Platyhelminthes (approximately 20,000 species); Nematoda (approximately 25,500 species); Annelida (approximately 16,500 species); Mollusca (approximately 93195 species); Arthropoda (approximately 1,156,000 species), and Echinodermata (approximately 7,000 species). Information regarding the presence of melatonin within the context of circadian rhythms in these phyla is very limited. To our knowledge, Porifera, Annelida, and Echinodermata have never been studied with respect to the presence of this indolamine within the context of circadian rhythm; despite their important phylogenetic position (see Table 1). In accordance with Tessmar and Raible [14], we argue that a re-focus on these species will be crucial to understand the main interactions and evolution of rhythms that govern a broad range of eukaryotes including the human species.

In Table 1, we show one example –if it exists– of the presence of melatonin within the context of circadian rhythms for the eight previously mentioned phyla. We also include other references corresponding to another species. If there are no studies with melatonin, we are also considering the presence of some of the precursors of melatonin, i.e. 5-HT, NAS, or the enzymes implicated in their respective synthesis, i.e. AA-NAT and HIOMT, whenever they appear within the context of circadian rhythms.

In invertebrates, 5-HT metabolism follows, as in vertebrates, two steps [7;11]: 5-HT is acetylated by the rate-limiting enzyme Arylalkylamine N-acetyl-transferase (AA-NAT) into N-acetyl-serotonin (NAS), which is then O-methylated by Hydroxyindole-O-methyl-transferase (HIOMT) into melatonin. We consider the presence of serotonin, NAS, or any of the enzymes implicated in melatonin synthesis as important because it cannot be excluded that many 5-HT-ir cells also express AA-NAT and HIOMT in order to produce NAS, and finally, melatonin. Of course, we consider it decisive to identify the presence of melatonin directly.

Biological Effects of Melatonin in Invertebrates

Physiological studies relative to the action of melatonin on circadian rhythms in invertebrates are truly scarce. It is possible, however, to propose that one of the main functions of melatonin is the day/night internal signaling associated with its absence or presence in plasma as well as seasonal signaling that includes its nocturnal peak duration [10;12].

Table 1.

Phylum and species	Rhythm	Employed method	Comment	Reference	Other references.
Porifera	To our knowledge, there are no studies on this phylum				
Cnidaria *Rennilla köellikeri*	Daily variations of melatonin were shown for 12 consecutive months of sampling (April 1995 to March 1996). Significant differences were found to exist between day and night values only in May and July. The highest mean value occurring during the day phase in both cases. However, the profiles of melatonin activity differ even between these 2 months, displaying significant but also inconsistent night or day peaks. Consequently, no daily rhythmic pattern of melatonin content emerged. In this case melatonin is not a daily photoperiodic messenger but may instead act as a seasonal marker for reproduction	RIA	It is accepted that Cnidaria possess the most ancient nervous system. Research on melatonin in these animals may provide important clues in evolutionary implications about the role of melatonin as the circadian hormone	(34)	To our knowledge there are no more references
Platyhelminthes *Dugesia japonica*	NAT, HIOMT, and melatonin levels exhibit a significant daily variation, peaking at the mid-dark time	HPLC	Data demonstrate that the planarian synthesizes melatonin through the same pathways as those in the majority of vertebrates and that melatonin synthesis fluctuates in a circadian manner. It is strongly suggested that the planarian contains a circadian clock controlling melatonin synthesis	(35)	(35-37)
Nematoda *Caenorhabditis elegans*	A rhythmic pattern of melatonin levels was observed, with higher levels toward the middle of the night	RIA	*C. elegans* provides an excellent model for genetics and neurobehavioral studies, and because its mutant availability and ease of culture, it could be used as a novel model for circadian studies	(38)	To our knowledge there are no more references

Table 1. (Continued)

Annelida	To our knowledge there are no studies in this phylum				
Mollusca *Octopus vulgaris*	Daily fluctuations were observed of melatonin levels in hemolymph, retina, and nervous system-related structures.	HPLC	Information regarding melatonin production in mollusks is very limited; however, some data suggest that melatonin might play a fundamental role in the transduction of the dark/light cycle information for adjustments of rhythmic events	(39)	(40;41)
Arthropoda *Procambarus clarkii*	Immunoreactivity to melatonin was detected in all samples assayed. Concentration ranged from 30-- 1813 pg/eyestalk depending on the time of eyestalk removal. Highest levels of the hormone were detected during the dark phase showing a pronounced peak at 20 hours circadian time	RIA	Unquestionably, Arthropoda is the most studied phylum of all invertebrate phyla. As we can see in "other references" there are many crustaceans in which melatonin has been detected: crabs, lobsters and prawns. Also we can account for a several species of insects including *Periplaneta americana, Musa autumnalis,* and *Drosophila.* Although the peak of melatonin generally occurs at night there are some cases, as *Macrobrachium rosenbergii* and *Nephrops Norvegicus*, for example in which the melatonin peak occurs during day	(42)	(22;26; 35;43-50)
Echino-dermata	Echinoderms and Chordates belong to the same monophyletic taxon, the Deuterostomia. Despite significant differences in body plan organization, both phyla share more common traits than was previously thought. However, despite this important fact, to our knowledge, Echinodermata has never been studied regarding to melatonin.				

Of course, we cannot ignore others effects of melatonin exerted in invertebrates, such as a potent antioxidant, a co-factor for specific enzymes, or a neuromodulator. These and other related effects reported in invertebrates [9;13-22].

If we focus on the circadian physiological effects produced by melatonin in invertebrates, we incredibly we find studies carried out in Arthropoda in solely two subphyla: Crustacea and Hexapoda. Unfortunately, the possible roles of melatonin in Arthropoda temporal organization are unclear.

In the crayfish *Procambarus clarkii*, our laboratory team noted a change in the electrical response to light in retinal photoreceptors, namely, the receptor potential, when the isolated eyestalk is perfused with melatonin: receptor potential amplitude decreases and its duration increases significantly. We propose that knowledge of the action of exogenous melatonin on photoreceptor cells must be helpful in understanding some of the mechanisms underlying the circadian rhythmicity due to the important role of photoreceptor cells in the organization of the circadian system. Ten years later, we found that the magnitude of electrical response to light by melatonin depends on the circadian time of the hormone application [23;24]. One hundred nM of melatonin during subjective day produces a greater effect than during subjective night. We also also found that the indole has an effect on the circadian rhythm of sensitivity to light (electroretinogram, ERG): a single dose of the hormone is able to shift the phase of the rhythm according to the hour of application and is capable of synchronizing the rhythm when a periodic dose is applied. We also hypothesized that melatonin acts as a non-photic synchronizer on effectors and on pacemakers of ERG circadian rhythm and that, as in vertebrates, it is in charge of sending a signal of darkness to the ERG circadian system.

Tilden *et al.* [25] also studied the effect of melatonin on the circadian motor rhythm of the crayfish *Procambarus clarkii* and found some differences in this effect attributable to the season of the year. In the early spring, control crayfish were significantly more active during mid-to-late photophase than during scotophase; glucose and lactate levels were both significantly higher during the active phase. When melatonin was injected at the onset of scotophase, it caused a significant nocturnal rise followed by a diurnal decrease in activity. Glucose was higher in scoto- and lower in photophase than control levels, though overall glucose levels were remained lower in scoto- than in photophase. Lactate levels in melatonin-treated crayfish were in phase with activity levels, with a significant increase in scotophase. During the late summer, control crayfish were significantly more active in scotophase, and glucose and lactate levels were also higher in scotophase. In the early summer, control crayfish exhibited higher activity levels at 12:00 and 21:00 h than at 15:00 and 18:00 h; melatonin had different effects on locomotor activity when injected at different times of the day. Melatonin significantly increased crayfish motor activity during mid-photophase (12:00 h and 15:00 h); it had no effect at late photophase (18:00 h) and reduced activity in early scotophase (21:00 h).

The effect of melatonin on locomotor rhythm also has been studied in the fiddler crab *Uca pugilator* [25]. Control crabs have low activity during early photophase, high activity at mid-photophase, increasing activity during the first scotophase trial, and decreasing activity during the second scotophase trial. Melatonin injection increased activity levels at some specific intervals: it did not influence activity levels injected during early photophase activity or in the early scotophase activity decline but, significantly, activity increases when melatonin is injected during the mid-photophase activity and early scotophase activity incline. A similar study were made by Tilden *et al* in the green shore crab *Carcinus maenas* [25]. Similar results were obtained in *Uca pugilator*: melatonin significantly increased activity during the mid-photophase and early scotophase.

In 2001, Tildet *et al.* published the effect of melatonin on hemolymph glucose and lactate levels in the fiddler crabs *Uca pugilator* [26]. In intact crabs, glucose and lactate levels cycled simultaneously, with peaks occurring during early and late photophase. Melatonin caused a shift in the glucose and lactate cycles, with a sole peak occurring close to mid-photophase.

To our knowledge the physiological effects of melatonin in insects were reported in the last decade of the past century by Gao and Hardie [27]. In this work, the authors investigated the possible role of melatonin in the pea aphid *Acyrthosiphon pisum*, a holocyclic species. Under long-day (summer) conditions virginoparae undergo asexual or parthenogenetic reproduction, while under short-day conditions (autumn) the appearance of males and sexual females (oviparae) is induced, which produce diapausing eggs after mating. Pea aphids were fed an artificial diet containing various concentrations of melatonin. Under long-day conditions (16 h light: 8 h dark), their progeny included males and virginoparous/oviparous (asexual/sexual) intermediate females, which normally occurs only in short days or *ca.* critical night-length. Melatonin is a hormone typically produced during the dark phase and the duration of the melatonin peak is a signal that provides many animals with an endocrine indication of night- length. Based on this concept, exogenous melatonin administered for several hours prior to lights-off might imitate the putative endogenous melatonin peak, thus resulting in a long night or a short day. This is because the authors proposed that melatonin may be involved in photoperiodic response.

In 2001, Yamando *et al.* found that the locomotor activity of *Acheta domesticus* became more synchronous in Light–dark (LD) cycles, *i.e.* it exhibited a smaller variance around the mean, as the concentration of melatonin in drinking water increased [28]. The ratio of night activity to total activity was increased and the acrophase was delayed by melatonin drinking. It was also observed that activity decreases in LD cycles as the melatonin concentration increases. The number of activity bouts in the free-running rhythm in Dark-dark (DD), however, was not influenced by the melatonin concentration. The most apparent effect of melatonin on activity in LD cycles appears to be the elimination of the day-time activity. Not only did melatonin eliminate day-time activity to supply better synchronization in LD cycles, the free-running rhythm was also affected, which tended to be more synchronized: activity became higher as the melatonin concentration increased. The amplitude of free-running rhythms also increased as the melatonin concentration increased, even at 100 μg melatonin /ml, although the amplitude in DD was lower than that in LD cycles.

To our knowledge, these are no additional works performed in invertebrates relative to establishing the biological effects of melatonin in these corresponding species. Overall, melatonin may be involved in the transmission of environmental timing information from the eyestalks to locomotors or sensitivity to light centers. Probably, transmission of information is not linear in the sense that melatonin also possesses the ability to modify the working order of one of the structures in charge of transmitting input signals: the eyestalk and, particularly the reticular photoreceptors. Studies also demonstrate the importance of the seasonal rhythms.

Mechanism of Action of Melatonin in Invertebrates

Liposoluble melatonin has been endowed with very special physicochemical properties: it is able to cross all biological barriers and enters easily into the compartment of every cell. Manyof the actions of melatonin also are mediated by G-protein-coupled receptors, MT1 and MT2, or indirectly by nuclear orphan receptors from the RORα/RZR family. It is also know that melatonin binds to the quinone reductase II enzyme, previously defined as the MT3 receptor. Melatonin receptor agonists and antagonists have an exciting future in that they could define the multiple mechanisms by which melatonin modulates the complexity of such a wide variety of physiological and pathological processes [29-32].

In general, it appears that melatonin acts as a fine tuner of organism physiology. The molecule can be a highly efficient electron donor; thus, it can repair biomolecules damaged by radicals and catalyse one-electron reactions, thereby increasing energy metabolism efficiency. From an evolutionary point of view, melatonin may have evolved at the time when photosynthetic organisms began to produce large amounts of oxygen and others cells began to rely on this oxygen [8;10]. This property appears to have the primary function of melatonin, utilized by organisms for trapping dangerous radicals resulting from both irradiation and metabolism. Because photoprotection is related with the light sensitivity of melatonin in the presence of cellular photocatalysts, this particular property should have rendered this indolamine suitable as a chemical mediator of darkness that can be employedused for purposes of circadian and annual rhythmicities.

To our knowledge, in only one work, the effect of some agonists and antagonists of melatonin within the context of circadian systems has been proved. Menadoza-Vargas et al. attempted to determine whether MT2 melatonin receptors regulate the melatonin-produced effect in the Receptor potential (RP) of the crayfish photoreceptor cells [23]. These authors carried out two series of experiments, at Circadian times (CT) 6 and CT 18, which included the following: (1) application of the MT2 receptor selective agonist 8-M-PDOT and antagonist DH97, and (2) the specific binding of [(125)I]-melatonin in eyestalk membranes. The amount of 10 nM of 8-M-PDOT exerts a similar effect on the RP amplitude of that produced. 1 nM DH97 abolished the effect produced by the hormone and 8-M-PDOT. Binding of [(125)I]-melatonin was saturable and specific. Scatchard analysis revealed an affinity constant Kd of 1.1 nM and a total number of binding sites of 6 fmol/mg protein at CT 6, and a Kd of 1.46 nM and Bmax of 7 fmol/mg protein at CT 18. These results indicate that the effect of melatonin is through MT2-like melatonin receptors and that the kinetics of the complex receptor-molecule depends on circadian time.

There are other works within different context from that of the circadian systems that were carried out in ivertebrates. For example, some authors examined the effects of melatonin and its receptor antagonists on various behaviors in Caenorhabditis elegans [21]. Exogenously applied melatonin specifically decreased locomotion rates in 15-min treatments, suggesting that melatonin directly regulates neural activities for locomotion. This melatonin signaling functions through MT1-like melatonin receptors, because the MT1/2 receptor antagonist luzindole effectively blocked the effect of melatonin on locomotion, while the MT2-specific antagonist 4-Phenyl-2-propionamidotetralin (4-P-PDOT) and the MT3-selective antagonist prazosin had no effect. Alternatively, long-term treatment with prazosin specifically altered homeostatic states of the worm, suggesting another melatonin-signaling pathway through MT3-like receptors. Other authors show that luzindole, a proven melatonin antagonist in vertebrates, has the same function in Periplaneta americana and Uca pugilator, respectively [16;33].

Conclusion

As in vertebrates, melatonin in invertebrates is a fundamental molecule able to carry information about both circadian and annual cyclicities. In all organisms that have been studied, melatonin is nearly exclusively synthesized during the night and mediates information concerning the temporal position and the duration of darkness.

Why has melatonin acquired this function during evolution? At present we do not know, but evolutive aspects of melatonin can be considered and justified because there is evidence of its presence in invertebrates and even in unicellular such as the dinoflagellate *Gonyaulax poliedra*.

Another indisputable thought is that our understanding of melatonin's biological functions and its physiological significance, particularly within the context of circadian rhythms, remain in substantially expansion.

We must compare the information obtained from vertebrates and invertebrates in order to show similarities and differences with the hope of learning more about the action of melatonin, a very-well known circadian hormone.

Acknowledgments

This work was supported by DGAPA grant IN228011.

References

[1] Peirson SN, Thompson S, Hankins MW, Foster RG. Mammalian photoentrainment: results, methods, and approaches. *Methods Enzymol.* 2005;393:697-726.

[2] Dibner C, Schibler U, Albrecht U. The mammalian circadian timing system: organization and coordination of central and peripheral clocks. *Annu. Rev. Physiol.* 2010;72:517-49.

[3] Barclay JL, Tsang AH, Oster H. Interaction of central and peripheral clocks in physiological regulation. *Prog. Brain Res.* 2012;199:163-81.

[4] Gwinner E, Brandstatter R. Complex bird clocks. *Philos. Trans R. Soc. Lond B. Biol. Sci.* 2001 Nov 29;356(1415):1801-10.

[5] Arechiga H, Fernandez-Quiroz F, Fernandez de MF, Rodriguez-Sosa L. The circadian system of crustaceans. *Chronobiol. Int.* 1993 Feb;10(1):1-19.

[6] Rodriguez-Sosa L, Calderon-Rosete G, Flores G. Circadian and ultradian rhythms in the crayfish caudal photoreceptor. *Synapse* 2008 Sep;62(9):643-52.

[7] Strauss J, Dircksen H. Circadian clocks in crustaceans: identified neuronal and cellular systems. *Front Biosci.* 2010;15:1040-74.

[8] Hardeland R, Balzer I, Poeggeler B, Fuhrberg B, Uria H, Behrmann G, et al. On the primary functions of melatonin in evolution: mediation of photoperiodic signals in a unicell, photooxidation, and scavenging of free radicals. *J. Pineal. Res.* 1995 Mar;18(2):104-11.

[9] Hardeland R, Coto-Montes A, Poeggeler B. Circadian rhythms, oxidative stress, and antioxidative defense mechanisms. *Chronobiol. Int.* 2003 Nov;20(6):921-62.

[10] Poeggeler B. Introduction. Melatonin and the light-dark zeitgeber in vertebrates, invertebrates and unicellular organisms. *Experientia* 1993 Aug 15;49(8):611-3.

[11] Vivien-Roels B, Pevet P, Masson-Pevet M, Canguilhem B. Seasonal variations in the daily rhythm of pineal gland and/or circulating melatonin and 5-methoxytryptophol concentrations in the European hamster, Cricetus cricetus. *Gen. Comp. Endocrinol.* 1992 May;86(2):239-47.

[12] Hardeland R. Melatonin, hormone of darkness and more: occurrence, control mechanisms, actions and bioactive metabolites. *Cell Mol. Life Sci.* 2008 Jul;65(13):2001-18.

[13] Anisimov VN, Popovich IG, Zabezhinski MA, Anisimov SV, Vesnushkin GM, Vinogradova IA. Melatonin as antioxidant, geroprotector and anticarcinogen. *Biochim. Biophys. Acta* 2006 May;1757(5-6):573-89.

[14] Bonilla E, Medina-Leendertz S, Diaz S. Extension of life span and stress resistance of Drosophila melanogaster by long-term supplementation with melatonin. *Exp. Gerontol.* 2002 May;37(5):629-38.
[15] Bustos-Obregon E, Gonzalez JR, Espinoza O. Melatonin as protective agent for the cytotoxic effects of diazinon in the spermatogenesis in the earthworm Eisenia foetida. *Ital J. Anat. Embryol.* 2005;110(2 Suppl 1):159-65.
[16] Cary GA, Cuttler AS, Duda KA, Kusema ET, Myers JA, Tilden AR. Melatonin: neuritogenesis and neuroprotective effects in crustacean x-organ cells. *Comp. Biochem. Physiol. A Mol. Integr. Physiol.* 2012 Apr;161(4):355-60.
[17] Izmaylov DM, Obukhova LK. Geroprotector effectiveness of melatonin: investigation of lifespan of Drosophila melanogaster. *Mech.* Ageing Dev. 1999 Jan 15;106(3):233-40.
[18] Maciel FE, Geihs MA, Monserrat JM, Nery LE. Antioxidant defense system rhythms in crustaceans and possible roles for melatonin. *Front Biosci.* (Elite Ed) 2010;2:1448-59.
[19] Maciel FE, Ramos BP, Geihs MA, Vargas MA, Cruz BP, Meyer-Rochow VB, et al. Effects of melatonin in connection with the antioxidant defense system in the gills of the estuarine crab Neohelice granulata. *Gen. Comp. Endocrinol.* 2010 Jan 15;165(2):229-36.
[20] Niva CC, Takeda M. Effects of photoperiod, temperature and melatonin on nymphal development, polyphenism and reproduction in Halyomorpha halys (Heteroptera: Pentatomidae). *Zoolog. Sci.* 2003 Aug;20(8):963-70.
[21] Tanaka D, Furusawa K, Kameyama K, Okamoto H, Doi M. Melatonin signaling regulates locomotion behavior and homeostatic states through distinct receptor pathways in Caenorhabditis elegans. *Neuropharmacology* 2007 Jul;53(1):157-68.
[22] Withyachumnarnkul B, Pongsa-Asawapaiboon A, Ajpru S, Siamwalla P, Trakulrungsi W, Samritthong C. Continuous light increases N-acetyltransferase activity in the optic lobe of the giant freshwater prawn Macrobrachium rosenbergii de Man (Crustacea: Decapoda). *Life Sci.* 1992;51(19):1479-84.
[23] Mendoza-Vargas L, Solis-Chagoyan H, Benitez-King G, Fuentes-Pardo B. MT2-like melatonin receptor modulates amplitude receptor potential in visual cells of crayfish during a 24-hour cycle. *Comp. Biochem. Physiol. A Mol. Integr. Physiol.* 2009 Dec;154(4):486-92.
[24] Solis-Chagoyan H, Mendoza-Vargas L, Fuentes-Pardo B. Melatonin modulates the ERG circadian rhythm in crayfish. *Comp. Biochem. Physiol. A Mol. Integr. Physiol.* 2008 Apr;149(4):373-9.
[25] Tilden AR, Brauch R, Ball R, Janze AM, Ghaffari AH, Sweeney CT, et al. Modulatory effects of melatonin on behavior, hemolymph metabolites, and neurotransmitter release in crayfish. *Brain Res.* 2003 Dec 5;992(2):252-62.
[26] Tilden AR, Alt J, Brummer K, Groth R, Herwig K, Wilson A, et al. Influence of photoperiod on N-acetyltransferase activity and melatonin in the fiddler crab Uca pugilator. *Gen. Comp. Endocrinol.* 2001 Jun;122(3):233-7.
[27] Hardie J, Gao N. Melatonin and the pea aphid, Acyrthosiphon pisum. *J. Insect. Physiol.* 1997 Jul;43(7):615-20.
[28] Yamano HO, Matsushita HO, Yanagiwara S. Plasma concentration of rabeprazole after 8-week administration in gastroesophageal reflux disease patients and intragastric pH elevation. *J. Gastroenterol. Hepatol.* 2008 Apr;23(4):534-40.

[29] Dubocovich ML, Delagrange P, Krause DN, Sugden D, Cardinali DP, Olcese J. International Union of Basic and Clinical Pharmacology. LXXV. Nomenclature, classification, and pharmacology of G protein-coupled melatonin receptors. *Pharmacol. Rev.* 2010 Sep;62(3):343-80.

[30] Slominski RM, Reiter RJ, Schlabritz-Loutsevitch N, Ostrom RS, Slominski AT. Melatonin membrane receptors in peripheral tissues: distribution and functions. *Mol. Cell. Endocrinol.* 2012 Apr 4;351(2):152-66.

[31] Tan DX, Manchester LC, Terron MP, Flores LJ, Tamura H, Reiter RJ. Melatonin as a naturally occurring co-substrate of quinone reductase-2, the putative MT3 melatonin membrane receptor: hypothesis and significance. *J. Pineal. Res.* 2007 Nov;43(4):317-20.

[32] Zlotos DP. Recent progress in the development of agonists and antagonists for melatonin receptors. *Curr. Med. Chem.* 2012;19(21):3532-49.

[33] Richter K, Peschke E, Peschke D. A neuroendocrine releasing effect of melatonin in the brain of an insect, Periplaneta americana (L.). *J. Pineal. Res.* 2000 Apr;28(3):129-35.

[34] Mechawar N, Anctil M. Melatonin in a primitive metazoan: seasonal changes of levels and immunohistochemical visualization in neurons. *J. Comp. Neurol. 1997* Oct 20;387(2):243-54.

[35] Itoh MT, Igarashi J. Circadian rhythm of serotonin levels in planarians. *Neuroreport* 2000 Feb 28;11(3):473-6.

[36] Morita M, Best JB. Electron microscopic studies of planarian regeneration. II. Changes in epidermis during regeneration. *J. Exp. Zool.* 1974 Mar;187(3):345-73.

[37] Morita M, Hall F, Best JB, Gern W. Photoperiodic modulation of cephalic melatonin in planarians. *J. Exp. Zool.* 1987 Mar;241(3):383-8.

[38] Migliori ML, Romanowski A, Simonetta SH, Valdez D, Guido M, Golombek DA. Daily variation in melatonin synthesis and arylalkylamine N-acetyltransferase activity in the nematode Caenorhabditis elegans. *J. Pineal. Res.* 2012 Aug;53(1):38-46.

[39] Munoz JL, Lopez Patino MA, Hermosilla C, Conde-Sieira M, Soengas JL, Rocha F, et al. Melatonin in octopus (Octopus vulgaris): tissue distribution, daily changes and relation with serotonin and its acid metabolite. J. Comp. Physiol. A Neuroethol. Sens. Neural Behav. *Physiol.* 2011 Aug;197(8):789-97.

[40] Abran D, Anctil M, Ali MA. Melatonin activity rhythms in eyes and cerebral ganglia of Aplysia californica. Gen Comp Endocrinol 1994 Nov;96(2):215-22.

[41] Blanc A, Vivien-Roels B, Pevet P, Attia J, Buisson B. Melatonin and 5-methoxytryptophol (5-ML) in nervous and/or neurosensory structures of a gastropod mollusc (Helix aspersa maxima): synthesis and diurnal rhythms. *Gen. Comp. Endocrinol.* 2003 Apr;131(2):168-75.

[42] Balzer I, Hardeland R. Circadian rhythmicity in the stimulation of bioluminescence by biogenic amines and MAO inhibitors in Gonyaulax polyedra. *Int. J. Biometeorol.* 1991 Mar;34(4):231-4.

[43] Amherd R, Hintermann E, Walz D, Affolter M, Meyer UA. Purification, cloning, and characterization of a second arylalkylamine N-acetyltransferase from Drosophila melanogaster. *DNA Cell Biol.* 2000 Nov;19(11):697-705.

[44] Bembenek J, Sehadova H, Ichihara N, Takeda M. Day/night fluctuations in melatonin content, arylalkylamine N-acetyltransferase activity and NAT mRNA expression in the CNS, peripheral tissues and hemolymph of the cockroach, Periplaneta americana. *Comp. Biochem. Physiol. B Biochem. Mol. Biol.* 2005 Jan;140(1):27-36.

[45] Itoh MT, Hattori A, Nomura T, Sumi Y, Suzuki T. Melatonin and arylalkylamine N-acetyltransferase activity in the silkworm, Bombyx mori. *Mol. Cell Endocrinol.* 1995 Nov 30;115(1):59-64.

[46] Itoh MT, Nomura T, Sumi Y. Hydroxyindole-O-methyltransferase activity in the silkworm (Bombyx mori). *Brain Res.* 1997 Aug 8;765(1):61-6.

[47] Markowska M, Bentkowski P, Kloc M, Pijanowska J. Presence of melatonin in Daphnia magna. *J. Pineal. Res.* 2009 Mar;46(2):242-4.

[48] Menesatti P, Aguzzi J, Costa C, Garcia JA, Sarda F. A new morphometric implemented video-image analysis protocol for the study of social modulation in activity rhythms of marine organisms. *J. Neurosci. Methods* 2009 Oct 30;184(1):161-8.

[49] Pablos MI, Agapito MT, Gutierrez R, Recio JM, Reiter RJ, Barlow-Walden L, et al. Melatonin stimulates the activity of the detoxifying enzyme glutathione peroxidase in several tissues of chicks. J Pineal Res 1995 Oct;19(3):111-5.

[50] Wetterberg L, Hayes DK, Halberg F. Circadian rhythm of melatonin in the brain of the face fly, Musca autumnalis De Geer. *Chronobiologia* 1987 Oct;14(4):377-81.

In: New Developments in Melatonin Research
ISBN: 978-1-62618-843-3
Editors: D.Acuña-Castroviejo, I.Rusanova, G.Escames

Chapter 3

The Scotophase Rise in Plasma Melatonin in *Rana* Tadpoles and Frogs Comes from the Pineal Gland and the Eyes, whereas the Gut does not Appear to Contribute to Circulating Melatonin

Mary L. Wright, Amy L. Wickett, Nils Pilotte, Lara Demoracski, Melanie Joy, Jill M. Bigos and Shaun E. Richardson*
Biology Department, College of Our Lady of the Elms, Chicopee, MA, US

Abstract

The origin of circulating melatonin has been studied in *Rana catesbeiana* tadpoles and *Rana pipiens* frogs on a 12L:12D cycle. Previous work had indicated that in tadpoles the eyes were a significant source of scotophase plasma melatonin, so we investigated the contribution of the pineal gland in tadpoles and the eyes and the pineal gland in frogs. The findings showed that in both larvae and adults the pineal gland and lateral eyes secrete nearly equal amounts of melatonin into the blood as determined by destruction of the pineal gland and eye extirpation. Pinealectomy and ophthalmectomy together reduce the mid-scotophase blood plasma level to that of photophase, so that the scotophase rise in melatonin is solely due to secretion of the pineal gland and the eyes. These procedures singly or in combination do not change the low mid-photophase level of plasma melatonin. The tadpole digestive tract was studied as a possible source of the photophase, and residual scotophase, plasma melatonin. The gut was found to contain a high level of melatonin, not changed by pineal and eye removal. However, gut extirpation did not change the plasma melatonin level in photophase or scotophase. The findings indicate

* E-mail: wrightm@elms.edu. Phone: (413) 265-2298.

that while the pineal gland and the eyes are the major sources of scotophase plasma melatonin in larval and adult frogs, there is a low level of blood melatonin coming from elsewhere, and that the source of this melatonin is not the gut.

Introduction

Melatonin acts as a link between environmental lighting conditions and the internal state of the organism. As such, the highest concentration is secreted during darkness, thus entraining circadian organization and rhythms of behavior and physiology. Many organs of amphibian larvae and adults contain melatonin. In addition to the plasma [1], pineal gland [2], lateral eyes [3], Harderian glands [4], and digestive tract [5] of adults, melatonin has been found in embryonic Rana pipiens, and in the plasma, eyes, pineal, thyroid, gills, intestine (gut), limb, tail and fat body [6;7] of the anuran larva. In addition to its well-known regulation of circadian periodicity, melatonin is a powerful antioxidant [8;9] and may have many other functions in various tissues. In the eyes, for example, melatonin has local effects on photoreceptors and pigment granules [10;11]. Melatonin has been detected in the gut of vertebrates ranging from fish to mammals[12], where it may modulate physiological processes such as digestion and absorption, the production of gut hormones and mucus, ion transport, and gut motility [13]. Melatonin might also play a role in the hormonal control of amphibian metamorphosis since it antagonizes the thyroid and significantly declines in concentration in the plasma at the metamorphic climax, when the thyroid hormone rises [14;15].

Melatonin is secreted mainly by the pineal gland in mammals, since the eyes do not release the hormone into the plasma [16]. Melatonin synthesis in the pineal gland is controlled by the suprachiasmatic nucleus of the hypothalamus with light input from the eyes [17]. In contrast, nonmammalian vertebrates have light-sensitive pineals often associated with accessory organs such as the parapineal (frontal organ in amphibians) which is also light sensitive [18]. In addition, deep brain photoreceptors have also been identified [19]. Thus, light perception in nonmammals is more complex and there may be other sources than the pineal for circulating melatonin.

Little is known about the origin of circulating melatonin in amphibians. Pinealectomy (PX) in *Ambystoma* (an urodele amphibian) lowers scotophase plasma melatonin by approximately 55% [1], indicating that a substantial portion of the night peak of melatonin in the plasma comes from the pineal gland, but also that there must be other melatonin-producing sites contributing to the blood level. Direct experimental evidence of an ocular contribution to circulating melatonin in amphibians comes from the demonstration that opthalmectomy (EX) in *Rana pipiens* and *Rana catesbeiana* tadpoles and froglets significantly reduces circulating melatonin [15]. This effect is independent of the light dark cycle and the developmental stage, and is primarily due to a reduction in the scotophase peak of plasma melatonin after EX. PX, EX, or the combined operations (PXEX) abolish day-night changes in Japanese newts [20]. However, there is no difference in plasma melatonin among the three procedures, and the scotophase peak is significantly lower than the control only in the pinealectomized group. Taken together, the findings above suggest that most of the scotophase peak of plasma melatonin comes from the eyes and the pineal gland, but that there must also be other source (s) of blood melatonin. It is not yet clear how active the pineal gland might be in anuran larvae, however, nor how much eyes and pineal contribute to plasma melatonin in anuran adults. Although melatonin has been identified in the gut of both larval and adult amphibians as indicated above, it is not clear if gut melatonin is produced there or if it is secreted into the blood.

The goal of the present work was to ascertain the contribution to plasma melatonin of the pineal gland in anuran larvae, and both the eyes and the pineal gland in the adult frog. In addition, we wanted to determine if the gut was also a contributor to circulating melatonin. To these ends, eyes, pineal gland, and both together were removed in frogs, and PX and PXEX done in tadpoles, and melatonin in the plasma was assessed. In another experiment, tadpoles underwent a combined PXEX procedure to lower plasma melatonin, and gut melatonin was assayed. If gut melatonin fluctuates with changes in plasma melatonin, it might indicate that the concentration of melatonin in the gut only reflects how much is taken up from the plasma. A unique gut extirpation (GX) procedure was then used in tadpoles to determine if the gut contributes to circulating melatonin. Pigmentation changes after all the surgeries were also observed since EX tadpoles darkened considerably in previous work [15].

Materials and Methods

Animals

Rana catesbeiana tadpoles and female *Rana pipiens* frogs were obtained from Connecticut Valley Biological Supply Co. (Southampton, MA, USA) and were maintained at 22° C on a 12L:12D cycle (L onset at 0800 h) in light and temperature controlled incubators. Newly acquired animals were acclimated to the LD cycle for a week or longer before an experiment. The tadpoles were kept in 10% Holtfreter's solution occasionally supplemented by spring water, which was changed three times weekly. They were given washed, canned spinach once a day early in the photophase. Tadpoles were staged according to Taylor and Kollros [21], and were in prometamorphosis at the beginning of the experiments. Frogs were kept individually in 2 gallon plastic tanks with a water bowl available and fed *Tenebrio* larvae three times a week. All experiments were performed in accordance with the NIH Guide for the Care and Use of Laboratory Animals and were approved by the IACUC at the College of Our Lady of the Elms.

Pinealectomy and Ophthalmectomy

Animals were kept at 8 or 12^{0} C for 24 h prior to PX operations. In animals undergoing both PX and EX, the operations were done on the same day, PX first. In addition to cold treatment, animals were anesthetized by immersion in 0.1% MS 222. Tadpoles and frogs were kept moist in 10% Holtfreter's solution during the operation, supported by kimwipes. The pineal gland was cauterized by inserting a hot needle dorsally through the skull. In the case of frogs and older tadpoles, skin and skull were removed before cauterization due to the thickness of the skull bones. Eyes were removed (EX) by penetrating the skin under the eye with watchmaker's forceps, severing the optic nerve, and gently pulling out the eye. After the operations, animals were returned to the cold incubator for another 24 h to minimize blood loss and discomfort as they recovered from the anesthesia and surgery.

Previous dissection of representative specimens, as well as the location of the frontal organ (brow spot), allowed for a precise measure of the location of the pineal region from the surface, even though the pineal glands were too small to see. In other work removing the pineal region for melatonin assay, histological studies confirmed the location of the pineal. Accuracy of the procedure was also indicated by the change of operated animals to a dark pigmentation following a successful operation. Finally, the pineal area was dissected out of control tadpoles, and those which had undergone both EX and PX, and analyzed for melatonin content according to procedures below. In the pineal area of control tadpoles there was 1951.00 +- 262.23 pg/g melatonin (n = 6) whereas in tadpoles that had undergone PX, there was only 193.27 +- 68.89 pg/g melatonin (n = 6). The results (p = 0.002) showed that comparatively little melatonin remained in the pineal region of the brain after PX, confirming the accuracy of the procedure. In PX and EX experiments, the controls were anesthetized, but did not receive sham operations. A preliminary experiment in tadpoles showed that there was no significant difference in plasma melatonin between untouched controls (30.57 +- 8.29 pg/ml; n = 8) and sham-operated controls (35.99 +- 6.40 pg/ml; n = 10) which had undergone combined PXEX operation procedures without removal or destruction of organs. In frogs, untouched control values (114.77 +- 39.67; n=9) were likewise not significantly different from sham-operated controls (75.34 +- 22.58; n = 11).

Gut Extirpation

Three days prior to surgery, tadpoles were placed in a suspension of 0.85% sulfadiazine (Sigma) in order to sterilize the intestine since the tadpoles consume the suspension. At this time, other feeding was discontinued. Tadpoles were kept at 8° C for 24 h prior to the operations, and anesthetized by 0.1% MS 222 just before surgery. The long, coiled intestine of the tadpole was removed from the stomach to the colon by gently pulling it out through an approximately 5 mm incision on the ventrolateral side of the animal and then cutting it off, a procedure which resulted in very little bleeding. In these experiments, control tadpoles were anesthetized and a ventrolateral incision was made into the body cavity, although the intestine was not disturbed or removed. Tadpoles were again returned to a cold incubator for 24 h for recovery. Neither control nor GX tadpoles were fed in the days after the operations. Tadpoles have large fat bodies which nourish them during starvation as previous studies have shown [7].

Tissue Collection Procedures

Melatonin was sampled at 1300 and 0100 hr on a 12L:12D cycle in most experiments. Previous work sampling 6 times in 24 hr confirmed that plasma melatonin is low throughout the photophase and highest during the scotophase at 0100 hr on a 12L:12D cycle [15]. In all of the tadpole experiments, 1300 and 0100 hr data were collected on the same day. Because of the difficulty of getting enough frogs at one time, 1300 and 0100 hr data were taken on separate days several weeks apart. Animals were anesthetized in 0.1% MS 222 and after dissection of the heart, blood was pipetted from the heart into siliconized microcentrifuge tubes. In most cases, the blood of one animal constituted a sample, but in a very few instances it was necessary to pool the blood of two animals in order to get the required volume for the melatonin assay. After centrifugation, the plasma was stored at -20°. Gut pieces measuring 6 mm were cut from the central region of the intestine, cleaned of any food residue, weighed, and frozen at -20° C. Before the assay, gut pieces were partially defrosted and homogenized with a glass rod in 500 μl of 0.7% saline. Following homogenization, the mixture was centrifuged to remove all solids and the supernatant was collected and frozen at -20° C. When the protocol called for a collection during the scotophase, room lights were turned out, and animals were handled under a dim red light.

Radioimmunoassay for Melatonin

Melatonin in the plasma was assayed directly, without extraction, using a human melatonin kit obtained from IBL America (Minneapolis, MN, USA). The plasma was enzyme-treated prior to the assay to free the hormone from albumin and other binding proteins. Gut supernatants and pineal area were assayed without enzyme treatment since these tissues had been homogenized in a saline solution. Assays were described, and validated for use with amphibian plasma and some tissues, in Wright et al. [14;22]. The assay was further validated for use with pineal area and gut samples. The means of the slopes of the inhibition curves generated from serially diluted homogenate supernatants of pineal area (-2.1574) and gut (-2.1080) samples using a logit curve fit were not significantly different from the slope of the curves constructed from kit-supplied melatonin standards (-2.0140). The intra- and inter-assay coefficients of variation were 8.1 and 16.1%, respectively. Tubes were counted in a Packard RIASTAR gamma counter with a counting efficiency greater than 80%. The calculations producing the standard curve and sample hormone content were performed by computer using manufacturer-installed software.

Statistics

Results were analyzed by ANOVA followed by Duncan's multiple range test, or t test, as appropriate. Differences were considered to be significant if $P<0.05$.

Results

The first experiment was designed to determine the contribution of the pineal gland to circulating melatonin in the tadpole and also to see if a combination of EX and PX would reduce blood melatonin to daytime levels. Since the contribution of the eyes to plasma melatonin had been studied previously [15], EX alone was not included. None of the surgeries affected photophase melatonin (Figure 1), suggesting that the eyes and pineal gland are not its source. However PX reduced the nighttime peak of plasma melatonin by approximately one-half whereas PXEX lowered the night peak to daytime levels (Figure 1). Thus, the scotophase rise in plasma melatonin comes from the eyes and the pineal gland. Several supplementary experiments were also done on tadpoles which confirmed the drastic drop in circulating melatonin in scotophase after PXEX (Table 1).

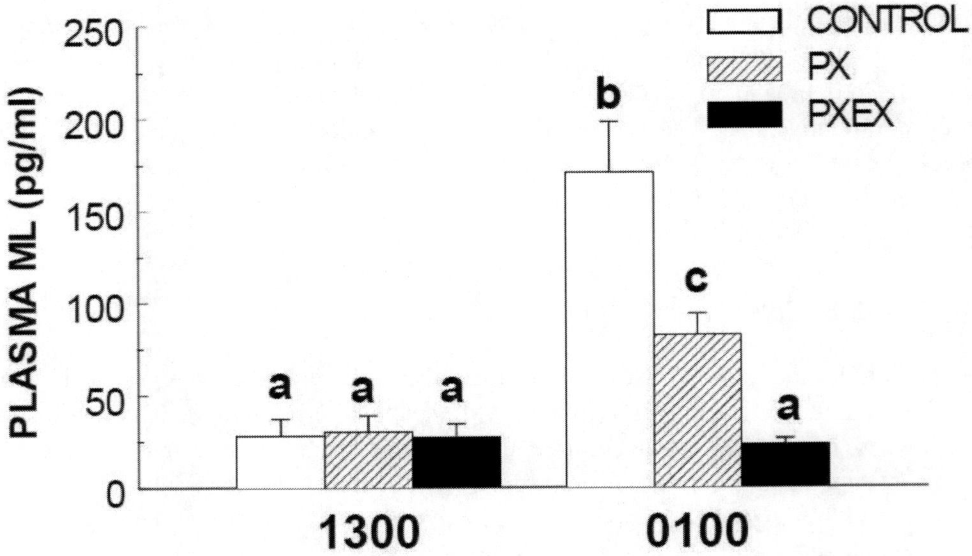

Figure 1. Plasma melatonin (mean +- S.E.) in tadpoles 14 d after PX or PXEX. N = 5 - 9 samples per group. ANOVA $p < 0.0001$. Means with different letters are significantly different with Duncan's Multiple Range test.

Frogs were studied in the next experiment to determine if the origin of plasma melatonin was similar in the adult. Since EX had not been studied in frogs, a group which had only the eyes removed was also included. As in tadpoles, photophase plasma melatonin was not changed by PX, EX, or PXEX whereas in scotophase, PX and EX alone reduced the melatonin level to slightly less than one-half of the control (Figure 2). PXEX lowered mid-dark melatonin to daytime levels, although the differences between PX, EX or PXEX were not significantly different. The findings indicated that as in tadpoles the pineal gland and the eyes produce the scotophase rise in plasma melatonin, and that there was no fundamental difference before and after metamorphosis.

One possible source of daytime and residual nighttime plasma melatonin is the gut. Since removal of the gut in tadpoles is easier than in frogs, and tadpoles recover more easily, the subsequent experiments utilized tadpoles. Gut melatonin was measured in mid-light and mid-dark in control and PXEX tadpoles (Figure 3). The gut contained a high concentration of melatonin (average of 1300 and 0100 hr values = 835.92+-162.02 pg/g intestine), which did not exhibit a circadian rhythm since the levels in photophase and scotophase were the same in both the controls and the PXEX groups. Additional experiments (data not shown) confirmed the lack of rhythmicity in gut melatonin.

PXEX did not affect the melatonin level at either time of day, suggesting that gut melatonin may be synthesized in situ and not taken up from the plasma.

Finally, the effect on circulating melatonin of removing the gut in tadpoles was ascertained (Figure 4). N GX had no effect on either photophase or scotophase plasma melatonin concentrations. Thus it does not appear that the digestive tract is the source of daytime plasma melatonin or of the residual scotophase plasma melatonin remaining after PXEX. Interestingly, there was a small piece of gut regenerated in the longer experiments to connect the two cut ends of the digestive tract.

The skin darkened to some extent in both tadpoles and frogs after removal of pineal or eyes, with animals showing this feature to varying degrees. PXEX resulted in extreme darkening of all animals, while GX did not alter the pigmentation in tadpoles.

Table 1. Supplementary experiments with tadpoles showing the decrease in plasma melatonin after PXEX[1]

		1300	0100
Exp. 1	Control PXEX	13.81+-3.94[a] (4) 12.72+-3.40[a] (4)	48.62+-17.64[b] (4) 6.50+-2.19[a] (5)
Exp. 2	Control PXEX	-------	254.06+-132.89[a] (4) 16.09+-2.50[b] (7)
Exp. 3	Control PXEX	--------	168.87+-35.46[a] (4) 12.83+-2.56[b] (4)

[1] Means (+-SEM). The numbers in parentheses indicate the number of samples. Different letters indicate significant differences (P<0.05) within each experiment.

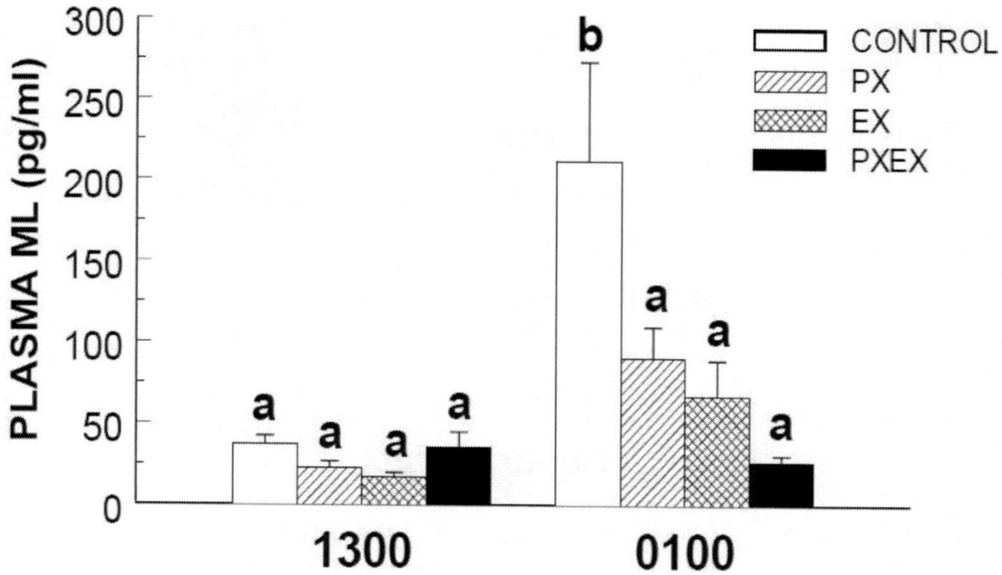

Figure 2. Plasma melatonin (mean +- S.E.) in adult frogs 7 d after surgery. N = 5 - 6 samples per group except for 4 samples in control 0100 and 3 samples in EX 0100. ANOVA p < 0.0001. Means with different letters are significantly different with Duncan's Multiple Range test.

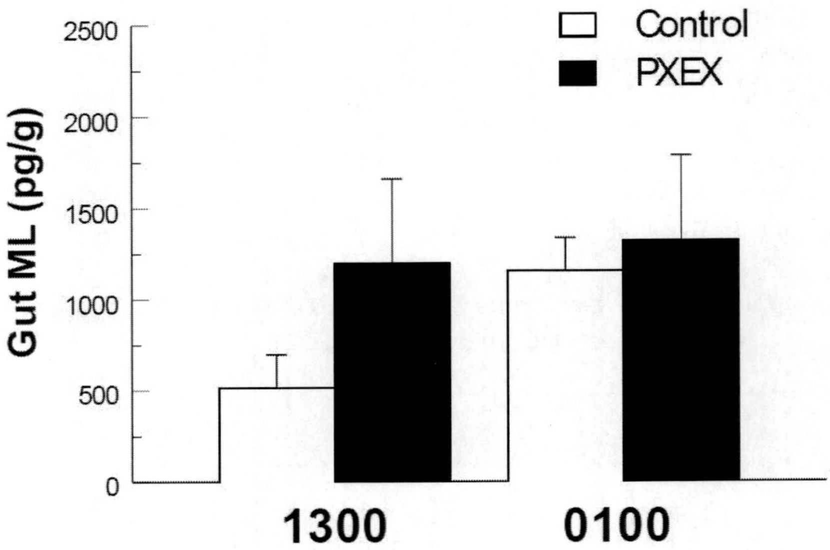

Figure 3. Gut melatonin (mean +- S.E.) in control and PXEX tadpoles 26 d after surgery. N = 5 samples per group. There were no significant differences.

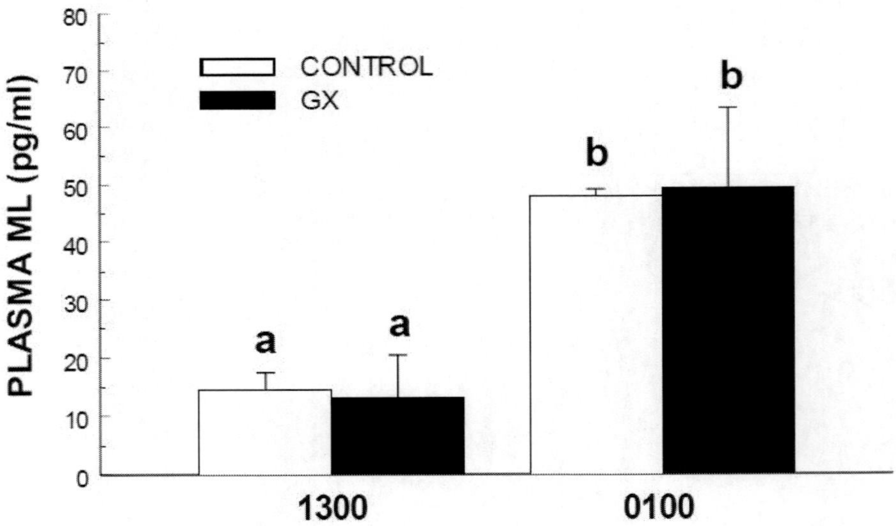

Figure 4. Plasma melatonin (mean +- S.E.) in tadpoles seven days after gut removal. N = 7 - 9 samples per group. ANOVA p = .0029. Means with different letters are significantly different with Duncan's Multiple Range test.

Discussion

In tadpoles, PX reduced scotophase plasma melatonin to about one-half of the control level, while PXEX reduced it an average of approximately 90% in the various experiments reported here, bringing it to about the photophase level. In a previous paper [15] EX reduced mid-scotophase plasma melatonin an average of 78% in several experiments comparable in LD cycle and other characteristics to the ones reported here. Similar results were found in frogs, where mid-scotophase plasma melatonin was reduced 69% by EX, 57% by PX, and 87% by PXEX.

Thus, it appears that both the eyes and the pineal gland contribute to nighttime circulating melatonin in both larvae and adults, and that these organs together are responsible for the scotophase peak. The findings also show that there is a baseline level of plasma melatonin present in both day and night, which does not derive from either the pineal or the eyes. These results on anuran larvae and adults are essentially in agreement with Gern and Norris [1] who did PX in Ambystoma, and Chiba et al. [20] who utilized PX, EX, and PXEX on the Japanese newt, except that Chiba et al. did not find a significant decrease in scotophase plasma melatonin after EX. The observations that melatonin is higher in the eyes than in the pineal gland in frogs, and melatonin circadian rhythms in the plasma are synchronized more to ocular melatonin profiles than to those of the pineal [2] are in agreement with a contribution of the eyes to blood melatonin. An ocular contribution to circulating melatonin has also been found in Japanese quail [23] and in the pigeon [24].

Bayarri et al. [25] had similar results to ours in sea bass, but attributed the decrease in blood melatonin after EX to the hypothesis that the pineal gland needs the eyes for proper melatonin output rather than that the eyes contribute to blood melatonin. This conclusion came from the finding that cutting the optic nerve had the same effect as EX in lowering plasma melatonin. This interpretation does not explain how PXEX reduces scotophase melatonin significantly more than PX alone. If the pineal gland were the sole source of circulating melatonin, PX should decrease the melatonin level to the same extent as PXEX, yet that was not the case in the present work or in Bayarri et al. [25].

Although PX was not done, Martinez-Chavez and Migaud [26;27] found that EX completely suppressed the scotophase rise in plasma melatonin, yet also attributed this to the pineal gland being dependent on the eyes for proper output. On the other hand, Kezuka et al. [28] found that EX had no effect on plasma melatonin in the goldfish. The origin of blood melatonin may differ in fish and amphibians. It has been hypothesized that there might be different roles for the eyes in the circadian physiology of various groups of fish [27].

The gut has a relatively high level of melatonin, which could be taken up from the blood rather than synthesized in the gut. If it was derived mainly from the circulation, gut melatonin would be expected to decrease proportionately to plasma melatonin after PXEX, but it did not. Since the level of melatonin in the gut did not fluctuate with the level in the plasma, melatonin must be synthesized in situ in the tadpole gut. In rats [29] and pigeons [30], pinealectomy does not affect the level of melatonin in gut tissues although it reduces plasma melatonin.

Our findings are in agreement with compelling evidence from other vertebrates that melatonin is made in the gut. For example, melatonin and the chief enzymes responsible for its synthesis, are localized in the enterochromaffin cells of the mucosa [12] together with the melatonin precursor, serotonin [31]. The level of melatonin differs in various parts of the gut [5;13], suggesting independent synthesis.

Gut melatonin was not significantly higher in the dark than in the light, indicating that the dial rhythm of melatonin in the plasma is not found in tadpole gut tissues. It is not yet clear if gut melatonin synthesis or secretion in other vertebrates shows circadian rhythmicity [13;32], but no diurnal variation was found in the digestive tract of the rat [33], nor was there diurnal variation of the enzyme N-acetyltransferase in the rat intestine [29]. There was no circadian rhythm of melatonin in the gill, small intestine and kidney of three fish species, except for the gill in sea bream [34]. In many mammals, only retina and pineal gland exhibit circadian rhythms of melatonin production [35], and that may be true of amphibians as well.

There was residual melatonin in the plasma of tadpoles and frogs after PXEX. It is unlikely that the residual scotophase melatonin came from an incomplete PX. Care was taken to remove the entire pineal area including the frontal organ which lies under a nonpigmented area on the surface called the brow spot [36].

The brain also contains melatonin [37] and this probably explains the melatonin left in extracts of the pineal area after PX as described in the Materials and Methods. Kezuka et al. [28] found melatonin remaining in the blood of goldfish and Bayarri et al. [25] in the plasma of sea bass after PXEX and in both cases it was suggested that it may have come from the gut. Many indirect experiments indicate that at least some of the residual melatonin found in the plasma after PX comes from the gastrointestinal tract, mainly in mammals [12]. However, in the present work the gut was removed in what, to our knowledge, is the first experiment of its kind. Yet GX did not affect the level of blood melatonin in photophase or scotophase, indicating that in amphibians it is not likely that the gut contributes to plasma melatonin. Although the long coiled tadpole intestine, by far the longest part of the digestive tract in the larva, was removed and not the larval stomach and short colon, it seems that there would be at least some reduction in plasma melatonin after the surgery if the gut secreted into the blood.

The photophase and residual scotophase (after PXEX) melatonin was at a fairly constant low level, which might indicate it is not from the gut, since gut melatonin has been reported to fluctuate with the diet or digestive activity [12]. The source of photophase and residual scotophase blood melatonin still has to be determined.

Both tadpoles and frogs darkened considerably after PXEX, even more than with PX or EX alone. Darkening after similar surgeries was also noted in sea bass [25]. EX-induced darkening did not appear to be due to an increase in α- melanotropin (α-MSH) since the pituitary content of this hormone in darkened tadpoles did not change [15]. Melatonin has been associated with tadpole lightening [38], so it is possible that a decrease in melatonin after PX, EX, or PXEX might cause darkening, especially since melatonin has been reported to antagonize the action of α-MSH [39]. Since plasma melatonin decreased more after PXEX than after PX or EX alone, it might be expected that PXEX animals would be the darkest, as they were. Loss of light perception by lateral eyes and/or the light-sensitive pineal might also be involved since amphibians regulate coloration by background [40].

Conclusion

The scotophase rise in circulating melatonin originates from the pineal gland and the eyes in both anuran larvae and adults. The gut contains a high level of melatonin which lacks day-night rhythmicity. Gut removal failed to affect the level of photophase or scotophase plasma melatonin. Therefore, in the species studied the photophase and residual (after PXEX) scotophase plasma melatonin does not come from the gut. The pronounced darkening of the skin of both larvae and adults after PXEX might be due to loss of the lightening action of melatonin, or to loss of light perception by eyes and pineal producing dark background adaptation.

Acknowledgment

The authors thank Brian Cunniff, Amanda Guyette, and Jessica Payne for technical assistance in the experiments. This research was supported by NSF grant IBN-0236251.

References

[1] Gern W. A, Norris DO. Plasma melatonin in the neotenic tiger salamander (Ambystoma tigrinum): effects of photoperiod and pinealectomy. *Gen. Comp. Endocrinol.* 1979 Aug;38(4):393-8.

[2] Delgado M. J, Vivien-Roels B. Effect of environmental temperature and photoperiod on the melatonin levels in the pineal, lateral eye, and plasma of the frog, Rana perezi: importance of ocular melatonin. *Gen. Comp. Endocrinol.* 1989 Jul; 75 (1):46-53.

[3] Pang S. F, Shiu S. Y, Tse S. F. Effect of photic manipulation on the level of melatonin in the retinas of frogs (Rana tigrina regulosa). *Gen. Comp. Endocrinol.* 1985 Jun;58(3):464-70.

[4] d'Istria M, Monteleone P, Serino I, Chieffi G. Seasonal variations in the daily rhythm of melatonin and NAT activity in the Harderian gland, retina, pineal gland, and serum of the green frog, Rana esculenta. *Gen. Comp. Endocrinol.* 1994 Oct; 96 (1):6-11.

[5] Bubenik G. A, Pang S. F. Melatonin levels in the gastrointestinal tissues of fish, amphibians, and a reptile. *Gen. Comp. Endocrinol*. 1997 Jun; 106 (3): 415-9.

[6] Wright M. L, Shea T. A, Visconti R. F, Ramah B. L, Francisco L. L, Scott J. L, et al. Melatonin in anuran development and metamorphosis. In: Haldar, C, Singaravel, M, Pandi-Perumal, S. R, Cardinali, D. P, editors. Experimental Endocrinology and Reproductive Biology. Enfield, NH USA:Science Publishers;2008;211-25.

[7] Wright M. L, Richardson S. E, Bigos J. M. The fat body of bullfrog (Lithobates catesbeianus) tadpoles during metamorphosis: changes in mass, histology, and melatonin content and effect of food deprivation. *Comp. Biochem. Physiol. A Mol. Integr. Physiol*. 2011 Dec; 160 (4): 498-503.

[8] Bettahi I, Pozo D, Osuna C, Reiter R. J, Acuna-Castroviejo D, Guerrero J. M. Melatonin reduces nitric oxide synthase activity in rat hypothalamus. *J. Pineal Res.* 1996 May;20(4):205-10.

[9] Karbownik M, Reiter R. J. Antioxidative effects of melatonin in protection against cellular damage caused by ionizing radiation. *Proc. Soc. Exp. Biol. Med.* 2000 Oct; 225 (1):9-22.

[10] Besharse J. C, Dunis D. A. Methoxyindoles and photoreceptor metabolism: activation of rod shedding. *Science.* 1983 Mar 18; 219 (4590): 1341-3.

[11] Tosini G. Melatonin circadian rhythm in the retina of mammals. *Chronobiol. Int.* 2000 Sep;17(5):599-612.

[12] Bubenik G. A. Gastrointestinal melatonin: localization, function, and clinical relevance. *Dig. Dis. Sci*. 2002 Oct; 47 (10): 2336-48.

[13] Motilva V, Cabeza J, Alarcon dlL. New issues about melatonin and its effects on the digestive system. *Curr. Pharm. Des*. 2001 Jul; 7 (10): 909-31.

[14] Wright M. L, Duffy J. L, Guertin C. J, Alves C. D, Szatkowski M. C, Visconti P. F. Developmental and diel changes in plasma thyroxine and plasma and ocular melatonin in the larval and juvenile bullfrog, Rana catesbeiana. *Gen. Comp. Endocrinol.* 2003 Feb; 130 (2):120-8.

[15] Wright M. L, Francisco L. L, Scott J. L, Richardson S. E, Carr J. A, King A. B, et al. Effects of bilateral and unilateral ophthalmectomy on plasma melatonin in Rana tadpoles and froglets under various experimental conditions. *Gen. Comp. Endocrinol.* 2006 Jun;147(2):158-66.

[16] Tosini G, Fukuhara C. Photic and circadian regulation of retinal melatonin in mammals. *J. Neuroendocrinol.* 2003 Apr;15(4):364-9.

[17] Meissl H. Photic regulation of pineal function. Analogies between retinal and pineal photoreception. *Biol. Cell.* 1997 Dec;89(9):549-54.

[18] Oksche A. Survey Of The Development And Comparative Morphology Of The Pineal Organ. *Prog. Brain Res.* 1965; 10:3-29.

[19] Foster R. G, Soni B. G. Extraretinal photoreceptors and their regulation of temporal physiology. *Rev. Reprod.* 1998 Sep; 3 (3):145-50.

[20] Chiba A, Hattori A, Iigo M. Daily and circadian variations of the pineal and ocular melatonin contents and their contributions to the circulating melatonin in the Japanese newt, Cynops pyrrhogaster. *Zoolog. Sci.* 2005 Jan; 22 (1):65-70.

[21] Taylor A. C, Kollros J. J. Stages in the normal development of Rana pipiens larvae. *Anat. Rec.* 1946 Jan;94:7-23.

[22] Wright M. L, Proctor K. L, Alves C. D. Hormonal profiles correlated with season, cold, and starvation in Rana catesbeiana (bullfrog) tadpoles. *Comp. Biochem. Physiol. C Pharmacol. Toxicol. Endocrinol.* 1999 Sep; 124 (1): 109-16.

[23] Underwood H, Binkley S, Siopes T, Mosher K. Melatonin rhythms in the eyes, pineal bodies, and blood of Japanese quail (Coturnix coturnix japonica). *Gen. Comp. Endocrinol.* 1984 Oct;56(1):70-81.

[24] Foà A, Menaker M. Contributions of pineal and retinae to the circadian rhythms of circulating melatonin in pigeons. *J. Comp. Physiol.* 1988 Jan;164A(1):25-30.

[25] Bayarri M. J, Rol de Lama M. A, Madrid J. A, Sanchez-Vazquez F. J. Both pineal and lateral eyes are needed to sustain daily circulating melatonin rhythms in sea bass. *Brain Res.* 2003 Apr 18; 969 (1-2):175-82.

[26] Martinez-Chavez C. C, Migaud H. Retinal light input is required to sustain plasma melatonin rhythms in Nile tilapia Oreochromis niloticus niloticus. *Brain Res.* 2009 May 7; 1269:61-7.

[27] Migaud H, Davie A, Martinez Chavez C. C, Al-Khamees S. Evidence for differential photic regulation of pineal melatonin synthesis in teleosts. *J. Pineal Res.* 2007 Nov;43(4):327-35.

[28] Kezuka H, Iigo M, Furukawa K, Aida K, Hanyu, I. Effects of photoperiod, pinealectomy, and opthalmectomy on circulating melatonin rhythms in the goldfish, Carassius auratus. *Zoolog. Sci.* 1992 May;9(5):1047-53.

[29] Bubenik G. A, Brown G. M. Pinealectomy reduces melatonin levels in the serum but not in the gastrointestinal tract of rats. *Biol. Signals.* 1997 Jan; 6(1):40-4.

[30] Vakkuri O, Rintamaki H, Leppaluoto J. Plasma and tissue concentrations of melatonin after midnight light exposure and pinealectomy in the pigeon. *J. Endocrinol.* 1985 May; 105 (2):263-8.

[31] Bubenik G. A, Ball R. O, Pang S. F. The effect of food deprivation on brain and gastrointestinal tissue levels of tryptophan, serotonin, 5-hydroxyindoleacetic acid, and melatonin. *J. Pineal. Res.* 1992 Jan; 12 (1): 7-16.

[32] Huether G. The contribution of extrapineal sites of melatonin synthesis to circulating melatonin levels in higher vertebrates. *Experientia.* 1993 Aug 15;49(8):665-70.

[33] Bubenik G. A. Localization of melatonin in the digestive tract of the rat. Effect of maturation, diurnal variation, melatonin treatment and pinealectomy. *Horm. Res.* 1980;12(6):313-23.

[34] Kulczykowska E, Kalamarz H, Warne J. M, Balment R. J. Day-night specific binding of 2-[125I]iodomelatonin and melatonin content in gill, small intestine and kidney of three fish species. *J. Comp. Physiol.* B 2006 May; 176 (4):277-85.

[35] Slominski A, Tobin D. J, Zmijewska M. A, Wortsman J, Paus R. Melatonin in the skin: synthesis, metabolism and functions. *Trends Endocrinol. Metab.* 2008 Jan; 19 (1): 17-29.

[36] Eakin R. M. Photoreceptors In The Amphibian Frontal Organ. *Proc. Natl. Acad. Sci. U S A.* 1961 Jul; 47 (7):1084-8.

[37] Hardeland R. Melatonin metabolism in the central nervous system. *Curr. Neuropharmacol.* 2010 Sep; 8 (3):168-81.

[38] Charlton H. M. The pineal gland and color change in *Xenopus laevis* Daudin. *Gen. Comp. Endocrinol.* 1966 Oct; 7 (2):384-97.

[39] Filadelfi A. M, Castrucci A. M. Comparative aspects of the pineal/melatonin system of poikilothermic vertebrates. *J. Pineal Res.* 1996 May; 20 (4):175-86.

[40] Camargo C. R, Visconti M. A, Castrucci AM. Physiological color change in the bullfrog, Rana catesbeiana. *J. Exp. Zool.* 1999 Feb 1; 283 (2): 160-9.

In: New Developments in Melatonin Research ISBN: 978-1-62618-843-3
Editors: D.Acuña-Castroviejo, I.Rusanova, G.Escames © 2013 Nova Science Publishers, Inc.

Chapter 4

Development of Novel Melatoninergics as Circadian Rhythm Sleep Disorder Therapeutics

King Hang Chan, Annie Suet Ting Cheung, Maurice Kwok Chung Ho and Yung Hou Wong*

Biotechnology Research Institute, Molecular Neuroscience Center, State Key Laboratory of Molecular Neuroscience, Division of Life Science, The Hong Kong University of Science and Technology, Hong Kong, China

Abstract

Sleep disorders are an amalgam of complex neurophysiological and psychological disturbances which are globally prevalent and cause significant socio-behavioral and economic burden. Circadian rhythm sleep disorders (CRSDs) are a subfamily of sleep disorders related to extrinsic (jet lag, shift works) and intrinsic (delayed or advance sleep phase syndromes) disturbances of the onset/offset, duration and regularity of sleep. Melatonin is an endogenous neurohormone well-known for its regulatory actions on circadian rhythm. The level of circulatory melatonin is synchronized with the onset of darkness in a normal diurnal cycle, and one of the roles of melatonin is to act as a signal for the body to sleep through its multiple central and peripheral actions. Melatoninergics have recently been adopted as medications for CRSDs because of their effectiveness in resetting the onset of sleep and they appear to have minimal unwanted side effects. Although melatonin has been commonly adopted as an over-the-counter sleeping pill, the major limitations for the use of melatonin as an effective therapeutic agent are its short half-life *in vivo* and poor oral bioavailability. Multiple molecular binding sites of melatonin have been identified, including two subtypes of G protein-coupled receptors (GPCRs), quinone reductase 2, and isoforms of nuclear ROR/RXR receptors, which

* Corresponding author: Yung Hou Wong. Biotechnology Research Institute, Hong Kong University of Science and Technology, Clear Water Bay, Kowloon, Hong Kong, China. Tel: (852) 2358 7328; Fax: (852) 2358 1552. Email: boyung@ust.hk.

account for the ubiquitous actions of melatonin in additional to its intrinsic antioxidant property. It is believed that most of the melatonin-induced physiological responses are mediated through the two subtypes of cell surface-expressing GPCRs. Drug discovery and development programs have been directed at identifying chemical molecules that bind to the two melatonin receptor subtypes. However, all of the melatoninergics in the market act on both subtypes of melatonin receptors without significant selectivity. The quest of developing melatoninergics with desired target specificity, tissue distribution and bioavailability has been continuing for the past decades. This chapter will first give a brief account on the structural diversity of melatoninergics that has been developed for therapeutic uses. Secondly, the discovery of subtype-selective melatoninergics with different chemical scaffolds will be illustrated with a focus on their pharmacological and pharmacokinetics competencies, followed by a discussion on the highly potent and subtype-selective novel melatoninergics that have recently been identified in our laboratory. Concluding remarks will be made on the pros and cons of the therapeutic uses of melatoninergics in CRSDs and the potential applications in other categories of sleep disorders.

Keywords: Circadian rhythm sleeps disorders, melatonin receptors

Introduction

Definition and Classification of Circadian Rhythm Sleep Disorders

According to the second edition of the International Classification of Sleep Disorders (ICSD-2), circadian rhythm sleep disorders (CRSDs) are defined as "a persistent or recurrent pattern of sleep disturbance primarily due to alterations in the circadian timekeeping system or a misalignment between the endogenous circadian rhythm and exogenous factors that affect the timing or duration of sleep" [1]. Classification of CRSDs has been formulated into 9 possible diagnoses of clinical interests, which can be generally differentiated into primary and secondary CRSDs based on the different etiological factors. There are 4 types of primary CRSDs which are caused by the disturbances of the internal system of circadian rhythm, including: (1) delayed sleep phase type, (2) advanced sleep phase type, (3) irregular sleep-wake pattern type and (4) non-24-h sleep-wake type. Another 4 types induced by external social or environmental factors are known as secondary CRSDs, including: (5) jet lag type, (6) shift work type, (7) disease-associated type, and (8) drug or substance abuse-related type. Other cases that meet the general diagnostic criteria for CRSDs but do not fall into any specific classifications are regarded as (9) CRSD Not Otherwise Specified (NOS).

The 6 most common CRSDs will be briefly described below to illustrate the characteristics of CRSDs. Delayed sleep phase disorder (DSPD) and advanced sleep phase disorder (ASPD) are both characterized by a displacement of the sleep period with regard to the desired sleeping time. DSPD typically occurs in adolescents and affects individuals with difficulty in initiating sleep and awakening at the desired clock time. ASPD is frequently associated with the elderly and results in an early sleep onset as well as early spontaneous awakening in the morning. Genetic factors involving the polymorphisms of the "clock genes" that generate the intrinsic circadian rhythm are known to be associated with both DSPD and

ASPD [2;3]. Irregular sleep-wake rhythm (ISWR) is easily recognized by its disorganized and variable episodes of sleep/awake patterns. The total sleep time of the ISWR patients may be comparable to normal subjects, but is usually broken up into several short blocks within the 24-hour day, and often, the timing of sleep and wakefulness varies from day to day. Non-24-hour sleep-wake syndrome (also dubbed free-running disorder) is highly prevalent in the blind [4]. These patients have longer intrinsic circadian period similar to those normal subjects in time-free environments, which are related to the absence of entrainment due to the lack of light-dark external time cue. Shift work disorder (SWD) and jet lag disorder (JLD) are due to a voluntary or imposed shift in the timing of sleep that exceeds the limits of circadian adaption, thus causing a misalignment between the circadian system and the desired sleeping time. SWD affects night-shift or early morning-shift workers where their working hours coincide with the habitual sleep period. They are influenced by excessive sleepiness and reduced alertness at work as a result of shortened sleep time and inadequate sleep quality. JLD is a consequence of rapid travel across multiple time zones, generating symptoms of insomnia, excessive sleepiness, impaired alertness and gastrointestinal illness. This type of disorder usually lasts for a few days and its severity depends on the direction of travel as well as the number of time zones crossed.

Therapeutic Approaches for CRSDs

In general, clinical treatments for CRSDs fall into three major categories: (1) prescribed sleep/wake scheduling, (2) circadian phase shifting, and (3) medications to promote sleep or wakefulness [5]. These treatments have been applied to different disorders of CRSDs based on their correlation with the mechanisms and symptoms of the specific disorders.

Prescribed sleep/wake scheduling has been mainly employed to cope with shift work disorders. Circadian phase shifting is usually achieved by timed exposure of either light or melatonin, which acts by synchronizing the endogenous circadian system to the desired sleep schedule [6-8]. Phototherapy has been demonstrated to be effective in ASPD using evening light therapy as well as in DSPD with light exposure at the desired waking up time [5]. Appropriate exposure to intense light or light avoidance also aids in resynchronizing the biological clock in patients with JLD and SWD [9]. Nonetheless, the applications of prescribed sleep/wake schedule and circadian phase shifting encounter some difficulties in implementation, for example, the incorporation of bright light into the work environment for the treatment of SWD is found to be inconvenient. Furthermore, treatment protocols with standard parameters have not yet been established for both timed light and melatonin treatments. It should be noted that optimization of light intensity and duration of light treatment for phototherapy as well as the scheduling and dosing of melatonin administration is required for effective outcomes on CRSDs [10].

The use of melatonin or, more recently, melatoninergic agonists are promising therapeutic options for the treatment of several CRSDs, though melatonin has not been approved by the United States Food and Drugs Administration (USFDA) as a drug. A general formulation of 3 mg of melatonin is widely available as nutritional supplement in the United States for producing pharmacological melatonin levels in the circulation [11]. Melatonin administered late in the afternoon could advance the sleep phase in individuals with DSPD and entrain totally blind people with FRD receiving sustained treatment [4;5]. Melatonin also reduces jet lag symptoms when applied at bedtime on the first nights after arrival following a rapid travel across multiple time zones [12]. Although melatonin represents one of the most adoptable treatment options for most of the CRSDs, the therapeutic use of melatonin as an oral drug is limited by a number of factors including its unfavorable pharmacokinetic properties and non-specific actions with other potential binding sites. The high first-pass metabolism and a short *in vivo* half-life of less than 30 minutes contribute to the poor bioavailability of melatonin after oral administration. Furthermore, the non-specific binding of melatonin to multiple melatonin receptors may produce potential unwanted side effects [13].

Sleep disorders are also often treated with benzodiazepine- or non-benzodiazepine-based hypnotics. To relieve the symptom of insomnia, hypnotic drugs have been employed to counteract the unwanted alertness whereas stimulants have been applied to relieve the symptom of excessive sleepiness. Specifically, benzodiazepine hypnotic agents, such as flurazepam, temazepam and triazolam, have been used for jet lag-induced insomnia and for daytime sleep in night shift workers [11;14]. Caffeine has been employed in JLD and SWD patients [15;16]. Modafinil ((±)-2-(benzhydrylsulfinyl)acetamide) has been approved by USFDA for treating necrolepsy and improving alertness in shift workers while at work [17]. Major drawbacks of these sedatives and analeptics are their non-specific effects on multiple brain regions such as the emotional centers [18], as well as the medial frontopolar and anterior cingulated cortex [19], and they may cause severe undesirable side-effects such as anxiety, depression and hypertension which are also unfavorable for treating CRSDs.

Melatonin and Melatonin Receptors

Melatonin

Melatonin (*N*-acetyl-5-methoxytryptamine) was first purified and characterized from the bovine pineal gland extract by the dermatologist Aaron Lerner in 1958. This indole hormone is broadly distributed in diverse flora and fauna from bacteria, plants to animals. Chemically, melatonin is a potent free radical scavenger and regulator of redox-active enzymes in many plants, while in animals and humans, it is an important hormone with renowned regulatory roles in mammalian circadian rhythm [20]. Melatonin is primarily secreted by the pineal gland, and many extrapineal tissues, including the retina [21], brain, thymus, platelets [22], bone marrow cells [23], the gastrointestinal tract [24], skin [25] and lymphocytes [26]. The mean production rate of endogenous melatonin in human is 28.8 micrograms/day and active concentrations of melatonin range from subnanomolar to millimolar doses depending on its actions [27].

A Chronobiotic

The primary roles of melatonin in circadian phase readjustment, sleep initiation and support of sleep maintenance are largely mediated by the membrane receptors and to these effects, melatonin has been widely used in the treatment of chronobiological disorders such as seasonal affective disorders, insomnia and sleep disorders caused by blindness, shift work and jet lag [28-31]. In both nocturnal and diurnal species, melatonin is produced by the pineal gland during the dark phase at night and its production is acutely suppressed by light. Once produced, melatonin is released into the bloodstream and the cerebrospinal fluids without storage, and is rapidly distributed to most tissues in the body [32]. Melatonin has a short half-life of less than 30 minutes and is quickly cleared from the circulation, the plasma melatonin level, therefore, is low during the day and high during the night, exhibiting circadian periodicity. With the continuing output of the pineal gland, melatonin circulates in a physiologically active concentration at night [33] and induces the nocturnal melatonin signal that encodes time of day and length of day information to the central biological clock [34].

The biosynthesis of melatonin begins with the acetylation of serotonin by the arylalkylamine-*N*-acetyltransferase (AANAT) producing *N*-acetylserotonin, which is metabolized into melatonin by the hydroxyindole-*O*-methyltransferase (HIOMT) [35]. The biosynthesis and secretion of pineal melatonin is strictly controlled by the suprachiasmatic nucleus (SCN) of the hypothalamus and is synchronized with the environmental light dark cycle. Light signal perceived by the retinal ganglion cells is transmitted to the SCN via the retino-hypothalamic tract (RHT) [36] to trigger the release of glutamate and pituitary adenylyl cyclase activating polypeptide (PACAP), which elicit phase shifts in the SCN circadian rhythm [37]. The SCN subsequently conveys the signal to the pineal gland to regulate melatonin production through the paraventricular nucleus, the intermediolateral cell column and the superior cervical ganglion [38]. In the absence of light, the postganglionic sympathetic fibers from the superior cervical ganglion activate the pineal β-adrenergic receptors through the release of norepinephrine and trigger the production of cAMP, which stimulates the melatonin-synthesizing enzyme AANAT expression and phosphorylation via protein kinase A. These processes are inversely affected by the exposure of light, which the pineal AANAT production is quickly terminated and subjected for degradation. Hence, when SCN activity is inhibited during the dark phase, the endogenous melatonin level increases through the upregulation of melatonin production and inhibits SCN neuronal firing in a feedback mechanism to promote sleep [39]. While during the light phase of the photoperiod, SCN suppresses the sympathetic output to the pineal gland with increased activity and reduced sleep propensity.

Administration of melatonin to elderly human subjects and Alzheimer's diseases patients, whom have been found to exhibit reduced expression of MT_2 receptors [40], has gained promising results in sleep improvement [41]. Melatonin also helps regulate normal sleep patterns for insomniac patients with psychiatric disorders, such as bipolar, depression, anxiety and schizophrenia.

Is Possibly More than a Chronobiotic?

Besides circadian rhythm, an immense diversity of physiological and pathophysiological processes are actually regulated by melatonin, including retinal physiology, seasonal reproductive cycles, cancer development and growth, immune modulation, antioxidation and free radical scavenging, mitochondrial respiration, cardiovascular function, bone metabolism, intermediary metabolism and gastrointestinal physiology [34;42;43]. Hence, melatonin was suggested to have a variety of clinical applications such as inhibiting the proliferation of various types of cancer cells [44] and exhibiting immunomodulatory properties [45]. As a potent antioxidant and free radical scavenger, melatonin offers neuroprotective and anti-inflammatory effects to neuronal cells from free radical and neurotoxin-induced damage and displays potential therapeutic benefits in treating neurodegenerative diseases including Parkinson's disease, Alzheimer's disease, muscular sclerosis, stroke and neuroendocrine disorders [46-50].

G Protein-Coupled Melatonin Receptors

Melatonin exerts most of its major physiological actions by interacting with seven-transmembrane G protein-coupled melatonin receptors besides its free radical scavenging property. The first melatonin receptor was cloned from *Xenopus laevis* immortalized melanophore mRNAs which was expressed only in non-mammalian species [51]. Subsequently, cDNAs encoding two different forms of human melatonin receptors have been cloned and denoted as types 1 and 2 melatonin receptors (MT_1 and MT_2, respectively) [52;53]. The binding characteristics of the two receptor subtypes are similar, exhibiting subnanomolar affinities for melatonin [54]. MT_1 and MT_2 are separately mapped to chromosome 4q35.1 and 11q21-22, respectively, and encoding two proteins with 350 and 365 amino acids, respectively [53;55], sharing 55% overall identity and 70% within membrane domains [56]. Like many other G protein-coupled receptors (GPCRs), melatonin receptors are potentially glycosylated at their extracellular N-termini, and protein kinase C (PKC), casein kinase 1 and 2, and protein kinase A (PKA) phosphorylation sites are found in the intracellular C-terminal tails [54], which are involved in the functional regulations. An orphan GPCR GPR50 shares 45% amino acid sequence identity with MT_1 and MT_2 [57], but its function is poorly understood. In fact, GPR50 does not bind melatonin at all. Intriguingly, co-expression studies showed that GPR50 dimerizes with either MT_1 or MT_2 and inhibits agonist binding of the MT_1 but not MT_2 and prevents the recruitment of intracellular signaling partners such as G proteins and β-arrestins to the receptor dimmers [58].

Both MT_1 and MT_2 are found in neuronal and peripheral tissues with non-identical distributions [43;59]. MT_1 and MT_2 are found in the suprachiasmatic nucleus (SCN) at high densities [60] and their expression levels are synchronized with the diurnal rhythm [61]. In addition to the SCN, MT_1 has been detected in the cerebellum [62], hippocampus [63], ovary [64], testis [65], mammary gland [44], retina [66], coronary blood vessels and aorta [67], liver and kidney [68], skin [69] and in T and B lymphocytes [70]. Functional MT_2 receptors are mainly localized in the brain [54], MT_2 are also found to be expressed in the lung [68], arteries and heart, myometrium and granulose cells [71], duodenum [72], adipocytes [73] and the immune system [54;74].

Functionally, MT_1 and MT_2 have distinctive physiological roles. For example, MT_1 mediates melatonin-regulated cardiac vasoconstriction [60;75;76], whereas MT_2 activation dilates cardiac vessels and modulates inflammatory as well as immune responses [77;78]. The use of subtype-selective antagonists and transgenic animals has further demonstrated the different pathways mediated by the two receptor subtypes. MT_1 knockout mice have improper sensorimotor gating and depression, indicating that the MT_1 signaling is critical for normal brain function [79]. Another behavioral effect reported in knockout mice study is a deficit in memory based on the elevated plus-maze test in MT_2 knockout mice [80;81]. However, the two receptors have been suggested to act in a complementary way in the SCN to modulate the body's circadian rhythms as well as the sleep-wake cycle. Studies in mice showed that the neuronal firing in the SCN is suppressed by MT_1 thereby implicating MT_1 in sleep promotion [60]. A more recent study showed that the MT_1 may also modulate biological clock-related gene expressions as the expression of most clock genes is reduced in the pituitary of MT_1 knockout mice but not in MT_2 knockout mice [82]. On the other hand, it has been shown that the phase advancement of rat SCN neuronal firing is mediated by MT_2, hence implying its role in causing phase-shifting of the circadian rhythmic activity of SCN neurons [75]. These effects have been confirmed for MT_1 on SCN slices by pharmacological experiments [60] or by *in vivo* treatment with the MT_2 selective antagonist 4P-PDOT for MT_2 [39].

Discovery and Development of Melatoninergics

The high affinity of melatonin toward its receptors and its natural occurrence in human body substantiate its safe and extensive usage in various treatment paradigms of CRSDs despite of its unfavorable pharmacokinetic properties. Long-releasing formulation of melatonin such as Circadin® has been developed to provide a more reliable and prolonged effect, which has been adopted in treating aged insomnia patients [83]. However, the corresponding efficacy of sleep-promoting effect is still lower than benzodiazepine-based hypnotics. It is hoped that novel therapeutic melatoninergics with longer life time but retaining a similar receptor binding characteristics as melatonin will eventually emerge. Early classes of melatoninergics agonists such as 2-iodomelatonin and 2-phenylmelatonin [84;85] were therefore developed. Bioisosteric replacements of the melatonin structure have also been widely adopted resulting in numerous non-indoleamine melatoninergics with heterocyclic scaffolds appearing in the literature. The ever-growing list includes indane, naphthalene, benzoxazole and benzofuran, fluroene, carbazole, quinoline, isoquinoline, benzopyran, benzothiazole, benzoxazine, benzothiazine, benzoxadole, azaindole, benzylpiperidine, biphenyl, pyridine, aryloxyanilide and phenylpropylamide [86-88].

Current Achievements in Therapeutic Melatoninergics

A couple of indole-based compounds have therefore been developed with modifications on the major metabolically-labile sites on melatonin. TIK-301 (or LY 156735; β-methyl-6-chloromelatonin) is an early example of melatoninergics closely resembling melatonin with slightly higher affinity toward MT_2 and resistant to 6-hydroxylation by cytochromes [89]. It has only modest sleep-promoting effect [90], and more interestingly, it shows antagonistic activity toward 5-hydroxyltryptamine $(5\text{-HT})_{2B}$ and 5-HT_{2C} receptors [91]. The opposite daily rhythmic occurrence of melatonin and 5-HT in human body and their apparent counteracting physiological consequences may actually favor the sedative effect of TIK-301, and hence it has been prescribed as an antidepressant. TIK-301 has reached Phase II trials [89] and it has been demonstrated to reduce sleep latency in patients with primary insomnia but marginal in healthy subjects at high doses of 20-100 mg [90]. At lower doses (5 mg), TIK-301 effectively causes phase-shifting of the circadian clock but only with moderate hypnotic effects [92].

Other therapeutic melatoninergics that are structurally diverse from the indoleamine scaffold of melatonin have also been developed. Ramelteon ((*S*)-*N*-[2-(1,6,7,8-tetrahydro-2*H*-indeno-[5,4-*b*]furan-8-yl)ethyl]propionamide) is among the first successful case of therapeutic melatoninergics in the drug market. It resembles a structure with the 5-methoxyl group of melatonin being cyclized to form the indane structure which prevents degradation by demethylation and hence prolongs its half-life time.

A group of investigational melatoninergics have recently been introduced by replacing the *N*-acetyl group on the acetamide chain of melatonin with aromatic substitutes, forming a series of novel pyrone amides and esters with high affinity to both receptor subtypes as well as potential strong free radical scavenging property. The corresponding comenamides and comanilamides are the two groups with the most effective biological activity. In additional to the typical melatoninergics effects, these compounds also show potential anxiolytic and neuroprotective effects which are believed to be attributed by the pyrone group.

Tasimelteon (BMS-214,778 or VEC-162; *N*-([1*R*,2*R*)-2-(2,3-dihydro-1-benzofuran-4-yl)cyclopropyl]methyl)propanamide)) is an investigational therapeutic melatoninergic under Phase III clinical trial with multiple variations on the overall structure as melatonin [93]. By mimicking the indane structure of Ramelteon, a dihydrobenzofuran scaffold is linked to the ethylamidomethyl chain by a cyclopropyl ring. The *in vivo* half-life is much longer than melatonin and it is metabolized by a completely different mechanism [94]. Oral administration of up to 100 mg of Tasimelteon significantly promotes the readjustment of circadian phase advance in a dose-dependent manner, and reduces the phase shift-induced extension of sleep latency to non-awake and to persistent sleep [93;94]. It has also been reported that Tasimelteon can improve insomnia symptoms in individuals with genetically-associated DSPS having a polymorphism of variable number of tandem repeats in the clock gene *per3*. Tasimelteon has also been shown to have antidepressive effects in rodents [93].

Several compounds with the replacement of the 5-membered ring of the indole scaffold with a 6-atom structure and alterations of the alkylamide chain have also been successfully made as investigational drug candidates. Agomelatine (*N*-[2-(7-methoxynaphthalen-1-yl)ethyl]acetamide) is actually a naphthalene-based compound with fair melatoninergic agonist activity, and, like TIK-301, it has been marketed as an antidepressant due to its antagonistic activity toward 5-HT_{2C} receptor. AH-001 (2-acetamido-8-methoxytetralin) and AH-017 (2-chloroacetamido-8-methoxytetralin) have been generated with modest MT_2 selectivity [95]. Rodents kept in constant darkness will spontaneously and continuously shift the occurrence of activity period earlier due to the lack of light cue. Melatonin administration further advances this phase-shifting phenomenon. The MT_2-selective AH-017 can mimic the effect of melatonin, but its analog AH-001 cannot do so [95].

The physiological effects of synthetic melatoninergics may deviate from melatonin in particular aspects, which is also dependent on the experimental conditions. An example is GR 196429 ((*N*-[2-[2,3,7,8-tetrahydro-1*H*-furo(2,3-*g*)indol-1-yl]ethyl]acetamide)), a non-selective potent melatoninergics agonist which inhibits cAMP production in recombinant system and Ca^{2+}-dependent dopamine release in rabbit retina like melatonin [96]. Administration of GR 196429 to rats kept in constant darkness causes an opposite action of phase delay instead of advancement as melatonin or AH-017. Moreover, GR 196429 can increase the amplitude of the rhythmic activity and cause remarkable broadenings of the nocturnal melatonin peak, an observation somewhat contrasting to melatonin [95]. Contrarily,

GR 196429 induces phase advance of neuronal firing in rat SCN slides [96]. It can also elicit arterial vasoconstriction in rats, which is known to be an MT_1-dependent response [97].

UCM765 (*N*-[2-[3-methoxyphenyl)phenylamino]ethyl]acetamide) is a relatively simple *N*-phenylaniline-based compound which preferentially binds MT_2 with an affinity of 2 orders of magnitudes higher than to MT_1 [98;99]. It decreases sleep latency, increases slow-wave sleep duration and the latency to REM sleep but not the duration [83;98]. These effects were sensitive to the blockade by MT_2-selective antagonist 4P-PDOT (4-phenyl-2-propionamido-tetralin) [100]. A metabolically more stable analog UCM924 (*N*-[2-[3-bromophenyl)-(4-fluorophenyl)amino]ethyl]-acetamide) has also been developed without compromising the binding affinity. An interesting trend could be seen in the development of therapeutic melatoninergics. While TIK-301, GR 196429 and tasimelteon are equally potent to both receptor subtypes, AH-017, UCM765 and UCM924 show 1-2 orders of higher affinities toward MT_2 than MT_1. In fact, their MT_2 selectivity are believed to be more favorable for reentrainment of the circadian rhythm and alleviation of symptoms related to shifted or poorly coupled circadian oscillations.

Structure-Activity Relationship

Despite its potential therapeutic value in treating circadian rhythm disorders, melatonin is ineffective in clinical use for its short half-life, thus prompting the development of melatoninergic ligands that mimic the actions of melatonin with improved potency and specificity. A diverse array of synthetic melatoninergic ligand from different structural scaffolds has been developed and their receptor affinity, intrinsic activity, subtype selectivity and metabolism were studied in relation to their chemical design. Abundant information has been drawn from both non-selective and selective melatoninergic ligands to rationalize their structure activity relationships and provide new insights into the development of new class melatoninergic therapeutic agents.

Determinants of Functionality and Affinity

Previous studies of structure-activity relationship have revealed that the 3-acylaminoethyl chain and 5-methoxy groups of melatonin are the crucial components in receptor binding; removal of either the acylaminoethyl chain or the methoxy group would lead to significant loss of receptor affinity [84;101]. The conformation of the amide terminal group on the acylaminoethyl chain appears to modulate ligand affinity on the melatonin receptors. Extending the acetyl group to propionyl endowed the compound with higher binding affinity and potency, but substituents higher than butyryl or composed of branched structure have an adverse effect on the affinity. There have been reports that substitutions with cyclopropyl-carbonyl or cyclobutylcarbonyl group would shift the intrinsic activity from agonist to antagonist [102;103]. The relative distance of the amide group and the methoxyl group is also critical for ligand-receptor interaction. Melatonin analogs with the methoxyl group moving to positions 4, 6 or 7 exhibited reduced affinity, indicating that 5-methoxyl group is optimal for receptor binding [102;104]. Replacement of the 5-methoxyl group by hydrogen, hydroxyl or alkoxy groups also decreased affinity, while halogen substituents are well tolerated and retained both affinity and intrinsic activity [105]. Affinity of melatonin can be further enhanced by substituting a halogen, methyl or a phenyl group at the C2 position of the indole ring. These substituents are likely interacting with an auxiliary binding subdomain in the receptor [106;107]. Furthermore, it has been subsequently revealed that the indole scaffold does not actually play a major role in the receptor binding. Either shifting the position of the nitrogen atom in the pyrrolidine ring or replacing indole with other aromatic fragments does not generally affect the receptor affinity [96;98]. Variations of scaffolds like indane and naphthalene have been widely adopted in the design of new classes of melatoninergics, such as Ramelteon and agomelatin. With the appropriately positioned acylaminoethyl and methoxy groups, these bioisosteres have demonstrated potent melatoninergic activity similar to indole-based derivatives [102;104].

There are other ways to modify the receptor affinity of melatoninergics besides introducing substitutions on the main scaffold. A novel series of substituted *N*-[3-(3-methoxyphenyl)propyl]amides were identified in our laboratory displaying superb binding affinities toward human MT_2, and MT_1 to a lesser extent [108]. Similar to melatonin, a terminal simple alkyl group (up to propyl) attached on the propylamide chain progressively improves the intrinsic activity, whereas a terminal phenyl substitute is devoid of any binding. Particularly, introduction of a 3'-methoxyl group to the benzyloxyl substitute incorporated at C6 position of the phenylpropylamide scaffold (analogous to C2 position of melatonin) dramatically enhances binding affinity toward MT_2 but not MT_1. The simplicity of such monocyclic compounds to retain potent melatoninergic activity is not surprising, because Tasimelteon (with the loss of the 5-membered ring as compared with melatonin but retaining the alkylamide chain) has been shown to be more flexible. Furthermore, unpublished results in our laboratory indicate that a 3'-methoxybenzyloxyl group linked with a bicyclic scaffold without the protruding alkylamide chain can still bind MT_2 at modest to high affinity when compared with melatonin, and these compounds are basically inactive toward MT_1. The physiological significance of such exclusively MT_2-selective compounds awaits further studies.

Determinants of Receptor Subtype Selectivity

With a great variety of subtype-selective melatoninergics having been developed from various chemical scaffolds, here we summarize the key structural features conveying the subtype selectivity. An interesting observation is that much more MT_2-selective compounds are identified than MT_1-selective ones. Luzindole (2-benzyl-*N*-acetyltryptamine) and 5-methoxyluzindole are among the early identified melatoninergics showing modest MT_2 selectivity. The incorporation of 2-benzyl group appears to reduce binding affinity at the MT_1, leading to MT_2 selectivity [109]. Similarly, analogs like N 0889 (2-benzyl-*N*-propionyl-acetyltryptamine) and DH97 (*N*-pentanoyl-2-benzyltryptamine) also endowed with higher affinity for MT_2 receptor with $K_i(MT_1)/K_i(MT_2)$ ratio ranging from 31- to 89-fold [109;110]. Further variations of the 2-benzyl group have been made by cyclization to constrain its orientation, yielding tetracyclic compounds like K185 (*N*-butanoyl-2-(5,6,7-trihydro-11-methoxybenzo[3,4]cyclohept[2,1-*a*]indol-13-yl)ethanamine) and IIK7 (*N*-butanoyl-2-(2-methoxy-6*H*-isoindolo[2,1-*a*]indol-11-yl)ethanamine), which also exhibited 90- and 132-fold higher affinity for the MT_2 than for the MT_1 receptor, respectively [111]. The role of an aromatic group right next to the alkylamide chain in subtype selectivity is further supported by other melatoninegics with non-indole scaffolds. Binding affinity of 4P-PDOT (4-phenyl-2-propionamidotetralin), S 24773 (*N*-{2-[3-(3-aminophenyl)-7-methoxy-1-naphthyl] ethyl} acetamide), S 24014 (*N*-[2-(2-(3-methoxybenzyl)5-methoxybenzo(*b*)furan-3-yl)ethyl] acetamide) and S 28407 (*N*-[2-(7-methoxy-3-phenyl-1,2,3,4-tetrahydronaphthalen-1-yl)ethyl] cyclobutyl carboxamide) display over 100-fold preferences toward MT_2 receptor [56; 112;113]. The case of investigational melatoninergics with *N*-phenylaniline scaffold like UCM765 and UCM924 represents another variation of structural scaffold possessing two aromatic cores that confer MT_2 selectivity [98;100]. Notably, a 3'-methoxyl group attached to the benzyl substitute further enhances the MT_2 selectivity. It is also manifested in melatoninergics with a simple scaffold such as phenylpropylamides, where MT_2 selectivity can be amplified up to 10^5 folds [108].

Discovery of MT-selective compounds is unexpectedly rare. A bulky substituent replacing the 5-methoxy group of melatonin or its naphthalenic analog gives rise to a series of modestly MT_1-selective compounds. A key feature is that most of them are dimeric derivatives resembling two molecules of S 20098 (*N*-(2-[7-methoxy-1-naphthalenyl] ethyl)acetamide) attached to both ends of a polymethylene chain [112]. The length of the linking chain can vary from 2 to 8, but 3 gives the highest selectivity ratio. Functional characterization of one of these dimeric melatoninergics reveals its antagonistic activity with approximately 40-fold MT_1 selectivity. Another MT_1-selective ligand, S 25567 (*N*-[2-(6-hexyloxy-3,4-dihydro-2*H*-chromen-4-yl)ethyl]acetamide), is not a dimeric derivative but bears a long hexyloxyl chain at C6 position of a chromene scaffold [56], and it is a partial agonist only.

Improvements of Metabolic Stability and Bioavailability

Circulating melatonin is subjected to rapid cytochrome P450-mediated degradation in the liver and exhibits a biphasic elimination pattern with a first-order elimination half-life of 2 minutes. Metabolite profiling unveiled that the C6 position of melatonin is the major metabolic soft spots in the structure and is hydroxylated during the extensive hepatic first pass metabolism [114]. In order to improve the metabolic stability and suitability of melatoninergics for insomnia treatment, several indolic analogs were first synthesized by introducing different substituents at the 6-position. 6-chloromelatonin has been shown to prevent hydroxylation at the 6-position, however, the substitution also greatly reduced the receptor affinity by over 100-fold [115]. TIK-301 is a 6-chlorinated melatonin derivative with a (*R*)-β-methyl group incorporated at the acylaminoethyl chain. While retaining high binding affinity towards MT_1 and MT_2, this synthetic melatoninergic agonist largely prevents the conversion to its analogue of 6-hydroxymelatonin and displays an extended half-life in circulation [89].

In addition to the C6 position, C2 and C3 of melatonin are also susceptible to cytochrome mediated *O*-dealkylation, which promotes pyrrole ring cleavage and the formation of kynuramine analogs [116]. Considering the dispensability of the pyrrole ring nitrogen in receptor binding, non-indolic melatonin receptor agonists have been developed with the ring nitrogen removed [117] or reduction of C2 and C3 positions [115]. Saturation of the 5-membered and 6-membered ring in indane and naphthalene derivatives avoids prevailing ring cleavage and the formation of kynuramine-like analogs. 5-methoxy group of melatonin plays an important role in affinity and functionality; therefore, it is crucial to prevent the substituent being attacked by catabolic enzymes. Integrating the methoxyl group into a dihydrofuran ring has shown to be an effective approach in preventing hydroxylation at this particular site of melatonin. The dihydrofuran structure is also preferred in indole, indane derivatives and other newly developed melatonin receptor agonists, such as GR 196429, Ramelteon and Tasimelteon.

Our laboratory has recently developed a series of 3-methoxylphenylpropyl amide derivatives that displayed extraordinary MT_2 selectivity by incorporating substituted benzyloxyl groups at 6-position [108]. These compounds were, however, subjected to rapid cytochrome P450-mediated degradation in rat and human liver microsomes *in vivo* with a shorter half-life compared to that of melatonin [118]. Metabolite profiling unveiled that C6-ether linkage and methoxyl substituents were likely the major metabolic soft spots in their structures, which provided important information for further improvement of their structural stability. To protect the selectivity conferring benzyloxyl substituent, the C6-ether linkage was replaced by alkyl group and led to a substantially divergent metabolism. Our preliminary results suggest, while retaining its potency and selectivity, the substituted 3-methoxyl-phenylpropyl amide exhibited extended half-life with hydroxylation being observed at all ring systems.

Pros and Cons of the Therapeutic Uses of Subtype-Selective Melatoninergics in CRSDs

Although none of the available subtype-selective melatoninergics has so far gone to clinical stages, the attempts to develop subtype-selective melatonin receptor ligands for treating sleep disorders and CRSDs are actively being pursued. The use of subtype-selective melatonin receptor ligands in the treatment of CRSDs offers several advantages over melatonin or other melatonin agonists. Comparing their respective actions, melatonin acts on multiple melatonin binding sites, including MT_1 and MT_2 receptors, thus generating several physiological effects simultaneously. However, for subtype-selective melatoninergics which bind specifically to their targets, only the desired effects are produced. In particular, MT_1-selective agonists are expected to inhibit neuronal firing within the SCN while MT_2-selective agonists induce a phase shift of circadian clock. Both are devoid of the actions mediated by the other melatonin receptor subtype. The actions exerted by non-selective melatoninergics are multiple, unpredictable, and often associated with a high propensity for unwanted side effects. In contrast, actions produced by subtype-selective melatoninergics are more predictable and specific. The application of subtype-selective melatoninergics could thus eliminate the side effects or unfavorable interactions arising from the non-specific actions of melatonin to other possible binding sites, leading to the evolution of a safer therapeutic agent with an improved pharmacological profile.

To date, several subtype-selective melatoninergics have been developed but only limited studies regarding the effects of these ligands on sleep have been found. Two novel high affinity MT_2-selective agonists, IIK7 and UCM765, have been identified with data from animal studies investigating their effects on sleep. When administrated at an intraperitoneal dose of 10 mg/kg, IIK7 significantly reduced non-rapid eye movement (NREM) sleep onset latency in rats, without affecting neither the REM sleep onset latency and duration nor the electroencephalogram power spectra of NREM sleep [119]. These effects of IIK7 on sleep are consistent with those results after administration of melatonin or ramelteon at similar dosage [120]. This indicated the potential for IIK7 as a target specific therapeutic agent for treatment of insomnia, with minimal unpredictable side effects and similar sleep-promoting action as melatonin. The other MT_2-selective agonist, UCM765, also induced a significant decrease in NREM sleep onset latency and an increase in NREM sleep duration in rats at a subcutaneous dose of ≥40 mg/kg [99]. However, UCM765 also showed an inhibition on REM sleep by delaying the REM sleep onset latency, which was found to be as effective as diazepam. The high dose of UCM765 required for its sleep-promoting effects may be due to its low bioavailability caused by high first pass metabolism and a short half-life, as well as its vulnerability to oxidative metabolism in rat liver. Regarding the unfavorable pharmacokinetics of UCM765, attempts to identify the structures contributing to its metabolic liability were made and a relatively metabolic stable derivative was generated, namely UCM924 [99]. Similar binding profile to UCM765 was observed in this compound which indicated UCM924 could be an alternative to UCM765. Overall, the sleep-promoting actions of these two MT_2-selective agonists have implied their potential as a promising agent for the treatment of insomnia and led to the recognition for the role of MT_2 receptors in mediating the hypnotic effect of melatonin. However, several shortcomings regarding the metabolic stability and pharmacokinetic profile of these melatonin receptor subtype-selective compounds have limited their therapeutic potential for treatment of CRSDs. Further modifications to these compounds are needed to produce alternatives with enhanced properties and thus higher efficacy while at the same time, the development for high affinity MT_1- or MT_2-selective melatoninergics is in progress.

Therapeutic Potentials of Subtype-Selective Melatoninergics in Other Diseases

In additional to its well-known regulation on circadian rhythms, the involvement of melatonin has been demonstrated extensively in other various physiological functions, such as blood pressure control, immune system regulation and pain perception. Owing to the multifunctional properties of this hormone and the presence of its receptors in different areas of the central nervous system as well as in peripheral tissues, melatonin has been shown to play an important role in a variety of pathological conditions other than sleep disorders, including cardiovascular diseases, several types of cancers and the development of type 2 diabetes (T2D). Furthermore, the potential for the use of other melatoninergics, such as subtype-selective melatonin receptor ligands, as novel therapeutic agents in these pathological conditions is been increasingly recognized.

Among the proposed therapeutic applications of melatonin, its use as a potential antihypertensive agent not only alleviates hypertension, but also decreases the general cardiovascular risk. Increasing evidence has suggested an important role of melatonin in the regulation of blood pressure [121]. Animal and human studies both show a correlation of melatonin with blood pressure in the hypertensive pathologies [122;123]. Administration of melatonin in both hypertensive rats and humans was found to be effective in lowering the blood pressure [124-126]. Among the different possible mechanisms proposed for the anti-hypertensive effects of melatonin, activation of melatonin receptors located in parts of the central nervous system involved in the regulation of blood pressure has been suggested for its anti-hypertensive effects [127]. Furthermore, the control of vascular tone by the MT_2 receptors has been shown to produce beneficial effects to counteract hypertension by inducing vasodilation [128]. The melatonin receptor-mediated effects on the vascular tone have previously been established, with MT_1 receptors causing vasoconstriction and MT_2 receptors inducing vasodilation [129]. These opposing actions on the vascular tone by the two melatonin receptor subtypes bring out the shortcomings for the use of melatonin or other melatonin receptor agoinsts lacking subtype selectivity. Thus, subtype-selective melatoninergics, specifically MT_1-selective agonists, undoubtedly would be a better therapeutic agent for the treatment of hypertension.

One of the significant findings on melatonin is the discovery of its ability in inhibiting cell proliferation and also inducing apoptosis in a number of tumor cell lines [130]. The oncostatic effects of melatonin were also observed in murine tumoral models, demonstrating a reduction of carcinogenesis [131]. Several mechanisms have been proposed for melatonin's actions to counteract tumor growth. Interesting findings have indicated the activation of specific MT_1 melatonin receptors for its anti-estrogenic and anti-aromatase properties in several estrogen-dependent tumors, such as breast cancer and prostate cancer [132-134]. Furthermore, there was also evidence indicating the antimetastatic effects of melatonin possibly through MT_1 receptors in MCF-7 human breast cancer cells [135]. Taken together, these findings support MT_1-selective agonists as a promising strategy for inhibiting the proliferation of tumors, thereby offering a possible rationale for anti-cancer therapy. Since limited information exists for the role of MT_2 receptors in tumor growth, the effectiveness with the use of MT_2-selective agonists remains questionable. Additional studies are needed to elucidate the precise mechanisms involved in the regulation of tumor growth, particularly in proliferation, differentiation and metastasis.

Recent interests have arisen on the application of melatonin in the T2D treatment. Correlation of melatonin to T2D was first discovered in patients with high blood glucose levels and impaired insulin resistance, which they have high plasma insulin levels as well as decreased plasma melatonin levels [136;137]. Melatonin administration was able to reduce hyperinsulinemia and insulin resistance in human patients and diabetic rats [138;139]. The insulin-inhibiting effects of melatonin were demonstrated to be mediated by MT_2-selective receptors on the pancreatic β-cells [140]. Recently, genetic evidence has further suggested that MT_2 is a risk factor for the development of T2D. A common variant in MT_2 was found to be associated with an increased risk for T2D [141]. The potential for subtype-selective melatoninergics antagonists in the treatment of T2D should not be underestimated.

Conclusion

Melatonin has been recognized as a natural sleep-promoting agent for decades, and also a number of investigational therapeutic melatoninergics have just been successfully developed in the recent years. Diversifications of chemical structures have been explored to derive melatoninergics with better metabolic stability, bioavailability, binding affinity and subtype selectivity. In particular, subtype-selective melatoninergics are of emerging interest since they may offer a more promising therapeutic action toward specific types of CRSDs as well as other pathophysiological conditions that involve melatonin receptor-mediated mechanisms. There are still plenty of rooms for exploration of the unrevealed therapeutic potentials of novel melatoninergics with differential properties to the two major GPCR subtypes, not necessarily only selectivity in terms of affinity but also agonist/antagonist actions, receptor internalization or stabilization. Off-target effects of the current therapeutic melatoninergics have not been fully investigated, particularly against those that bind melatonin naturally, in order to make more effective and safer therapeutic agents for those suffering from CRSDs.

Acknowledgment

Studies by the authors are supported in part by the Hong Kong Jockey Club, Research Grant Council (HKUST 660108) and University Grant Council of Hong Kong (T13-607/12R).

References

[1] American Academy of Sleep Medicine. The international classification of sleep disorders : diagnostic & coding manual. Westchester, IL: American Academy of Sleep Medicine. 2005.

[2] Carpen Jd, Archer Sn, Skene Dj, Smits M, Von Sm. A Single-Nucleotide Polymorphism In The 5'-Untranslated Region Of The Hper2 Gene Is Associated With Diurnal Preference. *J Sleep Res* 2005;14(3):293-7.

[3] Xu Y, Padiath Qs, Shapiro Re, Jones Cr, Wu Sc, Saigoh N, Et Al. Functional Consequences Of A Ckidelta Mutation Causing Familial Advanced Sleep Phase Syndrome. *Nature* 2005;434(7033):640-4.

[4] Skene Dj, Arendt J. Circadian Rhythm Sleep Disorders In The Blind And Their Treatment With Melatonin. *Sleep Med* 2007;8(6):651-5.

[5] Sack Rl, Auckley D, Auger Rr, Carskadon Ma, Wright Kp, Jr., Vitiello Mv, Et Al. Circadian Rhythm Sleep Disorders: Part Ii, Advanced Sleep Phase Disorder, Delayed Sleep Phase Disorder, Free-Running Disorder, And Irregular Sleep-Wake Rhythm. An American Academy Of Sleep Medicine Review. *Sleep* 2007;30(11):1484-501.

[6] Czeisler Ca, Allan Js, Strogatz Sh, Ronda Jm, Sanchez R, Rios Cd, Et Al. Bright Light Resets The Human Circadian Pacemaker Independent Of The Timing Of The Sleep-Wake Cycle. *Science* 1986;233(4764):667-71.

[7] Lewy Aj, Sack Rl, Miller Ls, Hoban Tm. Antidepressant And Circadian Phase-Shifting Effects Of Light. *Science* 1987;235(4786):352-4.

[8] Lewy Aj, Ahmed S, Jackson Jm, Sack Rl. Melatonin Shifts Human Circadian Rhythms According To A Phase-Response Curve. *Chronobiol Int* 1992;9(5):380-92.

[9] Martinez D, Lenz Mc. Circadian Rhythm Sleep Disorders. *Indian J Med Res* 2010;131:141-9.

[10] Duffy Jf, Wright Kp, Jr. Entrainment Of The Human Circadian System By Light. *J Biol Rhythms* 2005;20(4):326-38.

[11] Sack Rl, Lewy Aj. Circadian Rhythm Sleep Disorders: Lessons From The Blind. *Sleep Med Rev* 2001;5(3):189-206.

[12] Herxheimer A, Petrie Kj. Melatonin For The Prevention And Treatment Of Jet Lag. *Cochrane Database Syst Rev* 2002;(2):Cd001520.

[13] Turek Fw, Gillette Mu. Melatonin, Sleep, And Circadian Rhythms: Rationale For Development Of Specific Melatonin Agonists. *Sleep Med* 2004;5(6):523-32.

[14] Benca Rm. Diagnosis And Treatment Of Chronic Insomnia: A Review. *Psychiatr Serv* 2005;56(3):332-43.

[15] Beaumont M, Batejat D, Pierard C, Van Bp, Denis Jb, Coste O, Et Al. Caffeine Or Melatonin Effects On Sleep And Sleepiness After Rapid Eastward Transmeridian Travel. *J Appl Physiol* 2004;96(1):50-8.

[16] Wyatt Jk, Cajochen C, Ritz-De Ca, Czeisler Ca, Dijk Dj. Low-Dose Repeated Caffeine Administration For Circadian-Phase-Dependent Performance Degradation During Extended Wakefulness. *Sleep* 2004;27(3):374-81.

[17] Walsh Jk, Randazzo Ac, Stone Kl, Schweitzer Pk. Modafinil Improves Alertness, Vigilance, And Executive Function During Simulated Night Shifts. *Sleep* 2004;27(3):434-9.

[18] Holbrook Am, Crowther R, Lotter A, Cheng C, King D. Meta-Analysis Of Benzodiazepine Use In The Treatment Of Insomnia. *Cmaj* 2000;162(2):225-33.

[19] Koppelstaetter F, Poeppel Td, Siedentopf Cm, Ischebeck A, Verius M, Haala I, Et Al. Does Caffeine Modulate Verbal Working Memory Processes? An Fmri Study. *Neuroimage* 2008;39(1):492-9.

[20] Kennaway Dj, Wright H. Melatonin And Circadian Rhythms. *Curr Top Med Chem* 2002;2(2):199-209.

[21] Tosini G, Menaker M. The Clock In The Mouse Retina: Melatonin Synthesis And Photoreceptor Degeneration. *Brain Res* 1998;789(2):221-8.

[22] Champier J, Claustrat B, Besancon R, Eymin C, Killer C, Jouvet A, Et Al. Evidence For Tryptophan Hydroxylase And Hydroxy-Indol-O-Methyl-Transferase Mrnas In Human Blood Platelets. *Life Sci* 1997;60(24):2191-7.

[23] Conti A, Conconi S, Hertens E, Skwarlo-Sonta K, Markowska M, Maestroni Jm. Evidence For Melatonin Synthesis In Mouse And Human Bone Marrow Cells. *J Pineal Res* 2000;28(4):193-202.

[24] Bubenik Ga. Gastrointestinal Melatonin: Localization, Function, And Clinical Relevance. *Dig Dis Sci* 2002;47(10):2336-48.

[25] Slominski A, Fischer Tw, Zmijewski Ma, Wortsman J, Semak I, Zbytek B, Et Al. On The Role Of Melatonin In Skin Physiology And Pathology. *Endocrine* 2005;27(2):137-48.

[26] Carrillo-Vico A, Calvo Jr, Abreu P, Lardone Pj, Garcia-Maurino S, Reiter Rj, Et Al. Evidence Of Melatonin Synthesis By Human Lymphocytes And Its Physiological Significance: Possible Role As Intracrine, Autocrine, And/Or Paracrine Substance. *Faseb J* 2004;18(3):537-9.

[27] Lane Ea, Moss Hb. Pharmacokinetics of melatonin in man: first pass hepatic metabolism. *J Clin Endocrinol Metab*1985;61(6):1214-6.

[28] Arendt J, Skene Dj. Melatonin As A Chronobiotic. *Sleep Med Rev* 2005;9(1):25-39.

[29] Cardinali Dp, Furio Am, Brusco Li. The Use Of Chronobiotics In The Resynchronization Of The Sleep/Wake Cycle. Therapeutical Application In The Early Phases Of Alzheimer's Disease. *Recent Pat Endocr Metab Immune Drug Discov* 2011;5(2):80-90.

[30] Dawson D, Armstrong Sm. Chronobiotics--Drugs That Shift Rhythms. Pharmacol Ther 1996;69(1):15-36.

[31] Touitou Y, Bogdan A. Promoting Adjustment Of The Sleep-Wake Cycle By Chronobiotics. *Physiol Behav* 2007;90(2-3):294-300.

[32] Cardinali Dp, Pevet P. Basic Aspects Of Melatonin Action. *Sleep Med Rev* 1998;2(3):175-90.

[33] Boutin Ja, Audinot V, Ferry G, Delagrange P. Molecular Tools To Study Melatonin Pathways And Actions. *Trends Pharmacol Sci* 2005;26(8):412-9.

[34] Pandi-Perumal Sr, Srinivasan V, Maestroni Gj, Cardinali Dp, Poeggeler B, Hardeland R. Melatonin: Nature's Most Versatile Biological Signal? *Febs J* 2006;273(13):2813-38.

[35] Wurtman Rj, Axelrod J. The Formation, Metabolism And Physiologic Effects Of Melatonin. *Adv Pharmacol* 1968;6(Pt A):141-51.

[36] Berson Dm, Dunn Fa, Takao M. Phototransduction By Retinal Ganglion Cells That Set The Circadian Clock. *Science* 2002;295(5557):1070-3.

[37] Hannibal J, Fahrenkrug J. Neuronal Input Pathways To The Brain's Biological Clock And Their Functional Significance. *Adv Anat Embryol Cell Biol* 2006;182:1-71.

[38] Buijs Rm, Hermes Mh, Kalsbeek A. The Suprachiasmatic Nucleus-Paraventricular Nucleus Interactions: A Bridge To The Neuroendocrine And Autonomic Nervous System. *Prog Brain Res* 1998;119:365-82.

[39] Gerdin Mj, Masana Mi, Rivera-Bermudez Ma, Hudson Rl, Earnest Dj, Gillette Mu, Et Al. Melatonin Desensitizes Endogenous MT2 Melatonin Receptors In The Rat Suprachiasmatic Nucleus: Relevance For Defining The Periods Of Sensitivity Of The Mammalian Circadian Clock To Melatonin. *Faseb J* 2004;18(14):1646-56.

[40] Savaskan E, Ayoub Ma, Ravid R, Angeloni D, Fraschini F, Meier F, Et Al. Reduced Hippocampal MT2 Melatonin Receptor Expression In Alzheimer's Disease. *J Pineal Res* 2005;38(1):10-6.

[41] Maurizi Cp. Alzheimer's Disease: Roles For Mitochondrial Damage, The Hydroxyl Radical, And Cerebrospinal Fluid Deficiency of Melatonin. *Med Hypotheses* 2001;57(2):156-60.

[42] Arendt J. Melatonin And Human Rhythms. *Chronobiol Int* 2006;23(1-2):21-37.

[43] Ekmekcioglu C. Melatonin Receptors In Humans: Biological Role And Clinical Relevance. *Biomed Pharmacother* 2006;60(3):97-108.

[44] Ram Pt, Dai J, Yuan L, Dong C, Kiefer Tl, Lai L, Et Al. Involvement Of The MT1 Melatonin Receptor In Human Breast Cancer. *Cancer Lett* 2002;179(2):141-50.

[45] Carrillo-Vico A, Reiter Rj, Lardone Pj, Herrera Jl, Fernandez-Montesinos R, Guerrero Jm, Et Al. The Modulatory Role Of Melatonin On Immune Responsiveness. *Curr Opin Investig Drugs* 2006;7(5):423-31.

[46] Bondy Sc, Sharman Eh. Melatonin and the Aging Brain. *Neurochem Int* 2007;50(4):571-80.

[47] De Ja, Korevaar Jc, Van Munster Bc, De Rooij Se. Effectiveness Of Melatonin Treatment On Circadian Rhythm Disturbances In Dementia. Are There Implications For Delirium? A Systematic Review. *Int J Geriatr Psychiatry* 2010;25(12):1201-8.

[48] Jan Je, Reiter Rj, Wong Pk, Bax Mc, Ribary U, Wasdell Mb. Melatonin Has Membrane Receptor-Independent Hypnotic Action On Neurons: An Hypothesis. J *Pineal Res* 2011;50(3):233-40.

[49] Larson Eb, Zollman Fs. The Effect Of Sleep Medications On Cognitive Recovery From Traumatic Brain Injury. *J Head Trauma Rehabil* 2010;25(1):61-7.

[50] Reiter Rj, Tan Dx, Manchester Lc, Tamura H. Melatonin Defeats Neurally-Derived Free Radicals And Reduces The Associated Neuromorphological And Neurobehavioral Damage. *J Physiol Pharmacol* 2007;58 Suppl 6:5-22.

[51] Ebisawa T, Karne S, Lerner Mr, Reppert Sm. Expression Cloning Of A High-Affinity Melatonin Receptor From Xenopus Dermal Melanophores. *Proc Natl Acad Sci U S A* 1994;91(13):6133-7.

[52] Reppert Sm, Weaver Dr, Ebisawa T. Cloning And Characterization Of A Mammalian Melatonin Receptor That Mediates Reproductive And Circadian Responses. *Neuron* 1994;13(5):1177-85.

[53] Reppert Sm, Godson C, Mahle Cd, Weaver Dr, Slaugenhaupt Sa, Gusella Jf. Molecular Characterization Of A Second Melatonin Receptor Expressed In Human Retina And Brain: The Mel1b Melatonin Receptor. *Proc Natl Acad Sci U S A* 1995;92(19):8734-8.

[54] Dubocovich Ml, Markowska M. Functional MT1 And MT2 Melatonin Receptors In Mammals. *Endocrine* 2005;27(2):101-10.

[55] Slaugenhaupt Sa, Roca Al, Liebert Cb, Altherr Mr, Gusella Jf, Reppert Sm. Mapping Of The Gene For The Mel1a-Melatonin Receptor To Human Chromosome 4 (Mtnr1a) And Mouse Chromosome 8 (Mtnr1a). *Genomics* 1995;27(2):355-7.

[56] Audinot V, Mailliet F, Lahaye-Brasseur C, Bonnaud A, Le Ga, Amosse C, Et Al. New Selective Ligands Of Human Cloned Melatonin MT1 And MT2 Receptors. Naunyn Schmiedebergs. *Arch Pharmacol* 2003;367(6):553-61.

[57] Reppert Sm, Weaver Dr, Ebisawa T, Mahle Cd, Kolakowski Lf, Jr. Cloning Of A Melatonin-Related Receptor From Human Pituitary. *Febs Lett* 1996;386(2-3):219-24.

[58] Levoye A, Dam J, Ayoub Ma, Guillaume Jl, Couturier C, Delagrange P, Et Al. The Orphan Gpr50 Receptor Specifically Inhibits MT1 Melatonin Receptor Function Through Heterodimerization. *Embo J* 2006;25(13):3012-23.

[59] Pandi-Perumal Sr, Trakht I, Srinivasan V, Spence Dw, Maestroni Gj, Zisapel N, Et Al. Physiological Effects Of Melatonin: Role Of Melatonin Receptors And Signal Transduction Pathways. *Prog Neurobiol* 2008;85(3):335-53.

[60] Liu C, Weaver Dr, Jin X, Shearman Lp, Pieschl Rl, Gribkoff Vk, Et Al. Molecular Dissection Of Two Distinct Actions Of Melatonin On The Suprachiasmatic Circadian Clock. *Neuron* 1997;19(1):91-102.

[61] Reiter Rj. Pineal Melatonin: Cell Biology Of Its Synthesis And Of Its Physiological Interactions. *Endocr Rev* 1991;12(2):151-80.

[62] Al-Ghoul Wm, Herman Md, Dubocovich Ml. Melatonin Receptor Subtype Expression In Human Cerebellum. *Neuroreport* 1998;9(18):4063-8.

[63] Savaskan E, Olivieri G, Meier F, Brydon L, Jockers R, Ravid R, Et Al. Increased Melatonin 1a-Receptor Immunoreactivity In The Hippocampus Of Alzheimer's Disease Patients. *J Pineal Res* 2002;32(1):59-62.

[64] Clemens Jw, Jarzynka Mj, Witt-Enderby Pa. Down-Regulation Of MT1 Melatonin Receptors In Rat Ovary Following Estrogen Exposure. *Life Sci* 2001 May;69(1):27-35.

[65] Frungieri Mb, Mayerhofer A, Zitta K, Pignataro Op, Calandra Rs, Gonzalez-Calvar Si. Direct Effect Of Melatonin On Syrian Hamster Testes: Melatonin Subtype 1a Receptors, Inhibition Of Androgen Production, And Interaction With The Local Corticotropin-Releasing Hormone System. *Endocrinology* 2005;146(3):1541-52.

[66] Scher J, Wankiewicz E, Brown Gm, Fujieda H. MT(1) Melatonin Receptor In The Human Retina: Expression And Localization. *Invest Ophthalmol Vis Sci* 2002;43(3):889-97.

[67] Ekmekcioglu C, Haslmayer P, Philipp C, Mehrabi Mr, Glogar Hd, Grimm M, Et Al. Expression Of The MT1 Melatonin Receptor Subtype In Human Coronary Arteries. *J Recept Signal Transduct Res* 2001;21(1):85-91.

[68] Naji L, Carrillo-Vico A, Guerrero Jm, Calvo Jr. Expression Of Membrane And Nuclear Melatonin Receptors In Mouse Peripheral Organs. *Life Sci* 2004;74(18):2227-36.

[69] Slominski A, Pisarchik A, Zbytek B, Tobin Dj, Kauser S, Wortsman J. Functional Activity Of Serotoninergic And Melatoninergic Systems Expressed In The Skin. *J Cell Physiol* 2003;196(1):144-53.

[70] Pozo D, Garcia-Maurino S, Guerrero Jm, Calvo Jr. Mrna Expression Of Nuclear Receptor Rzr/Roralpha, Melatonin Membrane Receptor MT, And Hydroxindole-O-Methyltransferase In Different Populations Of Human Immune Cells. *J Pineal Res* 2004;37(1):48-54.

[71] Soares Jm, Jr., Masana Mi, Ersahin C, Dubocovich Ml. Functional Melatonin Receptors In Rat Ovaries At Various Stages Of The Estrous Cycle. *J Pharmacol Exp Ther* 2003;306(2):694-702.

[72] Stebelova K, Anttila K, Manttari S, Saarela S, Zeman M. Immunohistochemical Definition Of MT(2) Receptors And Melatonin In The Gastrointestinal Tissues Of Rat. *Acta Histochem* 2010;112(1):26-33.

[73] Zalatan F, Krause Ja, Blask De. Inhibition Of Isoproterenol-Induced Lipolysis In Rat Inguinal Adipocytes In Vitro By Physiological Melatonin Via A Receptor-Mediated Mechanism. *Endocrinology* 2001;142(9):3783-90.

[74] Guerrero Jm, Reiter Rj. Melatonin-Immune System Relationships. *Curr Top Med Chem* 2002;2(2):167-79.

[75] Jin X, Von Gc, Pieschl Rl, Gribkoff Vk, Stehle Jh, Reppert Sm, Et Al. Targeted Disruption Of The Mouse Mel(1b) Melatonin Receptor. *Mol Cell Biol* 2003;23(3):1054-60.

[76] Masana Mi, Doolen S, Ersahin C, Al-Ghoul Wm, Duckles Sp, Dubocovich Ml, Et Al. MT(2) Melatonin Receptors Are Present And Functional In Rat Caudal Artery. *J Pharmacol Exp Ther* 2002;302(3):1295-302.

[77] Drazen Dl, Bilu D, Bilbo Sd, Nelson Rj. Melatonin Enhancement Of Splenocyte Proliferation Is Attenuated By Luzindole, A Melatonin Receptor Antagonist. *Am J Physiol Regul Integr Comp Physiol* 2001;280(5):R1476-R1482.

[78] Drazen Dl, Nelson Rj. Melatonin Receptor Subtype MT2 (Mel 1b) And Not MT1 (Mel 1a) Is Associated With Melatonin-Induced Enhancement Of Cell-Mediated And Humoral Immunity. *Neuroendocrinology* 2001;74(3):178-84.

[79] Weil Zm, Hotchkiss Ak, Gatien Ml, Pieke-Dahl S, Nelson Rj. Melatonin Receptor (MT1) Knockout Mice Display Depression-Like Behaviors And Deficits In Sensorimotor Gating. *Brain Res Bull* 2006;68(6):425-9.

[80] Dubocovich Ml, Hudson Rl, Sumaya Ic, Masana Mi, Manna E. Effect Of MT1 Melatonin Receptor Deletion On Melatonin-Mediated Phase Shift Of Circadian Rhythms In The C57bl/6 Mouse. *J Pineal Res* 2005;39(2):113-20.

[81] Larson J, Jessen Re, Uz T, Arslan Ad, Kurtuncu M, Imbesi M, Et Al. Impaired Hippocampal Long-Term Potentiation In Melatonin MT2 Receptor-Deficient Mice. *Neurosci Lett* 2006;393(1):23-6.

[82] Von Gc, Weaver Dr, Moek J, Jilg A, Stehle Jh, Korf Hw. Melatonin Plays A Crucial Role In The Regulation Of Rhythmic Clock Gene Expression In The Mouse Pars Tuberalis. *Ann N Y Acad Sci* 2005;1040:508-11.

[83] Hardeland R. Tasimelteon, A Melatonin Agonist For The Treatment Of Insomnia And Circadian Rhythm Sleep Disorders. *Curr Opin Investig Drugs* 2009;10(7):691-701.

[84] Dubocovich Ml, Takahashi Js. Use Of 2-[125i]Iodomelatonin To Characterize Melatonin Binding Sites In Chicken Retina. *Proc Natl Acad Sci U S A* 1987;84(11):3916-20.

[85] Nonno R, Lucini V, Pannacci M, Mazzucchelli C, Angeloni D, Fraschini F, Et Al. Pharmacological Characterization Of The Human Melatonin Mel1a Receptor Following Stable Transfection Into Nih3t3 Cells. *Br J Pharmacol* 1998;124(3):485-92.

[86] Hardeland R. Investigational Melatonin Receptor Agonists. *Expert Opin Investig Drugs* 2010;19(6):747-64.

[87] Mor M, Rivara S, Pala D, Bedini A, Spadoni G, Tarzia G. Recent Advances In The Development Of Melatonin MT(1) And MT(2) Receptor Agonists. *Expert Opin Ther Pat* 2010;20(8):1059-77.

[88] Zlotos Dp. Recent Progress In The Development Of Agonists And Antagonists For Melatonin Receptors. *Curr Med Chem 2012*;19(21):3532-49.

[89] Mulchahey Jj, Goldwater Dr, Zemlan Fp. A Single Blind, Placebo Controlled, Across Groups Dose Escalation Study Of The Safety, Tolerability, Pharmacokinetics And Pharmacodynamics Of The Melatonin Analog Beta-Methyl-6-Chloromelatonin. *Life Sci* 2004;75(15):1843-56.

[90] Zemlan Fp, Mulchahey Jj, Scharf Mb, Mayleben Dw, Rosenberg R, Lankford A. The Efficacy And Safety Of The Melatonin Agonist Beta-Methyl-6-Chloromelatonin In Primary Insomnia: A Randomized, Placebo-Controlled, Crossover Clinical Trial. *J Clin Psychiatry* 2005;66(3):384-90.

[91] Landolt Hp, Wehrle R. Antagonism Of Serotonergic 5-Ht2a/2c Receptors: Mutual Improvement Of Sleep, Cognition And Mood? *Eur J Neurosci* 2009;29(9):1795-809.

[92] Nickelsen T, Samel A, Vejvoda M, Wenzel J, Smith B, Gerzer R. Chronobiotic Effects Of The Melatonin Agonist Ly 156735 Following A Simulated 9h Time Shift: Results Of A Placebo-Controlled Trial. *Chronobiol Int* 2002;19(5):915-36.

[93] Rajaratnam Sm, Polymeropoulos Mh, Fisher Dm, Roth T, Scott C, Birznieks G, Et Al. Melatonin Agonist Tasimelteon (Vec-162) For Transient Insomnia After Sleep-Time Shift: Two Randomised Controlled Multicentre Trials. *Lancet* 2009;373(9662):482-91.

[94] Vachharajani Nn, Yeleswaram K, Boulton Dw. Preclinical Pharmacokinetics And Metabolism Of Bms-214778, A Novel Melatonin Receptor Agonist. *J Pharm Sci* 2003;92(4):760-72.

[95] Drijfhout Wj, De Vries Jb, Homan Ej, Brons Hf, Copinga S, Gruppen G, Et Al. Novel Non-Indolic Melatonin Receptor Agonists Differentially Entrain Endogenous Melatonin Rhythm And Increase Its Amplitude. *Eur J Pharmacol* 1999;382(3):157-66.

[96] Beresford Ij, Browning C, Starkey Sj, Brown J, Foord Sm, Coughlan J, Et Al. Gr196429: A Nonindolic Agonist At High-Affinity Melatonin Receptors. *J Pharmacol Exp Ther* 1998;285(3):1239-45.

[97] Lew Mj, Flanders S. Mechanisms Of Melatonin-Induced Vasoconstriction In The Rat Tail Artery: A Paradigm Of Weak Vasoconstriction. *Br J Pharmacol* 1999;126(6):1408-18.

[98] Rivara S, Mor M, Bedini A, Spadoni G, Tarzia G. Melatonin Receptor Agonists: Sar And Applications To The Treatment Of Sleep-Wake Disorders. *Curr Top Med Chem* 2008;8(11):954-68.

[99] Rivara S, Vacondio F, Fioni A, Silva C, Carmi C, Mor M, Et Al. N-(Anilinoethyl)Amides: Design And Synthesis Of Metabolically Stable, Selective Melatonin Receptor Ligands. *Chemmedchem* 2009;4(10):1746-55.

[100] Rivara S, Lodola A, Mor M, Bedini A, Spadoni G, Lucini V, Et Al. N-(Substituted-Anilinoethyl)Amides: Design, Synthesis, And Pharmacological Characterization Of A New Class Of Melatonin Receptor Ligands. *J Med Chem* 2007;50(26):6618-26.

[101] Sugden D, Pickering H, Teh MT, Garratt Pj. Melatonin Receptor Pharmacology: Toward Subtype Specificity. *Biol Cell* 1997;89(8):531-7.

[102] Garratt Pj, Travard S, Vonhoff S, Tsotinis A, Sugden D. Mapping The Melatonin Receptor. 4. Comparison Of The Binding Affinities Of A Series Of Substituted Phenylalkyl Amides. *J Med Chem* 1996;39(9):1797-805.

[103] Navajas C, Kokkola T, Poso A, Honka N, Gynther J, Laitinen Jt. A Rhodopsin-Based Model For Melatonin Recognition At Its G Protein-Coupled Receptor. *Eur J Pharmacol* 1996;304(1-3):173-83.

[104] Spadoni G, Bedini A, Diamantini G, Tarzia G, Rivara S, Lorenzi S, Et Al. Synthesis, Enantiomeric Resolution, And Structure-Activity Relationship Study Of A Series Of 10,11-Dihydro-5h-Dibenzo[A,D]Cycloheptene MT2 Receptor Antagonists. *Chemmedchem* 2007;2(12):1741-9.

[105] Mor M, Rivara S, Silva C, Bordi F, Plazzi Pv, Spadoni G, Et Al. Melatonin Receptor Ligands: Synthesis Of New Melatonin Derivatives And Comprehensive Comparative Molecular Field Analysis (Comfa) Study. *J Med Chem* 1998;41(20):3831-44.

[106] Spadoni G, Bedini A, Rivara S, Mor M. Melatonin Receptor Agonists: New Options For Insomnia And Depression Treatment. *Cns Neurosci Ther* 2011;17(6):733-41.

[107] Sugden D, Chong Nw, Lewis Df. Structural Requirements At The Melatonin Receptor. Br J Pharmacol 1995;114(3):618-23.

[108] Hu Y, Ho Mk, Chan Kh, New Dc, Wong Yh. Synthesis Of Substituted N-[3-(3-Methoxyphenyl)Propyl] Amides As Highly Potent MT(2)-Selective Melatonin Ligands. *Bioorg Med Chem Lett* 2010;20(8):2582-5.

[109] Dubocovich Ml, Masana Mi, Iacob S, Sauri Dm. Melatonin Receptor Antagonists That Differentiate Between The Human Mel1a And Mel1b Recombinant Subtypes Are Used To Assess The Pharmacological Profile Of The Rabbit Retina Ml1 Presynaptic Heteroreceptor. Naunyn Schmiedebergs *Arch Pharmacol* 1997;355(3):365-75.

[110] Teh MT, Sugden D. Comparison Of The Structure-Activity Relationships Of Melatonin Receptor Agonists And Antagonists: Lengthening The N-Acyl Side-Chain Has Differing Effects On Potency On Xenopus Melanophores. Naunyn Schmiedebergs. *Arch Pharmacol* 1998;358(5):522-8.

[111] Faust R, Garratt Pj, Jones R, Yeh Lk, Tsotinis A, Panoussopoulou M, Et Al. Mapping The Melatonin Receptor. 6. Melatonin Agonists And Antagonists Derived From 6h-Isoindolo[2,1-A]Indoles, 5,6-Dihydroindolo[2,1-A]Isoquinolines, And 6,7-Dihydro-5h-Benzo[C]Azepino[2,1-A]Indoles. *J Med Chem 2000*;43(6):1050-61.

[112] Descamps-Francois C, Yous S, Chavatte P, Audinot V, Bonnaud A, Boutin Ja, Et Al. Design And Synthesis Of Naphthalenic Dimers As Selective MT1 Melatoninergic Ligands. *J Med Chem* 2003;46(7):1127-9.

[113] Wallez V, Durieux-Poissonnier S, Chavatte P, Boutin Ja, Audinot V, Nicolas Jp, Et Al. Synthesis And Structure-Affinity-Activity Relationships Of Novel Benzofuran Derivatives As MT(2) Melatonin Receptor Selective Ligands. *J Med Chem* 2002;45(13):2788-800.

[114] Kopin Ij, Pare Cm, Axelrod J, Weissbach H. 6-Hydroxylation, The Major Metabolic Pathway For Melatonin. *Biochim Biophys Acta* 1960;40:377-8.

[115] Kennaway Dj, Hugel Hm, Clarke S, Tjandra A, Johnson Dw, Royles P, Et Al. Structure-Activity Studies Of Melatonin Analogues In Prepubertal Male Rats. *Aust J Biol Sci* 1988;41(3):393-400.

[116] Kveder S, Mcisaac Wm. The Metabolism Of Melatonin (N-Acetyl-5-Methoxy-tryptamine) And 5-Methoxytryptamine. *J Biol Chem* 1961;236:3214-20.

[117] Fukatsu K, Uchikawa O, Kawada M, Yamano T, Yamashita M, Kato K, Et Al. Synthesis Of A Novel Series Of Benzocycloalkene Derivatives As Melatonin Receptor Agonists. *J Med Chem* 2002;45(19):4212-21.

[118] Zhu J, Hu Y, Ho Mk, Wong Yh. 3-Methoxylphenylpropyl Amides As Novel Receptor Subtype-Selective Melatoninergic Ligands: Characterization Of Physicochemical And Pharmacokinetic Properties. *Xenobiotica* 2011;41(1):35-45.

[119] Fisher Sp, Sugden D. Sleep-Promoting Action Of Iik7, A Selective MT2 Melatonin Receptor Agonist In The Rat. *Neurosci Lett* 2009;457(2):93-6.

[120] Fisher Sp, Davidson K, Kulla A, Sugden D. Acute Sleep-Promoting Action Of The Melatonin Agonist, Ramelteon, In The Rat. *J Pineal Res* 2008;45(2):125-32.

[121] Arangino S, Cagnacci A, Angiolucci M, Vacca Am, Longu G, Volpe A, Et Al. Effects Of Melatonin On Vascular Reactivity, Catecholamine Levels, And Blood Pressure In Healthy Men. *Am J Cardiol* 1999;83(9):1417-9.

[122] Zanoboni A, Forni A, Zanoboni-Muciaccia W, Zanussi C. Effect Of Pinealectomy On Arterial Blood Pressure And Food And Water Intake In The Rat. *J Endocrinol Invest* 1978;1(2):125-30.
[123] Zeman M, Dulkova K, Bada V, Herichova I. Plasma Melatonin Concentrations In Hypertensive Patients With The Dipping And Non-Dipping Blood Pressure Profile. *Life Sci* 2005;76(16):1795-803.
[124] Cagnacci A, Cannoletta M, Renzi A, Baldassari F, Arangino S, Volpe A. Prolonged Melatonin Administration Decreases Nocturnal Blood Pressure In Women. *Am J Hypertens* 2005;18(12 Pt 1):1614-8.
[125] Holmes Sw, Sugden D. Proceedings: The Effect Of Melatonin On Pinealectomy-Induced Hypertension In The Rat. *Br J Pharmacol* 1976;56(3):360p-1p.
[126] Scheer Fa, Van Montfrans Ga, Van Someren Ej, Mairuhu G, Buijs Rm. Daily Nighttime Melatonin Reduces Blood Pressure In Male Patients With Essential Hypertension. *Hypertension* 2004;43(2):192-7.
[127] Paulis L, Simko F. Blood Pressure Modulation And Cardiovascular Protection By Melatonin: Potential Mechanisms Behind. *Physiol Res* 2007;56(6):671-84.
[128] Simko F, Pechanova O. Potential Roles Of Melatonin And Chronotherapy Among The New Trends In Hypertension Treatment. *J Pineal Res* 2009;47(2):127-33.
[129] Doolen S, Krause Dn, Dubocovich Ml, Duckles Sp. Melatonin Mediates Two Distinct Responses In Vascular Smooth Muscle. *Eur J Pharmacol* 1998;345(1):67-9.
[130] Cos S, Garcia-Bolado A, Sanchez-Barcelo Ej. Direct Antiproliferative Effects Of Melatonin On Two Metastatic Cell Sublines Of Mouse Melanoma (B16bl6 And Pg19). *Melanoma Res* 2001;11(2):197-201.
[131] Kubatka P, Bojkova B, Kalicka K, Chamilova M, Adamekova E, Ahlers I, Et Al. Preventive Effects Of Raloxifene And Melatonin In N-Methyl-N-Nitrosourea-Induced Mammary Carcinogenesis In Female Rats. *Neoplasma* 2001;48(4):313-9.
[132] Gonzalez A, Martinez-Campa C, Mediavilla Md, Alonso-Gonzalez C, Sanchez-Mateos S, Hill Sm, Et Al. Effects Of MT1 Melatonin Receptor Overexpression On The Aromatase-Suppressive Effect Of Melatonin In Mcf-7 Human Breast Cancer Cells. *Oncol Rep* 2007;17(4):947-53.
[133] Hill Sm, Frasch T, Xiang S, Yuan L, Duplessis T, Mao L. Molecular Mechanisms Of Melatonin Anticancer Effects. *Integr Cancer Ther* 2009;8(4):337-46.
[134] Kiefer T, Ram Pt, Yuan L, Hill Sm. Melatonin Inhibits Estrogen Receptor Transactivation And Camp Levels In Breast Cancer Cells. *Breast Cancer Res Treat* 2002;71(1):37-45.
[135] Cos S, Fernandez R, Guezmes A, Sanchez-Barcelo Ej. Influence Of Melatonin On Invasive And Metastatic Properties Of Mcf-7 Human Breast Cancer Cells. *Cancer Res* 1998;58(19):4383-90.
[136] Peschke E, Frese T, Chankiewitz E, Peschke D, Preiss U, Schneyer U, Et Al. Diabetic Goto Kakizaki Rats As Well As Type 2 Diabetic Patients Show A Decreased Diurnal Serum Melatonin Level And An Increased Pancreatic Melatonin-Receptor Status. *J Pineal Res* 2006;40(2):135-43.
[137] Peschke E, Stumpf I, Bazwinsky I, Litvak L, Dralle H, Muhlbauer E. Melatonin And Type 2 Diabetes - A Possible Link?. *J Pineal Res* 2007;42(4):350-8.

[138] Kadhim Hm, Ismail Sh, Hussein Ki, Bakir Ih, Sahib As, Khalaf Bh, Et Al. Effects Of Melatonin And Zinc On Lipid Profile And Renal Function In Type 2 Diabetic Patients Poorly Controlled With Metformin. *J Pineal Res* 2006;41(2):189-93.

[139] Nishida S, Segawa T, Murai I, Nakagawa S. Long-Term Melatonin Administration Reduces Hyperinsulinemia And Improves The Altered Fatty-Acid Compositions In Type 2 Diabetic Rats Via The Restoration Of Delta-5 Desaturase Activity. *J Pineal Res* 2002;32(1):26-33.

[140] Muhlbauer E, Albrecht E, Hofmann K, Bazwinsky-Wutschke I, Peschke E. Melatonin Inhibits Insulin Secretion In Rat Insulinoma Beta-Cells (Ins-1) Heterologously Expressing The Human Melatonin Receptor Isoform MT2. *J Pineal Res* 2011;51(3):361-72.

[141] Lyssenko V, Nagorny Cl, Erdos Mr, Wierup N, Jonsson A, Spegel P, Et Al. Common Variant In MTnr1b Associated With Increased Risk Of Type 2 Diabetes And Impaired Early Insulin Secretion. *Nat Genet* 2009;41(1):82-8.

In: New Developments in Melatonin Research ISBN: 978-1-62618-843-3
Editors: D.Acuña-Castroviejo, I.Rusanova, G.Escames © 2013 Nova Science Publishers, Inc.

Chapter 5

MT_3: The Other Melatonin Binding Site

Jean A. Boutin
Biotechnology, Molecular and Cellular Pharmacology,
Institut de Recherches SERVIER,
Croissy-sur-Seine, France

Abstract

Melatonin is a neurohormone synthesized at night by the pineal gland, in mammals. It circulates in the low nanomolar range, and is believed to relay central circadian information to peripheral organs.

Furthermore, melatonin has been described as having multiple activities, some of them at 'pharmacological' concentrations (micro-molar and beyond) that cannot be reached in natural conditions. To exert those activities, melatonin has three clearly described targets that translate the binding of the hormone into cellular signals. Those three targets are two GPCRs named MT_1 and MT_2, and a binding site originally described in hamster brains and inventively called MT_3. This binding site has some original features that have been precisely described in the literature. The present review deals with the progression of the knowledge of this binding site, with a focus on the experiments that led to the discovery of the enzyme hidden behind MT_3, namely QR2. Although research regarding QR2 is booming at the moment, the goal of the present review is to insist on the characterization(s) of the binding site, rather than provide a description of QR2. Indeed, this identification is one of the rare successes of reverse pharmacology. The detailed arguments on which we based our assumption that MT_3 was indeed QR2 will be described and discussed in the present review, highlighting the main points and the main discrepancies between the historical description of the MT_3 binding site and our observations about QR2.

The minimal role of melatonin in the biochemistry of QR2 will also be discussed. The meaning of this identification in pathophysiological terms will be briefly addressed in the conclusive remarks, particularly regarding the importance it may have for the near future.

Introduction

Melatonin is a neurohormone synthesized in the pineal gland in a circadian manner: it is produced at a high concentration at night, and at a low concentration during the day [1]. This compound, which is derived from the indole core of tryptophan, is believed to relay circadian information to peripheral organs. It has been clearly linked to seasonal rhythms, and therefore remains a key player in reproduction [2]. Historically, the question of how melatonin was transmitting its message to organs and cells remained open for quite a long time. There are literally hundreds of actions that are due to melatonin, suggesting that the number of pathways with which melatonin does interfere is enormous. Most of those actions have been covered by various reviews [3-23]. Some additional reviews have been published regarding melatonin receptor pharmacology, attempting mainly to survey the MT_1 and MT_2 receptor-mediated actions of the neurohormone [24-27]. Traditionally, one could separate the actions of melatonin at 'low' concentrations (*i.e.*, at physiologically achievable concentrations: in the nanomolar range) from those obtained at 'high' concentrations (*i.e.*, so-called pharmacological concentrations: in the micromolar range and greater) without presuming the possible higher concentrations at a local level in some tissues. Another view of this segregation might be that some targets of melatonin are modulated by the neurohormone at 'high' concentrations, and therefore might have modest affinities for melatonin, in which case only high concentrations would have actions with respect to those proteins.

After the pioneering works of Cohen *et al.* [28] in 1978, Niles *et al.* [29] in 1979, and Cardinali *et al.* [30] in 1979, several papers revealed the existence of binding site(s) in the membrane and/or cytoplasm of various organs of a variety of animals, including the brains of rat [31], cow [30], hamster [32], and chicken [33], as well as chicken retina [34].

Table 1 summarizes, in chronological order, the various attempts made to characterize the melatonin binding sites during the pre-cloning period (from approximately 1979 to 1992). Obviously, depending on the conditions, tissues, and subcellular preparations, those measures might have contained several of the melatonin binding sites – MT_1, MT_2, and/or MT_3. Interestingly, beyond a certain point, the binding site in the cytosol was disregarded if not entirely forgotten (see below), and reviews tend to address the membrane-bound binding sites exclusively (see, for instance, Dubocovich [35] and Kennaway *et al.* [36]). Some of the initial observations were based on the use of [^{3}H]-melatonin, and clearly demonstrated the plurality of the molecular (proteic) targets of melatonin, a feature that would thereafter be somewhat underregarded, particularly after the discovery of the 7-transmembrane domain, G-coupled receptors MT_1 and MT_2 [37, 38]. The conditions under which those cytosolic binding sites were described were nicely reported, but did not correspond in the authors' mind to melatonin receptor(s), which was(were) thought to be membrane-associated. Indeed, the use of iodinated melatonin, which was reported by at least four groups in 1986-1987 [32, 39-41] after the initial work of Vakkuri *et al.* [42, 43], provided a better tool in the search of those 7-transmembrane G-coupled melatonin receptors. Kennaway and Hugel questioned the use of this tool in a complete and interesting review [36]. If the availability of this radiolabeled compound changed the focus of the melatonin community from searching for the binding site(s) to characterizing the two GPCRs, it also resulted in an almost complete loss of interest in anything else other than those receptors.

Table 1. In search of the lost putative melatonin binding site – A chronological compilation

Authors	(Ref)	Year	Species	Organ	Cytosol or Membranes	Ligand	Affinity* (nM)	Bmax (fmol/mg protein)	Method
Cohen *et al.*	(28)	1978	Hamster	Ovary	Cytosol	[^{3}H]-melatonin	6.3	52	charcoal
			Hamster	Ovary	Cytosol	[^{3}H]-melatonin	550	420	charcoal
			Rat	Ovary	Cytosol	[^{3}H]-melatonin	NR	300-440	charcoal
			Human	Ovary	Cytosol	[^{3}H]-melatonin	NR	330	charcoal
			Hamster	Liver	Cytosol	[^{3}H]-melatonin	NR	150-1000	charcoal
			Rat	Liver	Cytosol	[^{3}H]-melatonin	NR	290	charcoal
Cardinali *et al.*	(30)	1979	Bovine	Brain	Membranes	[^{3}H]-melatonin	5**	20**	filtration
Vacas and Cardinali	(31)	1979	Hamster	Brain	Membranes	[^{3}H]-melatonin	34	53	filtration
			Rat	Brain	Membranes	[^{3}H]-melatonin	94	77	filtration
Niles *et al.*	(29)	1979	Rat	Brain	Cytosol	[^{3}H]-melatonin	8-300	60-1370	charcoal
Duncan *et al.*	(32)	1986	Hamster	Brain	Membranes	2-[^{125}I]-melatonin	4	109	filtration
Laudon and Zisapel	(39)	1986	Rat	Brain	Membranes	2-[^{125}I]-melatonin	38	81	filtration
Dubocovich and Takahashi	(34)	1987	Chicken	Retina	Membranes	2-[^{125}I]-melatonin	0.4	74	filtration

Table 1. (Continued)

Authors	(Ref)	Year	Species	Organ	Cytosol or Membranes	Ligand	Affinity* (nM)	Bmax (fmol/mg protein)	Method
Vanecek *et al.*	(152)	1987	Rat	Brain	Membranes	2-[^{125}I]-melatonin	0.02	8	filtration
Niles *et al.*	(40)	1987	Hamster	Brain	Membranes	2-[^{125}I]-melatonin	0.32	6	filtration
			Hamster	Brain	Membranes	2-[^{125}I]-melatonin	10	123	filtration
Pickering *et al.*	(33)	1988	Hamster	Hypothalamus	Membranes	2-[^{125}I]-melatonin	2	75	filtration
			Hamster	Testes	Membranes	2-[^{125}I]-melatonin	1	18	filtration
			Chicken	Brain	Membranes	2-[^{125}I]-melatonin	2	170	filtration
			Chicken	Retina	Membranes	2-[^{125}I]-melatonin	0.7	66	filtration
Duncan *et al.*	(67)	1988	Hamster	Brain	Membranes	2-[^{125}I]-melatonin	3.3	110	filtration
Anis *et al.*	(153)	1989	Hamster	Brain	Membranes	2-[^{125}I]-melatonin	60-230**	350-1200**	filtration
Duncan *et al.*	(63)	1989	Hamster	Hypothalamus	Membranes	2-[^{125}I]-melatonin	0.04	3	filtration
Pickering and Niles	(52)	1990	Hamster	Hypothalamus	Membranes	2-[^{125}I]-melatonin	1.8	75	filtration
Song *et al.*	(154)	1992	Duck	Kidney	Membranes	2-[^{125}I]-melatonin	0.04	6	filtration
Wang *et al.*	(155)	1992	Quail	Testes	Membranes	2-[^{125}I]-melatonin	0.05	3	filtration

Authors	(Ref)	Year	Species	Organ	Cytosol or Membranes	Ligand	Affinity* (nM)	Bmax (fmol/mg protein)	Method
Kennaway *et al.*	(69)	1994	Chicken	Brain	Membranes	2-[^{125}I]-melatonin	24	5***	filtration
			Chicken	Brain	Membranes	[^{3}H]-melatonin	125	5.5***	filtration
Molinari *et al.*	(70)	1996	Hamster	Brain	Membranes	2-[^{125}I]-MCANAT	0.1	3	filtration
			Mouse	Brain	Membranes	2-[^{125}I]-MCANAT	NR	1.3	filtration
			Guinea pig	Brain	Membranes	2-[^{125}I]-MCANAT	NR	0.4	filtration
			Rat	Brain	Membranes	2-[^{125}I]-MCANAT	NR	0.2	filtration
			Rabbit	Brain	Membranes	2-[^{125}I]-MCANAT	NR	0.3	filtration
			Chicken	Brain	Membranes	2-[^{125}I]-MCANAT	NR	0.3	filtration
			Chicken	Optic tectum	Membranes	2-[^{125}I]-MCANAT	NR	0.3	filtration
			Chicken	Retina	Membranes	2-[^{125}I]-MCANAT	NR	0.2	filtration
Paul *et al*	(66)	1999	Hamster	Kidney	Membranes	2-[^{125}I]-melatonin	1.9	90	filtration
			Hamster	Intestine	Membranes	2-[^{125}I]-melatonin	1.7	31	filtration
Nosjean *et al.*	(68)	2001	Hamster	Kidney	Homogenate	2-[^{125}I]-MCANAT	0.5	173	filtration

NR: Not reported.

*: All K_d data measured below 1 nM are likely MT_1 and/or MT_2. Data above 10 nM are likely MT_3.

**: The range describes a variety of conditions. See original publications for details.

***: fmol/10 mg wet tissue.

Nevertheless, the receptors were not cloned until 1994-1995 [37, 38], first from mice [44], and much later from various other species, including human [37, 45], ovine [37, 46, 47], hamster [48], and rat [49]. The lack of *ad hoc* tools (particularly a radiotracer that permitted the detection of putative soluble melatonin binding sites) considerably slowed the studies regarding the soluble binding site, which nearly disappeared from the literature during several years thereafter. However, a handful of groups continued to search for the nature of the extra binding sites [33, 50-55]. One of the most complete papers was a report by Acuna-Castroviejo *et al.* [56], in which the characteristics of a nuclear membrane melatonin binding site were described. It was not followed by the purification of the corresponding protein. Another work was published in 1994 [57] reporting a nuclear receptor that nicely rationalized the described genomic actions of melatonin [58].

According to the description, this nuclear receptor seemed unrelated to the one described by Acuna-Castroviejo *et al.* [56]. Similar experiments to those described by Becker-Andre *et al.* [57] were never repeated in the melatonin community, suggesting that the initial observation was artefactual. However, this work is continuously cited in the literature (see for instance Slominski *et al.* [59]).

The next melatonin binding site in line, known for quite some time, was the Mel1c receptor, which has been cloned in several species (*e.g.*, xenopus, zebrafish, chicken) [60]. This interesting receptor turned out to be orthologous to gpr50 [61], a human orphan 7-transmembrane receptor that is closely related to the MT_1 and MT_2 melatonin receptors [62], but has lost its capacity to bind melatonin over the course of evolution.

After this period, the melatonin community remained oriented towards describing the actions mediated by the classical MT_1 and MT_2 receptors. The existence of MT_3 remained controversial because the conditions under which it could be measured were non-classical: 4°C and very fast association/ dissociation kinetics [63, 64]. Nevertheless, under these conditions, a pharmacology profile of this binding site was published that clearly differed from the profiles of the canonical melatonin receptors. Of particular interest were the 'specific' ligand, MCA-NAT [64] (although specificity in the field of pharmacology is often a function of dose [65]) and the fact that, unlike MT_1 and MT_2, MT_3 bound prazosin [33, 52].

The Biochemistry and Pharmacology of MT_3

When we came across the body of work from the Dubocovich laboratory, which used pharmacological tools to define a 'new' binding site, MT_3, we were fascinated by the strangeness of its behavior [64]. It presented very fast equilibrium kinetics, in the 1- to 10-second range, and an affinity for melatonin that could be considered modest, in the 10-50 nM range. The best characterization used membranes or homogenates from hamster brain. Finally, the conditions under which those experiments were conducted were judged particular, as the filtration assay had to be diligently performed to catch such transient binding. We first attempted to repeat and broaden the pharmacological characterization of MT_3 [66]. We did repeat those data, and were able to further characterize the MT_3 binding site independent of the originating laboratory [67]. We later described this binding site in other tissues, such as intestine, and using 2-[^{125}I]-iodomelatonin [68]. We also employed a larger and different set of compounds, including but not limited to those described in earlier pharmacological profiles of MT_3 [67]. Finally, we found a dissociation constant, K_D, for the ligand in the nanomolar range, relatively close to the published literature on MT_3. Interestingly, at that stage, the K_i value of melatonin in this test was already in the 50 nM range, far from the K_D described for the classical MT receptor (*i.e.*, in the sub-nanomolar range). The low and transience affinity of the conditions under which the MT3 binding was measured should have alerted us to the possibility that this binding site might be an enzyme rather than a membrane-associated receptor (see also discussion in Kennaway and Hugel [36]). However, until much later, most of our actions were based on the fact that we were looking for a new member of the melatonin GPCR, in line with the plethoric family of serotonin GPCRs that had already been pharmacologically characterized.

The exact localization of this binding site was tentatively described in two nice papers [50, 52] using autoradiographic approaches. The papers reached two different conclusions that are confusing, and somewhat mutually exclusive. These studies employed different hamster strains: Djungarian (*Phodopus sungorus*) in Duncan *et al.* [50], and Syrian (*Mesocricetus auratus*in) in Pickering and Niles [52]. In their results sections, both papers stressed the fact that the main location was indeed membranous. In both cases, the experiments were described regarding membrane preparations, strongly suggesting that MT_3 could not be found anywhere else, in agreement with the previous indications of Dubocovich's laboratory that the MT_3 binding site should be membrane-associated (as it was – as already stated – *obviously* a new member of the GPCR family of proteins), as reviewed in [35, 64]. Historically, one must recall that the hamster was the main species in which this laboratory found the putative MT_3 receptor, albeit in various hamster strains. This species was also shown to possess only one (MT_1) of the classical melatonin GPCRs, while the MT_2 receptor gene was later shown to be interrupted by a stop codon [48]. Probably because [^{3}H]-melatonin was fading away as a tool in favor of the newly described 2-[^{125}I]-iodomelatonin, fewer and fewer experiments were conducted with the former, until it was no longer used for any type of experiment, with the sole exception of the Kennaway paper, in which a comparison was made between radioligands [69]. Nevertheless, the membranous nature of MT_3 was also based on a very strong paper from Dubocovich's laboratory [70] that precisely characterized the subcellular localization of the binding site using the newly described MT_3-specific iodo-melatonin analogue 5-methoxycarbonylamino-N-acetyltryptamine (MCA-NAT). This paper by Molinari *et al.* [70] nicely dissected the binding of the then newly synthesized 2-[^{125}I]-iodo-MCANAT to hamster brain membranes. Several lines of evidence clearly indicate that MT_3 is membrane-associated under those experimental conditions.

It remains curious that, by a twist of fate, the researchers in the domain suddenly – over a period of less than 10 years – turned from a whole cell search for this described and original MT_3 binding site to a membrane-bound MT_3 binding site, even though the pioneer paper of Cohen *et al.* [28] was still cited, and had shown that a cytosolic binding site of melatonin did exist. Furthermore, this last result was also somewhat confirmed by other techniques in other groups, including radiation inactivation [71], autoradiography [51], differential pharmacology (discovering that prazosin was a ligand of MT_3, although not of MT_1 or MT_2) [40], and pioneering attempts to affinity purify MT_3 [54, 55].

A technical limitation might also explain why this lack of interest in a cytoplasmic receptor arose. Indeed, binding by filtration assay was and still is a fairly routine technique, usually applied systematically to membrane-bound targets. Although it is true that using it on cytosolic material might be trickier, experimental solutions existed and could have been used to attempt to validate these alternative approaches. Indeed, those conditions were used for our independent validation of the MT_3 pharmacological characterization, which was conducted using a fast filtration assay [66].

Finally, several pharmacological papers [52, 66, 70, 72] in which the MT_3 binding sites was described with iodo-melatonin or iodo-MCA-NAT led to the accurate characterization of a binding site whose characteristics clearly differed from those of MT_1/MT_2 receptors.

Reverse Pharmacology

In a classic reverse pharmacological approach, we attempted to identify the protein responsible for the binding of MCA-NAT by using a derivative of this selective MT_3 compound and hamster kidneys as biological source [73]. Indeed, this later tissue was preferred over brain, because it was clearly stated by previous authors that kidneys were also a rich source of melatonin-derivative bindings [70]. The major discovery and description of MCA-NAT as an MT_3 tool and as an MT_3 radiolabelled ligand opened an experimental route for the identification of this protein (see above). We chose to synthetize a close analogue of MCA-NAT (namely, N-[2-(7-amino-1-naphthyl)ethyl]-acetamide), which was then immobilized to an affinity chromatography medium. Because the published arguments were in favor of a membrane-associated MT_3, the first purification step was a very mild solubilization of the homogenates using octylglucopyranoside detergent.

Afterwards, it was surprisingly easy to trap an almost pure protein onto the column, and to identify it by mass spectrometry [73] as quinone reductase 2 (QR2; for more information on this protein, see below and Vella *et al* [74]). In the same set of experiments, and previous to this key step in our understanding of MT_3, we assessed a methodology that permitted the analysis of MT_3 binding, taking into consideration the rapidity of its kinetics and its possible cytosolic nature.

The characterization of various tissues from various species for their MT_3 binding site-like capacity was also assessed at the same time [68], bolstering the hypotheses on which we built our approach: that numerous tissues contained this binding site, and that it was usually associated with soluble cytoplasmic tissue fractions.

In short, QR2 was an enzyme initially described with regard to its capacity to reduce menadione in the presence of non-canonical hydride donors, such as N-ribosyl-, N-methyl-, and N-phenyl-dihydronicotinamide [75, 76]. Several papers have described the characteristics of QR2 enzyme activity.

In 1990, Jaiswal *et al.* [77], in attempting to find isoforms of QR1, cloned a shorter-than-QR1 sequence with 47 amino acids missing from the C-terminus, and roughly 50% sequence homology to QR1 for the remaining of the amino acid sequence.

Talalay's group also cloned but thoroughly characterized the enzyme on the basis of Liao's initial works, and named the enzyme QR2 [78]. The actual function of this enzyme remained poorly documented thereafter. Several approaches closely documented the characteristics of the enzyme, including 1/ co-crystallization with the substrates menadione [79] and CB1954 [80], or with the inhibitors resveratrol [81], melatonin [82], and MCA-NAT [83]; 2/ detailed considerations of its catalytic activity [84]; and 3/ a close description of QR2 substrate and/or inhibitor behavior by mass spectrometry [85]. Pharmacological profiles [86, 87] and co-substrate specificity [88] were also reported in detail.

The enzyme was also described in several papers as forming complexes with p53 and nrf2 [89, 90]; however, that precious information was generally not further exploited.

During the years after this discovery, and despite the fact that – to our knowledge – no other laboratories had reported the same observation (that is, that MT_3 and QR2 were one and the same), we gathered more information strongly suggesting that QR2 was the missing MT_3. Chronologically, the data were as follows:

1. Cells such as HEK express a measurable MT_3 binding site only after (never before) the transfection of QR2 [73].
2. Organs from $QR2^{-/-}$ mice do not express a measurable amount of MT_3 binding sites, while wild type animals do express measurable MT_3 binding sites in control experiments conducted in the same conditions [91].
3. The pharmacology of MT_3 and of QR2 are similar if not identical, provided compounds in the MT_3 system were properly described [86, 87].
4. Co-crystallizations of QR2 with MCA-NAT, iodo-MCA-NAT, iodo-melatonin, and melatonin (all MT_3 compounds) have been reported, as have data regarding their affinities for QR2 [82, 83].

However, inhibitors of QR2 are not necessarily ligands of MT_3, and vice-versa [92]. Furthermore, QR2 is, *a priori*, not a membrane-associated protein [78], despite the observation that in overexpressing cells, membrane preparations express an antigen recognized by the anti-QR2 antibody (Moulharat, Ferry and Boutin, unpublished).

To speculate on these two points, it must be pointed out that the techniques used for the characterizations of the MT_3 binding [66, 93] and the QR2 inhibition [86, 87] are obviously different.

We attempted (unsuccessfully, so far) to describe QR2 binding by using pure enzyme in a soluble form. The main limitation of this approach is probably the minute amount of immobilized QR2 available for melatonin or resveratrol binding (less than 5%), a feature that is still being assessed in our laboratory. Furthermore, the question of the membrane-bound nature of MT_3, which is strongly suggested by the work of Dubocovich's group [64, 70, 94], remains open. Indeed, a close observation of the sequence of QR2 reveals a cryptic myristoylation site at the N-terminus (for details on myristoylation, see [95]).

The myristoylation of proteins is an event leading to their membrane association via a myristoyl group at the N-terminus of the protein. The fact that this type of cryptic site can be revealed by caspase digestion has been reported in the literature [96]. The experimental validation of this observation is under way in our laboratory.

Reverse pharmacology is an approach that has been used by several groups to find the molecular target(s) of various chemicals. It has been successfully used on several occasions, with resveratrol [97], chloroquin [98], and dabigatran (a thrombin inhibitor) [99]. In all of those cases, QR2 was identified as a major target of these compounds. This variety of compounds able to recognize the somewhat large cavity of QR2 may also signify, as for QR1 and in the UDP-glucuronosyltransferase and cytochrome P450 families, a particular capacity to recognize structurally diverse compounds, like the xenobiotics recognized by drug metabolism enzymes.

MT_3 and Chemistry

MT_3 chemistry has been visited in a couple of laboratories associated with either Dubocovich's or our laboratory. MCA-NAT, the first 'specific' MT_3 binder used after its discovery [70], formed the basis for the synthesis of new analogues. Additional exploration of its properties was performed using chemo-informatic tools [100]. This study provided a clear indication (if needed) that MT_3 was different from MT_1 and MT_2. On several occasions, we also attempted to bring new chemicals into the MT_3 pharmacological picture [101-104]. We [105] and others [106, 107] also attempted to model the MT_3 binding site, based on the ligands available in the literature.

Unfortunately, likely because the exact nature of the binding site was unknown, it was impossible to base a chemical program on the actual structure of the protein.

Therefore, an alternative route was chosen, namely gathering biophysical information about the relationship between the compounds and the protein. Hence, most of the information has been gained from analogues of active, often indole-derived chemicals, as in the case of MCA-NAT. The discovery of the protein nature of MT_3 (*i.e.*, QR2) implicated more and easier screens, either from large libraries of compounds [87, 93, 108, 109], from natural compounds (*e.g.*, casimiroin and derivatives [110, 111], resveratrol and analogues [112], flavonoids [86, 113] or phenazine derivatives [114]), from indolequinone derivatives [115] or from antimalarial drugs [84, 98]. Those compound potencies range from low nanomolar to high micromolar. The structures of those compounds are exemplified in Figure 1. It is clear that from an experimental perspective, the compounds from Boussard *et al.* [93] or from Mailliet *et al.* [92] proved to be among the most potent, and were active in various living systems [116, 117].

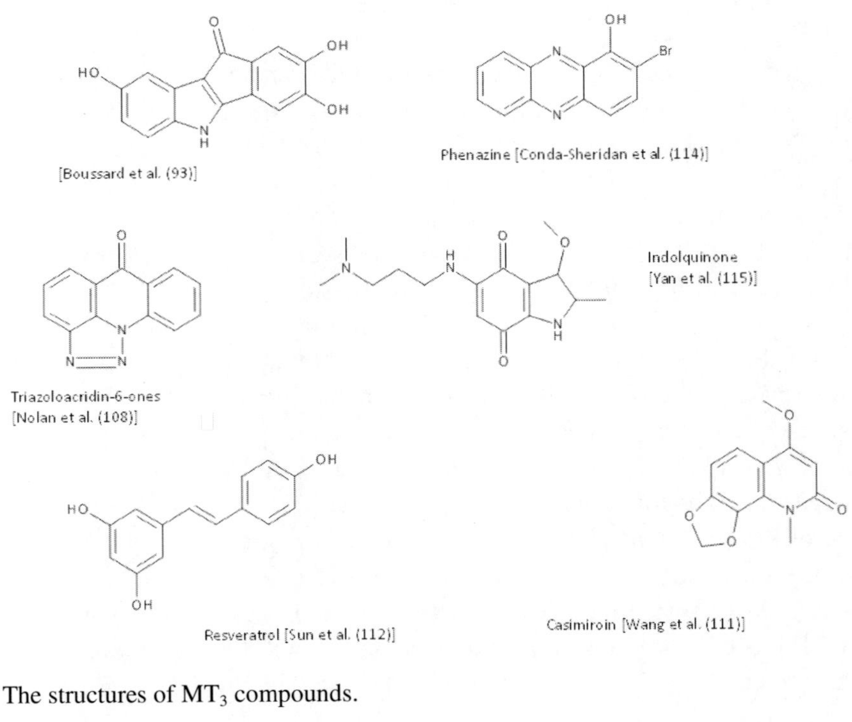

Figure 1. The structures of MT_3 compounds.

Non-Molecular Pharmacology

Obviously, it was on the basis of the pharmacology of compounds described as 'MT_3 ligands' that a pharmacological role for this target in various physio-pathological processes was hypothesized. The main features of the MT_3 compounds in various models are listed below. The intraocular pressure model and its behavior after MCA-NAT treatment are described in more detail in the final sub-section.

1. *Phosphoinositide hydrolysis*: Very early in the characterization of MT_3, it was reported that its activation was leading to the stimulation of phosphoinositide hydrolysis [118, 119] in chicken brain slices and a cell line (RPMI 1846), respectively. In the former paper, the authors determined that in this animal model (chicken brain), a series of melatoninergic compounds led to the breakdown of phosphoinositides with a rank order different from the rank order of the binding of those compounds at classical melatonin receptors [118]. In the latter publication, the action of a series of melatoninergic compounds correlated with the binding of those compounds to the hamster hypothalamus MT_3; hence, the cell line would express the MT_3 binding site [119].
2. *Leukocyte adhesion*: A clear paper by Lotufo *et al.* reported that N-acetylserotonin, a 'specific' MT_3 ligand, inhibits leukocyte adhesion, strongly suggesting (according to the authors) that MT_3 modulates leukocyte adhesion [120].
3. *Heart ischemia-reperfusion injury:* Lagneux *et al.* [121] nicely demonstrated that MCA-NAT administrated *in vivo* to rats 30 minutes prior to heart excision protected those hearts from ischemia-reperfusion injuries. These observations have been extended to other MT_3 compounds.
4. *Antidepressant activity*: MCA-NAT, administrated *in vivo*, decreased the immobilization time in the tail suspension test in a dose-dependent manner [122]. This activity is synonymous with anti-depressive capacity.
5. *MCA-NAT and retinal neurodevelopment in chicken*: In a straightforward paper, Sampaio [123] described how MCA-NAT enhances the cAMP level in chicken retina.
6. *Pain:* Ray *et al.* [124] evaluated the role of MT_3 in mediating the antinociceptive activity of melatonin. Although the description is interesting, the pharmacological evidence demonstrating this involvement remains limited, as it is based on correlations between various compounds, the specificity of some of which remains questionable.
7. *MT3 and intraocular pressure (IOP)*: Regarding the relative lack of specificity of MCA-NAT: In a series of very interesting papers, Pintor's group (see recent reviews [125-128]) dissected the mechanism by which MCA-NAT, a renowned MT_3 ligand, was able to reduce the intraocular pressure (IOP) [129-132]. Because the compound was originally qualified as "MT_3 specific" [70], it was believed that MCA-NAT was unable to touch any other targets, which is, after all, the core notion of specificity. Therefore, this enzyme being MT_3, and MT_3 being QR2, the action of MCA-NAT in this model ought to be mediated by this enzyme. The underlying hypothesis was that MCA-NAT would activate QR2, which would in turn reduce the IOP. One of the most impressive works in this series was an experiment by Alarma-Estramy *et al.*

[133], in which siRNA was used to decrease QR2 expression in rabbit eyes. This beautiful work demonstrated that despite the decrease of QR2 expression (and activity), MCA-NAT was still reducing the IOP. This finding definitely demonstrated that MCA-NAT was not acting through QR2 in this model to reduce IOP. Vincent *et al.* finally published a key paper describing the molecular pharmacology of the compound [65]. Indeed, although it is more active on MT_3 than many MT_1/MT_2 compounds are, MCA-NAT still presented affinity for those two 7-transmembrane melatonin receptors in the micromolar range, and was described as an agonist. Therefore, the possibility that MCA-NAT was acting through the classical MT receptors could not be ruled out, particularly given that MCA-NAT activity on MT receptors was antagonized by luzindole (a classical MT receptor antagonist), and that a paper from Tosini's group demonstrated very clearly that IOP was increased in mice lacking the MT_1 receptor [134]. New efforts were published by the same group regarding the finding of new molecules that were more MT_1/MT_2 oriented and loosely derived from the structure of melatonin [135]. Finally, the most recent paper from this group indicated that MCA-NAT is also a pharmacological ligand of carbonic anhydrases [136].

8. *Actions of QR2 inhibitors*: The reduction of QR2 activity (by means of shRNA transfection) in QR2-knockdown HT22 cells was correlated with a 50% reduction in menadione/BNAH-mediated toxicity, strongly suggesting that QR2 is central to the toxicity of menadione [137]. Finally, two observations are worth mentioning, although they were achieved recently in a system in which the core topic has evolved from MT_3 to QR2: the same compound S29434, in two different *in vivo* systems (memory impairment inhibition [116] and paraquat-induced toxicity inhibition [117]) has a very potent activity in preventing either memory loss or central nervous system paraquat toxicity. It seems that QR2 is pivotal in several processes associated with memory loss, neuron survival, and most generally in neurogenerative diseases, as hypothesized some time ago [138].

Sources of Misunderstanding and Confusion

The demonstration that MT_3 was most likely QR2 opened many roads of investigation, as it was important to understand the meaning of this identity. A clear view of this discovery was somehow hampered by confusion in the literature between different things: 1/ QR2 and NQO2 are considered the same. NQO2 is the historical name for mitochondrial complex I, also referred to as NADH:ubiquinone oxidoreductase (E.C. 1.6.5.3), (for details see [139]), while the EC number for QR2 (NRH:quinone reductase 2) is 1.10.99.2; and 2/ Despite a series of confusing reports [77, 140, 141], NADH (and NAPDH) are not co-substrates of QR2 [78]. It is somewhat interesting to note that despite the incapacity of QR2 to recognize NADH as an electron donor, its official name appears to be NAD(P)H dehydrogenase quinone 2 (Gene ID 4835, as provided by HGNC). Furthermore, and most importantly, because QR2 is (for historical reasons) a close relative of QR1, many scientists deduced that QR2, like QR1, was a detoxification enzyme (see for instance Testa [142]).

Practically speaking, rather little experimental evidence is available to demonstrate that QR2 is indeed an enzyme involved in phase I/II of drug metabolism, putting aside the sequence similarity of QR2 with QR1, the role of which is beyond doubt. It remains that the relative failure (toxicity?) of some kinase inhibitors was kindly attributed to the remarkable fact that those compounds, which are not pharmacologically 'specific' inhibitors, did inhibit QR2, as demonstrated by either catalytic activity inhibition or by co-crystallization [140, 141, 143-145]. In their discussions, the authors strongly suggested that if the compounds were toxic, it was likely because they potently inhibited QR2, 'this important enzyme of drug metabolism'.

In contrast, a large panel of compounds from the Pharmacopeia has been tested by CEREP as part of the BioPrint® program for possible binding to MT_3. Approximately 50 out of 2000 of those compounds present a high affinity (< 200 nM) in this binding model (J. Migeon, and T. Jean, personal communication, www.cerep.com). They range from clinically-used anti-hypertensive compounds to anti-proliferative and 5HT-3 antagonists. For most of these compounds (except the anticancer ones, albeit for other obvious reasons), no acute toxicity has been reported. These data strongly suggest that inhibiting QR2 has no obvious side effects.

Future, Hypotheses

Reasonable answers have not yet been found to a series of remaining questions. These questions fall into two groups: those directly linked to the MT_3/QR2 identity, and those linked more particularly to the activity of QR2, a subject that has stepped more and more out of the melatonin sphere, as melatonin – like resveratrol – was simply a tool that permitted us to gain a larger view of the role of this enzyme in different contexts. In this final section, some of the open questions remaining in this domain will be briefly addressed.

1. What exactly is QR2 doing? Why is the activity of this enzyme observed in different types of situations, particularly pathological ones? Why does QR2 appear to use very exotic reducing agents, such as N-ribosyl-, N-benzyl-, or N-methyldi-hydro-nicotinamide, as co-substrates? QR2 may be a sensor of the state of the cell. As such, it may be turned on whenever NADH catabolites (namely, N-ribosyl- and/or N-methyldihydronicotinamide) reach a level beyond a certain concentration, signaling a desperate situation for the cells (i.e., no remaining NADH). Does the fact that QR2 is also a major protein target of resveratrol [81] (another ubiquitous compound described with several pharmacological actions [146, 147]) tell us something about the role of this QR2 enzyme, even though one knows that resveratrol – like melatonin – interacts with many protein targets?
2. Do the co-substrates really derive from NADH degradation? When and how are they produced? Indeed, in resting cells, they are nearly absent [148]. In fact, several enzymes might very well play a role, such as the membrane-associated CD38 [149, 150]. The subsequent questions in this domain, which are currently being explored in our laboratory, comprise essentially: 1/ an understanding of the source of in cellulo

QR2 co-substrate(s) and the variations thereof; 2/ further exploration of the functional activity of QR2, particularly regarding (again in a cellular model) the QR2-dependent production of radical oxygen species; 3/ closer studies of the phenotype of $QR2^{-/-}$ animals, particularly in stress conditions; and 4/ the relevance of QR2 expression and activity to the metabolism of catechols, particularly dopaquinone.

Conclusion

It is fascinating to look at the 25 last years of research regarding that particularly elusive melatonin third binding site (MT_3). Indeed, we have evolved from a very academic search for new melatonin binding sites, to exploration of the pivotal role of a poorly known enzyme, the activity of which might very well be involved in several major pathological situations. Interestingly, the discrepancy between the inhibitory capacity of QR2 inhibitors and their capacity to bind to MT_3, or the capacity of MT_3 binders to inhibit QR2, has been intriguing since the first observations [92].

However, this discrepancy is not isolated in the literature; indeed, such discrepancies between inhibitory capacities and apparent affinities have been reported in several systems, particularly regarding insulin-regulated aminiopeptidase (IRAP), which turned out to be the angiotensin AT_4 receptor [151]. This finding is important and will help understand those discrepancies. Finally, a large body of evidence, including those particular observations, strongly suggests that inhibiting QR2 is not synonymous with toxicity, and that only very high concentrations of melatonin (*e.g.*, so-called "pharmacological concentrations", such as 100 μM and beyond) may inhibit QR2 activity.

Acknowledgment

Many people have been working on this subject for the last fourteen years. Chronologically, the main contributors were: Dr. Emmanuel Canet, Dr. Béatrice Guadiola-Lemaître, Dr. Philippe Delagrange, Dr. Pierre Renard, Dr. Pascal Paul, Dr. Olivier Nosjean, Dr. Gilles Ferry, Dr. Fanny Vella, Dr. François Mailliet, Dr. Florence Chatelain-Egger, Carine Saunier, Prof. Andrew Mesecar, Dr. Barbara Calamini, Dr. Scott Pegan, Prof. Françoise Nepveu, Dr. Karine Reybier, Prof. Rémi Quirion, Charles-Etienne Benoit, Dr. Bernard Marchand, Johann Stojko, Dr. Philippe Beauverger, Dr. Pascale Chomarat, Dr. Philippe Hennig, Dr. Sophie Bertin, Dr. Pierre-Hervé Lambert, Christine Ouvry, Dr. Francis Cogé, Sophie-Pénélope Guenin, Sabrina Hecht, Dr. Ludwig Vincent, Dr. Michael Spedding, Estelle Marcheteau, Sophie Coumailleau, Dr. Mathias Antoine, Sylvie Berger, and Natacha Moulharat.

References

[1] Arendt J. Melatonin. *Clin. Endocrinol.,* (Oxf), 1988,29:205-229.

[2] Reiter R. J. The pineal and its hormones in the control of reproduction in mammals. *Endocr. Rev.,* 1980,1:109-131.

[3] Ginter E, Simko V. Brown fat tissue - a potential target to combat obesity. *Bratisl. Lek. Listy*, 2012,113:52-56.

[4] Cutolo M, Buttgereit F, Straub R. H. Regulation of glucocorticoids by the central nervous system. *Clin. Exp. Rheumatol.*, 2011,29:S-22.

[5] Brigo F, Del F. A. Melatonin as add-on treatment for epilepsy. *Cochrane Database Syst. Rev.*, 2012,6:CD006967.

[6] Anderson G, Maes M. Melatonin: an overlooked factor in schizophrenia and in the inhibition of anti-psychotic side effects. *Metab. Brain Dis.,* 2012,27:113-119.

[7] Bagnaresi P, Nakabashi M, Thomas A. P, Reiter R. J, Garcia C. R. The role of melatonin in parasite biology. *Mol. Biochem. Parasitol.*, 2012, 181: 1-6.

[8] Blasiak J, Kasznicki J, Drzewoski J, Pawlowska E, Szczepanska J, Reiter R. J. Perspectives on the use of melatonin to reduce cytotoxic and genotoxic effects of methacrylate-based dental materials. *J. Pineal Res.,* 2011, 51: 157-162.

[9] Boga J. A, Coto-Montes A, Rosales-Corral SA, Tan D. X, Reiter R. J. Beneficial actions of melatonin in the management of viral infections: a new use for this "molecular handyman"? *Rev. Med. Virol.*, 2012.

[10] Bubenik G. A, Konturek S. J. Melatonin and aging: prospects for human treatment. *J. Physiol. Pharmacol.*, 2011,62:13-19.

[11] Cardinali D. P, Cano P, Jimenez-Ortega V, Esquifino A. I. Melatonin and the metabolic syndrome: physiopathologic and therapeutical implications. *Neuroendocrinology*, 2011,93:133-142.

[12] Carpentieri A, Diaz de B. G, Areco V, Peralta L. M, Tolosa de T. N. New perspectives in melatonin uses. *Pharmacol. Res.,* 2012,65:437-444.

[13] Desotelle J. A, Wilking M. J, Ahmad N. The Circadian Control of Skin and Cutaneous Photodamage(dagger). *Photochem. Photobiol.*, 2012.

[14] Escames G, Ozturk G, Bano-Otalora B, Pozo M. J, Madrid J. A, Reiter R. J, Serrano E, Concepcion M, Acuna-Castroviejo D. Exercise and melatonin in humans: reciprocal benefits. *J. Pineal Res.*, 2012,52:1-11.

[15] Greene M. W. Circadian rhythms and tumor growth. *Cancer Lett.,* 2012,318:115-123.

[16] Mozaffari S, Abdollahi M. Melatonin, a promising supplement in inflammatory bowel disease: a comprehensive review of evidences. *Curr. Pharm. Des.*, 2011,17:4372-4378.

[17] Nduhirabandi F, du Toit E. F, Lochner A. Melatonin and the metabolic syndrome: a tool for effective therapy in obesity-associated abnormalities? *Acta Physiol.* (Oxf), 2012,205:209-223.

[18] Reiter R. J, Tan D. X, Korkmaz A, Ma S. Obesity and metabolic syndrome: Association with chronodisruption, sleep deprivation, and melatonin suppression. *Ann. Med.*, 2011.

[19] Russcher M, Koch B, Nagtegaal E, van der Putten K, Ter W. P, Gaillard C. The role of melatonin treatment in chronic kidney disease. *Front Biosci.,* 2012,17:2644-2656.

[20] Santos C. M. New agents promote neuroprotection in Parkinson's disease models. *CNS Neurol. Disord. Drug Targets,* 2012,11:410-418.

[21] Srinivasan V, Pandi-Perumal S. R, Brzezinski A, Bhatnagar K. P, Cardinali D. P. Melatonin, immune function and cancer. *Recent Pat. Endocr. Metab. Immune Drug Discov.*, 2011,5:109-123.

[22] Turgut M, Kaplan S. Effects of melatonin on peripheral nerve regeneration. *Recent Pat. Endocr. Metab. Immune Drug Discov.,* 2011,5:100-108.

[23] Wang Y. M, Jin B. Z, Ai F, Duan CH, Lu Y. Z, Dong T. F, Fu Q. L. The efficacy and safety of melatonin in concurrent chemotherapy or radiotherapy for solid tumors: a meta-analysis of randomized controlled trials. *Cancer Chemother. Pharmacol.*, 2012,69:1213-1220.

[24] Jockers R, Maurice P, Boutin J. A, Delagrange P. Melatonin receptors, heterodimerization, signal transduction and binding sites: what's new? *Br. J. Pharmacol.*, 2008,154:1182-1195.

[25] Reppert S. M. Melatonin receptors: molecular biology of a new family of G protein-coupled receptors. *J. Biol. Rhythms*, 1997,12:528-531.

[26] Zlotos D. P. Recent Progress in the Development of Agonists and Antagonists for Melatonin Receptors. *Curr. Med. Chem.*, 2012.

[27] Boutin J. A, Audinot V, Ferry G, Delagrange P. Molecular tools to study melatonin pathways and actions. *Trends Pharmacol. Sci.,* 2005,26:412-419.

[28] Cohen M, Roselle D, Chabner B, Schmidt T. J, Lippman M. Evidence for a cytoplasmic melatonin receptor. *Nature,* 1978,274:894-895.

[29] Niles L. P, Wong Y. W, Mishra R. K, Brown G. M. Melatonin receptors in brain. *Eur. J. Pharmacol.,* 1979,55:219-220.

[30] Cardinali D. P, Vacas M. I, Boyer E. E. Specific binding of melatonin in bovine brain. *Endocrinology*, 1979,105:437-441.

[31] Vacas M. I, Cardinali D. P. Diurnal changes in melatonin binding sites of hamster and rat brains. Correlations with neuroendocrine responsiveness to melatonin. *Neurosci. Lett.,* 1979,15:259-263.

[32] Duncan M. J, Takahashi JS, Dubocovich M. L. Characterization of 2-[125I]iodomelatonin binding sites in hamster brain. *Eur. J. Pharmacol.*, 1986,132:333-334.

[33] Pickering D. S, Niles L. P. 2-[125I]iodomelatonin binding sites in hamster and chick exhibit differential sensitivity to prazosin. *J. Pharm. Pharmacol.,* 1989,41:356-357.

[34] Dubocovich M. L, Takahashi J. S. Use of 2-[125I]iodomelatonin to characterize melatonin binding sites in chicken retina. *Proc. Natl. Acad. Sci. U S A,* 1987,84:3916-3920.

[35] Dubocovich M. L. Pharmacology and function of melatonin receptors. *FASEB J.*, 1988,2:2765-2773.

[36] Kennaway D. J, Hugel H. M. Melatonin binding sites: are they receptors? *Mol. Cell Endocrinol.*, 1992,88:C1-C9.

[37] Reppert S. M, Weaver D. R, Ebisawa T. Cloning and characterization of a mammalian melatonin receptor that mediates reproductive and circadian responses. *Neuron,* 1994,13:1177-1185.

[38] Reppert S. M, Godson C, Mahle C. D, Weaver D. R, Slaugenhaupt S. A, Gusella J. F. Molecular characterization of a second melatonin receptor expressed in human retina and brain: the Mel1b melatonin receptor. *Proc. Natl. Acad. Sci. U S A,* 1995,92:8734-8738.

[39] Laudon M, Zisapel N. Characterization of central melatonin receptors using 125I-melatonin. *FEBS Lett.,* 1986,197:9-12.

[40] Niles L. P, Pickering D. S, Sayer B. G. HPLC-purified 2-[125I] iodomelatonin labels multiple binding sites in hamster brain. *Biochem. Biophys. Res. Commun.,* 1987, 147:949-956.

[41] Weaver D. R, Namboodiri M. A, Reppert S. M. Iodinated melatonin mimics melatonin action and reveals discrete binding sites in fetal brain. *FEBS Lett.,* 1988,228:123-127.

[42] Vakkuri O, Lamsa E, Rahkamaa E, Ruotsalainen H, Leppaluoto J. Iodinated melatonin: preparation and characterization of the molecular structure by mass and 1H NMR spectroscopy. *Anal. Biochem.,* 1984,142:284-289.

[43] Vakkuri O, Leppaluoto J, Vuolteenaho O. Development and validation of a melatonin radioimmunoassay using radioiodinated melatonin as tracer. *Acta Endocrinol. (Copenh),* 1984,106:152-157.

[44] Roca A. L, Godson C, Weaver D. R, Reppert S. M. Structure, characterization, and expression of the gene encoding the mouse Mel1a melatonin receptor. *Endocrinology,* 1996,137:3469-3477.

[45] Audinot V, Mailliet F, Lahaye-Brasseur C, Bonnaud A, Le GA, Amosse C, Dromaint S, Rodriguez M, Nagel N, Galizzi J. P, Malpaux B, Guillaumet G, Lesieur D, Lefoulon F, Renard P, Delagrange P, Boutin J. A. New selective ligands of human cloned melatonin MT1 and MT2 receptors. *Naunyn. Schmiedebergs Arch. Pharmacol.,* 2003, 367: 553-561.

[46] Mailliet F, Audinot V, Malpaux B, Bonnaud A, Delagrange P, Migaud M, Barrett P, Viaud-Massuard M. C, Lesieur D, Lefoulon F, Renard P, Boutin J. A. Molecular pharmacology of the ovine melatonin receptor: comparison with recombinant human MT1 and MT2 receptors. *Biochem. Pharmacol*., 2004,67:667-677.

[47] Coge F, Guenin S. P, Fery I, Migaud M, Devavry S, Slugocki C, Legros C, Ouvry C, Cohen W, Renault N, Nosjean O, Malpaux B, Delagrange P, Boutin J. A. The end of a myth: cloning and characterization of the ovine melatonin MT(2) receptor. *Br. J. Pharmacol.,* 2009, 158: 1248-1262.

[48] Weaver D. R, Liu C, Reppert S. M. Nature's knockout: the Mel1b receptor is not necessary for reproductive and circadian responses to melatonin in Siberian hamsters. *Mol. Endocrinol*., 1996, 10:1478-1487.

[49] Audinot V, Bonnaud A, Grandcolas L, Rodriguez M, Nagel N, Galizzi J. P, Balik A, Messager S, Hazlerigg D. G, Barrett P, Delagrange P, Boutin J. A. Molecular cloning and pharmacological characterization of rat melatonin MT1 and MT2 receptors. *Biochem. Pharmacol.,* 2008, 75: 2007-2019.

[50] Duncan M. J, Takahashi J. S, Dubocovich M. L. Characteristics and autoradiographic localization of 2-[125I]iodomelatonin binding sites in Djungarian hamster brain. *Endocrinology,* 1989,125:1011-1018.

[51] Williams L. M. Melatonin-binding sites in the rat brain and pituitary mapped by in-vitro autoradiography. J Mol Endocrinol, 1989,3:71-75.

[52] Pickering D. S, Niles L. P. Pharmacological characterization of melatonin binding sites in Syrian hamster hypothalamus. *Eur. J. Pharmacol*., 1990,175:71-77.

[53] Pickering D. S, Niles L. P. Pharmacological characterization of melatonin binding sites in Syrian hamster hypothalamus. *Eur. J. Pharmacol.,* 1990, 175: 71-77.

[54] Anis Y, Zisapel N. Affinity labeling of melatonin binding sites in the hamster brain. *Biochem. Biophys. Res. Commun.,* 1991, 178: 1147-1152.

[55] Laudon M, Zisapel N. Melatonin binding proteins identified in the rat brain by affinity labeling. *FEBS Lett.,* 1991,288:105-108.

[56] Acuna-Castroviejo D, Reiter R. J, Menendez-Pelaez A, Pablos M. I, Burgos A. Characterization of high-affinity melatonin binding sites in purified cell nuclei of rat liver. *J. Pineal. Res.,* 1994, 16:100-112.

[57] Becker-Andre M, Wiesenberg I, Schaeren-Wiemers N, Andre E, Missbach M, Saurat J. H, Carlberg C. Pineal gland hormone melatonin binds and activates an orphan of the nuclear receptor superfamily. *J. Biol. Chem.,* 1994,269:28531-28534.

[58] Reiter R. J, Oh CS, Fujimori O. Melatonin Its intracellular and genomic actions. *Trends Endocrinol. Metab.,* 1996,7:22-27.

[59] Slominski R. M, Reiter R. J, Schlabritz-Loutsevitch N, Ostrom R. S, Slominski A. T. Melatonin membrane receptors in peripheral tissues: distribution and functions. *Mol. Cell Endocrinol.,* 2012, 351: 152-166.

[60] Reppert S. M, Weaver D. R, Cassone V. M, Godson C, Kolakowski L. F, Jr. Melatonin receptors are for the birds: molecular analysis of two receptor subtypes differentially expressed in chick brain. *Neuron,* 1995,15:1003-1015.

[61] Dufourny L, Levasseur A, Migaud M, Callebaut I, Pontarotti P, Malpaux B, Monget P. GPR50 is the mammalian ortholog of Mel1c: evidence of rapid evolution in mammals. *BMC Evol. Biol.,* 2008,8:105.

[62] Reppert S. M, Weaver D. R, Ebisawa T, Mahle C. D, Kolakowski L. F, Jr. Cloning of a melatonin-related receptor from human pituitary. *FEBS Lett.,* 1996,386:219-224.

[63] Duncan M. J, Takahashi J. S, Dubocovich M. L. Characteristics and autoradiographic localization of 2-[125I]iodomelatonin binding sites in Djungarian hamster brain. *Endocrinology,* 1989,125:1011-1018.

[64] Dubocovich M. L. Melatonin receptors: are there multiple subtypes? *Trends Pharmacol. Sci.,* 1995,16:50-56.

[65] Vincent L, Cohen W, Delagrange P, Boutin J. A, Nosjean O. Molecular and cellular pharmacological properties of 5-methoxycarbonylamino-N-acetyltryptamine (MCA-NAT): a nonspecific MT3 ligand. *J. Pineal. Res.,* 2010,48:222-229.

[66] Paul P, Lahaye C, Delagrange P, Nicolas J. P, Canet E, Boutin J. A. Characterization of 2-[125I]iodomelatonin binding sites in Syrian hamster peripheral organs. *J. Pharmacol. Exp. Ther.,* 1999,290:334-340.

[67] Duncan M. J, Takahashi J. S, Dubocovich M. L. 2-[125I]iodomelatonin binding sites in hamster brain membranes: pharmacological characteristics and regional distribution. *Endocrinology,* 1988, 122: 1825-1833.

[68] Nosjean O, Nicolas J. P, Klupsch F, Delagrange P, Canet E, Boutin J. A. Comparative pharmacological studies of melatonin receptors: MT1, MT2 and MT3/QR2. Tissue distribution of MT3/QR2. *Biochem. Pharmacol.,* 2001,61:1369-1379.

[69] Kennaway D. J, Hugel H. M, Rowe S. A. Characterization of the chicken brain melatonin-binding protein using iodinated and tritiated ligands. *J. Pineal Res.,* 1994,17:137-148.

[70] Molinari E. J, North P. C, Dubocovich M. L. 2-[125I]iodo-5-methoxycarbonylamino-N-acetyltryptamine: a selective radioligand for the characterization of melatonin ML2 binding sites. *Eur. J. Pharmacol.,* 1996, 301: 159-168.

[71] Pickering D. S, Niles L. P, Jung C. Y. Molecular mass of the melatonin receptor in hamster hypothalamus and chicken retina. *Neuroscience Res. Comm.,* 1990,6:11-18.
[72] Kennaway D. J, Hugel H. M, Rowe S. A. Characterization of the chicken brain melatonin-binding protein using iodinated and tritiated ligands. *J. Pineal Res.,* 1994,17:137-148.
[73] Nosjean O, Ferro M, Coge F, Beauverger P, Henlin JM, Lefoulon F, Fauchere J. L, Delagrange P, Canet E, Boutin J. A. Identification of the melatonin-binding site MT3 as the quinone reductase 2. *J. Biol. Chem.,* 2000, 275:31311-31317.
[74] Vella F, Ferry G, Delagrange P, Boutin J. A. NRH:quinone reductase 2: an enzyme of surprises and mysteries. *Biochem. Pharmacol.,* 2005, 71:1-12.
[75] Liao S, Williams-Ashman H. G. Enzymatic oxidation of some non-phosphorylated derivatives of dihydronicotinamide. *Biochem. Biophys. Res. Commun.,* 1961,4:208-213.
[76] Liao S, Dulaney J. T, Williams-Ashman H. G. Purification and properties of a flavoprotein catalyzing the oxidation of reduced ribosyl nicotinamide. *J. Biol. Chem.,* 1962, 237:2981-2987.
[77] Jaiswal A. K, Burnett P, Adesnik M, McBride O. W. Nucleotide and deduced amino acid sequence of a human cDNA (NQO2) corresponding to a second member of the NAD(P)H:quinone oxidoreductase gene family. Extensive polymorphism at the NQO2 gene locus on chromosome 6. *Biochemistry,* 1990, 29:1899-1906.
[78] Zhao Q, Yang X. L, Holtzclaw W. D, Talalay P. Unexpected genetic and structural relationships of a long-forgotten flavoenzyme to NAD(P)H:quinone reductase (DT-diaphorase). *Proc. Natl. Acad. Sci. U S A,* 1997,94:1669-1674.
[79] Foster C. E, Bianchet M. A, Talalay P, Zhao Q, Amzel L. M. Crystal structure of human quinone reductase type 2, a metalloflavoprotein. *Biochemistry,* 1999,38:9881-9886.
[80] Fu Y, Buryanovskyy L, Zhang Z. Crystal structure of quinone reductase 2 in complex with cancer prodrug CB1954. *Biochem. Biophys. Res. Commun.,* 2005,336:332-338.
[81] Buryanovskyy L, Fu Y, Boyd M, Ma Y, Hsieh T. C, Wu J. M, Zhang Z. Crystal structure of quinone reductase 2 in complex with resveratrol. *Biochemistry,* 2004,43:11417-11426.
[82] Calamini B, Santarsiero B. D, Boutin J. A, Mesecar A. D. Kinetic, thermodynamic and X-ray structural insights into the interaction of melatonin and analogues with quinone reductase 2. *Biochem. J.,* 2008,413:81-91.
[83] Pegan S. D, Sturdy M, Ferry G, Delagrange P, Boutin J. A, Mesecar A. D. X-ray structural studies of quinone reductase 2 nanomolar range inhibitors. *Protein Sci.,* 2011,20:1182-1195.
[84] Kwiek J. J, Haystead T. A, Rudolph J. Kinetic mechanism of quinone oxidoreductase 2 and its inhibition by the antimalarial quinolines. *Biochemistry,* 2004,43:4538-4547.
[85] Antoine M, Marcheteau E, Delagrange P, Ferry G, Boutin J. A. Characterization of cofactors, substrates and inhibitor binding to flavoenzyme quinone reductase 2 by automated supramolecular nano-electroSpray ionization mass spectrometry. *Int. J. Mass Spec.,* 2012, 312: 87-96.
[86] Boutin J. A, Chatelain-Egger F, Vella F, Delagrange P, Ferry G. Quinone reductase 2 substrate specificity and inhibition pharmacology. *Chem. Biol. Interact,* 2005,151:213-228.

[87] Ferry G, Hecht S, Berger S, Moulharat N, Coge F, Guillaumet G, Leclerc V, Yous S, Delagrange P, Boutin J. A. Old and new inhibitors of quinone reductase 2. *Chem. Biol. Interact*, 2010,186:103-109.

[88] Knox R. J, Jenkins T. C, Hobbs S. M, Chen S, Melton R. G, Burke P. J. Bioactivation of 5-(aziridin-1-yl)-2,4-dinitrobenzamide (CB 1954) by human NAD(P)H quinone oxidoreductase 2: a novel co-substrate-mediated antitumor prodrug therapy. *Cancer Res.,* 2000,60:4179-4186.

[89] Gong X, Kole L, Iskander K, Jaiswal AK. NRH:quinone oxidoreductase 2 and NAD(P)H:quinone oxidoreductase 1 protect tumor suppressor p53 against 20s proteasomal degradation leading to stabilization and activation of p53. *Cancer Res.,* 2007, 67:5380-5388.

[90] Wang W, Jaiswal A. K. Nuclear factor Nrf2 and antioxidant response element regulate NRH:quinone oxidoreductase 2 (NQO2) gene expression and antioxidant induction. *Free Radic. Biol. Med.,* 2006, 40: 1119-1130.

[91] Mailliet F, Ferry G, Vella F, Thiam K, Delagrange P, Boutin J. A. Organs from mice deleted for NRH:quinone oxidoreductase 2 are deprived of the melatonin binding site MT3. *FEBS Lett.,* 2004, 578:116-120.

[92] Mailliet F, Ferry G, Vella F, Berger S, Coge F, Chomarat P, Mallet C, Guenin S. P, Guillaumet G, Viaud-Massuard M. C, Yous S, Delagrange P, Boutin JA. Characterization of the melatoninergic MT3 binding site on the NRH:quinone oxidoreductase 2 enzyme. *Biochem. Pharmacol.,* 2005, 71:74-88.

[93] Boussard M. F, Truche S, Rousseau-Rojas A, Briss S, Descamps S, Droual M, Wierzbicki M, Ferry G, Audinot V, Delagrange P, Boutin J. A. New ligands at the melatonin binding site MT(3). *Eur. J. Med. Chem.,* 2006, 41:306-320.

[94] Dubocovich M. L. Pharmacology and function of melatonin receptors. *FASEB J.,* 1988, 2:2765-2773.

[95] Boutin J. A. Myristoylation. *Cell Signal,* 1997, 9:15-35.

[96] Degli Esposti M., Ferry G, Masdehors P, Boutin JA, Hickman J. A, Dive C. Post-translational modification of Bid has differential effects on its susceptibility to cleavage by caspase 8 or caspase 3. *J. Biol. Chem.,* 2003, 278:15749-15757.

[97] Wang Z, Chen Y, Labinskyy N, Hsieh T. C, Ungvari Z, Wu J. M. Regulation of proliferation and gene expression in cultured human aortic smooth muscle cells by resveratrol and standardized grape extracts. *Biochem. Biophys. Res. Commun.,* 2006,346:367-376.

[98] Graves P. R, Kwiek J. J, Fadden P, Ray R, Hardeman K, Coley A. M, Foley M, Haystead TA. Discovery of novel targets of quinoline drugs in the human purine binding proteome. *Mol. Pharmacol.*, 2002,62:1364-1372.

[99] Michaelis S, Marais A, Schrey A. K, Graebner O. Y, Schaudt C, Sefkow M, Kroll F, Dreger M, Glinski M, Koester H, Metternich R, Fischer J. J. Dabigatran and dabigatran ethyl ester: potent inhibitors of ribosyldihydronicotinamide dehydrogenase (NQO2). *J. Med. Chem.,* 2012, 55:3934-3944.

[100] Jansen J. M, Copinga S, Gruppen G, Molinari E. J, Dubocovich M. L, Grol C. J. The high affinity melationin binding site probed with conformationally restricted ligand--I. Pharmacophore and minireceptor models. *Bioorg. Med. Chem.,* 1996,4:1321-1332.

[101] Leclerc V, Ettaoussi M, Rami M, Farce A, Boutin J. A, Delagrange P, Caignard D. H, Renard P, Berthelot P, Yous S. Design and synthesis of naphthalenic derivatives as new ligands at the melatonin binding site MT3. *Eur. J. Med. Chem.,* 2011,46:1622-1629.

[102] Ettaoussi M, Peres B, Klupsch F, Delagrange P, Boutin J. A, Renard P, Caignard D. H, Chavatte P, Berthelot P, Lesieur D, Yous S. Design and synthesis of benzofuranic derivatives as new ligands at the melatonin-binding site MT3. *Bioorg. Med. Chem.,* 2008,16:4954-4962.

[103] Du H, Wang J, Zhang X, Hu Z. A novel quantitative structure-activity relationship method to predict the affinities of MT3 melatonin binding site. *Eur. J. Med. Chem.,* 2008, 43:2861-2869.

[104] Hu Y, Ho M. K, Chan K. H, New D. C, Wong Y. H. Synthesis of substituted N-[3-(3-methoxyphenyl)propyl] amides as highly potent MT(2)-selective melatonin ligands. *Bioorg. Med. Chem. Lett.,* 2010, 20:2582-2585.

[105] Farce A, Dilly S, Sabaouinin A, Yous S, Berthelot P, Boutin J. A, Delagrange P, Renard P, Chavatte P. Three-dimensional quantitative structure-activity relationship of MT3 melatonin binding site ligands: a comparative molecular field analysis. *QSAR and combin. Sci.,* 2007, 26: 820-827.

[106] Ludwig C, Michiels P. J, Wu X, Kavanagh K. L, Pilka E, Jansson A, Oppermann U, Gunther UL. SALMON: solvent accessibility, ligand binding, and mapping of ligand orientation by NMR spectroscopy. *J. Med. Chem.*, 2008, 51:1-3.

[107] Nolan K. A, Caraher M. C, Humphries M. P, Bettley H. A, Bryce R. A, Stratford I. J. In silico identification and biochemical evaluation of novel inhibitors of NRH:quinone oxidoreductase 2 (NQO2). *Bioorg. Med. Chem. Lett.*, 2010,20:7331-7336.

[108] Nolan K. A, Humphries M. P, Barnes J, Doncaster J. R, Caraher M. C, Tirelli N, Bryce R. A, Whitehead R. C, Stratford I. J. Triazoloacridin-6-ones as novel inhibitors of the quinone oxidoreductases NQO1 and NQO2. *Bioorg. Med. Chem.,* 2010,18:696-706.

[109] Nolan K. A, Humphries M. P, Bryce R. A, Stratford I. J. Imidazoacridin-6-ones as novel inhibitors of the quinone oxidoreductase NQO2. *Bioorg. Med. Chem. Lett.,* 2010,20:2832-2836.

[110] Maiti A, Reddy P. V, Sturdy M, Marler L, Pegan S. D, Mesecar A. D, Pezzuto J. M, Cushman M. Synthesis of casimiroin and optimization of its quinone reductase 2 and aromatase inhibitory activities. *J. Med. Chem.,* 2009, 52:1873-1884.

[111] Wang M, Gao M, Miller K. D, Sledge G. W, Hutchins G. D, Zheng Q. H. Synthesis of carbon-11-labeled casimiroin analogues as new potential PET agents for imaging of quinone reductase 2 and aromatase expression in breast cancer. *Steroids,* 2010,75:967-973.

[112] Sun B, Hoshino J, Jermihov K, Marler L, Pezzuto J. M, Mesecar A. D, Cushman M. Design, synthesis, and biological evaluation of resveratrol analogues as aromatase and quinone reductase 2 inhibitors for chemoprevention of cancer. *Bioorg. Med. Chem.,* 2010,18:5352-5366.

[113] Dufour M, Yan C, Siegel D, Colucci M. A, Jenner M, Oldham N. J, Gomez J, Reigan P, Li Y, De Matteis CI, Ross D, Moody C. J. Mechanism-based inhibition of quinone reductase 2 (NQO2): selectivity for NQO2 over NQO1 and structural basis for flavoprotein inhibition. *Chembiochem.,* 2011, 12:1203-1208.

[114] Conda-Sheridan M, Marler L, Park E. J, Kondratyuk T. P, Jermihov K, Mesecar A. D, Pezzuto J. M, Asolkar R. N, Fenical W, Cushman M. Potential chemopreventive agents based on the structure of the lead compound 2-bromo-1-hydroxyphenazine, isolated from Streptomyces species, strain CNS284. *J. Med. Chem.,* 2010,53:8688-8699.

[115] Yan C, Dufour M, Siegel D, Reigan P, Gomez J, Shieh B, Moody C. J, Ross D. Indolequinone inhibitors of NRH:quinone oxidoreductase 2. Characterization of the mechanism of inhibition in both cell-free and cellular systems. *Biochemistry,* 2011,50:6678-6688.

[116] Benoit CE, Bastianetto S, Brouillette J, Tse Y, Boutin J. A, Delagrange P, Wong T, Sarret P, Quirion R. Loss of quinone reductase 2 function selectively facilitates learning behaviors. *J. Neurosci.,* 2010, 30:12690-12700.

[117] Janda E, Parafati M, Aprigliano S, Carresi C, Visalli V, Sacco I, Ventrice D, Mega T, Vadala N, Rinaldi S, Musolino V, Palma E, Gratteri S, Rotiroti D, Mollace V. The antidote effect of Quinone Oxidoreductase 2 (QR2) inhibitor on paraquat-induced toxicity in vitro and in vivo. *Br. J. Pharmacol.,* 2012.

[118] Popova J. S, Dubocovich M. L. Melatonin receptor-mediated stimulation of phosphoinositide breakdown in chick brain slices. *J. Neurochem.,* 1995, 64:130-138.

[119] Eison A. S, Mullins U. L. Melatonin binding sites are functionally coupled to phosphoinositide hydrolysis in Syrian hamster RPMI 1846 melanoma cells. *Life Sci.,* 1993,53:L393-L398.

[120] Lotufo C. M, Lopes C, Dubocovich M. L, Farsky S. H, Markus R. P. Melatonin and N-acetylserotonin inhibit leukocyte rolling and adhesion to rat microcirculation. *Eur. J. Pharmacol.,* 2001, 430:351-357.

[121] Lagneux C, Joyeux M, Demenge P, Ribuot C, Godin-Ribuot D. Protective effects of melatonin against ischemia-reperfusion injury in the isolated rat heart. *Life Sci.,* 2000,66:503-509.

[122] Oxenkrug G. F, Bachurin S. O, Prakhie I. V, Zefirov N. S. Quinone reductase 2 and antidepressant effect of melatonin derivatives. *Ann. N Y Acad. Sci.,* 2010, 1199:121-124.

[123] Sampaio L. F. An unexpected effect of 5-MCA-NAT in chick retinal development. *Int. J. Dev. Neurosci.,* 2009, 27:511-515.

[124] Ray M, Mediratta P. K, Mahajan P, Sharma K. K. Evaluation of the role of melatonin in formalin-induced pain response in mice. *Indian J. Med. Sci.,* 2004,58:122-130.

[125] Colligris B, Crooke A, Gasull X, Escribano J, Herrero-Vanrell R, Benitez-Del-Castillo J. M, Garcia-Feijoo J, Pintor J. Recent Patents and Developments in Glaucoma Biomarkers. *Recent Pat. Endocr. Metab. Immune Drug Discov.,* 2012.

[126] Crooke A, Huete-Toral F, Martinez-Aguila A, Colligris B, Pintor J. Ocular disorders and the utility of animal models in the discovery of melatoninergic drugs with therapeutic potential. *Expert Opin. Drug Discov.*, 2012.

[127] Crooke A, Colligris B, Pintor J. Update in glaucoma medicinal chemistry: emerging evidence for the importance of melatonin analogues. *Curr. Med. Chem.,* 2012,19:3508-3522.

[128] Alarma-Estrany P, Pintor J. Melatonin receptors in the eye: location, second messengers and role in ocular physiology. *Pharmacol. Ther.,* 2007, 113:507-522.

[129] Alarma-Estrany P, Crooke A, Peral A, Pintor J. Requirement of intact sympathetic transmission for the ocular hypotensive effects of melatonin and 5-MCA-NAT. *Auton. Neurosci.*, 2007,137:63-66.

[130] Andres-Guerrero V, Alarma-Estrany P, Molina-Martinez I. T, Peral A, Herrero-Vanrell R, Pintor J. Ophthalmic formulations of the intraocular hypotensive melatonin agent 5-MCA-NAT. *Exp. Eye Res.*, 2009,88:504-511.

[131] Pintor J, Martin L, Pelaez T, Hoyle C. H, Peral A. Involvement of melatonin MT(3) receptors in the regulation of intraocular pressure in rabbits. *Eur. J. Pharmacol.*, 2001,416:251-254.

[132] Pintor J, Pelaez T, Hoyle C. H, Peral A. Ocular hypotensive effects of melatonin receptor agonists in the rabbit: further evidence for an MT3 receptor. *Br. J. Pharmacol.*, 2003,138:831-836.

[133] Alarma-Estrany P, Crooke A, Pintor J. 5-MCA-NAT does not act through NQO2 to reduce intraocular pressure in New-Zealand white rabbit. *J. Pineal Res.*, 2009,47:201-209.

[134] Alcantara-Contreras S, Baba K, Tosini G. Removal of melatonin receptor type 1 increases intraocular pressure and retinal ganglion cells death in the mouse. *Neurosci. Lett.*, 2011,494:61-64.

[135] Alarma-Estrany P, Guzman-Aranguez A, Huete F, Peral A, Plourde R, Jr., Pelaez T, Yerxa B, Pintor J. Design of novel melatonin analogs for the reduction of intraocular pressure in normotensive rabbits. *J. Pharmacol. Exp. Ther.*, 2011,337:703-709.

[136] Crooke A, Huete-Toral F, Martinez-Aguila A, Martin-Gil A, Pintor J. Involvement of carbonic anhydrases in the ocular hypotensive effect of melatonin analogue 5-MCA-NAT. *J. Pineal Res.*, 2012,52:265-270.

[137] Chomarat P, Coge F, Guenin S. P, Mailliet F, Vella F, Mallet C, Giraudet S, Nagel N, Leonce S, Ferry G, Delagrange P, Boutin J. A. Cellular knock-down of quinone reductase 2: a laborious road to successful inhibition by RNA interference. *Biochimie*, 2007,89:1264-1275.

[138] Olakowska E, Marcol W, Kotulska K, Lewin-Kowalik J. The role of melatonin in the neurodegenerative diseases. *Bratisl. Lek. Listy.*, 2005, 106: 171-174.

[139] Walker J. E. The NADH:ubiquinone oxidoreductase (complex I) of respiratory chains. *Q. Rev. Biophys.*, 1992,25:253-324.

[140] Jamieson D, Tung A. T, Knox R. J, Boddy A. V. Reduction of mitomycin C is catalysed by human recombinant NRH:quinone oxidoreductase 2 using reduced nicotinamide adenine dinucleotide as an electron donating co-factor. *Br. J. Cancer*, 2006,95:1229-1233.

[141] Rix U, Hantschel O, Durnberger G, Remsing Rix L. L, Planyavsky M, Fernbach N. V, Kaupe I, Bennett K. L, Valent P, Colinge J, Kocher T, Superti-Furga G. Chemical proteomic profiles of the BCR-ABL inhibitors imatinib, nilotinib, and dasatinib reveal novel kinase and nonkinase targets. *Blood*, 2007,110:4055-4063.

[142] Testa B, Kramer S. D. The biochemistry of drug metabolism--an introduction: Part 2. Redox reactions and their enzymes. *Chem. Biodivers.*, 2007,4:257-405.

[143] Rix U, Remsing Rix L. L, Terker A. S, Fernbach N. V, Hantschel O, Planyavsky M, Breitwieser F. P, Herrmann H, Colinge J, Bennett K. L, Augustin M, Till J. H, Heinrich M. C, Valent P, Superti-Furga G. A comprehensive target selectivity survey of the

BCR-ABL kinase inhibitor INNO-406 by kinase profiling and chemical proteomics in chronic myeloid leukemia cells. *Leukemia,* 2010,24:44-50.

[144] Winger J. A, Hantschel O, Superti-Furga G, Kuriyan J. The structure of the leukemia drug imatinib bound to human quinone reductase 2 (NQO2). *BMC Struct. Biol.,* 2009,9:7.

[145] Bantscheff M, Eberhard D, Abraham Y, Bastuck S, Boesche M, Hobson S, Mathieson T, Perrin J, Raida M, Rau C, Reader V, Sweetman G, Bauer A, Bouwmeester T, Hopf C, Kruse U, Neubauer G, Ramsden N, Rick J, Kuster B, Drewes G. Quantitative chemical proteomics reveals mechanisms of action of clinical ABL kinase inhibitors. *Nat. Biotechnol.,* 2007,25:1035-1044.

[146] Pezzuto J. M. Resveratrol as an Inhibitor of Carcinogenesis. *Pharm. Biol.,* 2008, 46:443-573.

[147] Nakata R, Takahashi S, Inoue H. Recent advances in the study on resveratrol. *Biol. Pharm. Bull.,* 2012,35:273-279.

[148] Formentini L, Moroni F, Chiarugi A. Detection and pharmacological modulation of nicotinamide mononucleotide (NMN) in vitro and in vivo. *Biochem. Pharmacol.,* 2009,77:1612-1620.

[149] Grahnert A, Grahnert A, Klein C, Schilling E, Wehrhahn J, Hauschildt S. Review: NAD +: a modulator of immune functions. *Innate Immun.,* 2011, 17:212-233.

[150] Vaisitti T, Audrito V, Serra S, Bologna C, Brusa D, Malavasi F, Deaglio S. NAD+-metabolizing ecto-enzymes shape tumor-host interactions: the chronic lymphocytic leukemia model. *FEBS Lett.,* 2011, 585: 1514-1520.

[151] Lew R. A, Mustafa T, Ye S, McDowall S. G, Chai S. Y, Albiston A. L. Angiotensin AT4 ligands are potent, competitive inhibitors of insulin regulated aminopeptidase (IRAP). *J. Neurochem.,* 2003, 86:344-350.

[152] Vanecek J, Pavlik A, Illnerova H. Hypothalamic melatonin receptor sites revealed by autoradiography. *Brain Res.,* 1987, 435: 359-362.

[153] Anis Y, Nir I, Zisapel N. Diurnal variations in melatonin binding sites in the hamster brain: impact of melatonin. *Mol. Cell. Endocrinol.,* 1989, 67: 121-129.

[154] Song Y, Ayre E. A, Pang S. F. The identification and characterization of 125I-labelled iodomelatonin-binding sites in the duck kidney. *J. Endocrinol.,* 1992,135:353-359.

[155] Wang Z. P, Cheng K. M, Brown G. M, Pang C. S, Pang S. F. Characterization of 2-[125I]iodomelatonin-binding sites in quail testes at mid-light and mid-dark. *Neurosci. Lett.,* 1992,146:195-198.

In: New Developments in Melatonin Research ISBN: 978-1-62618-843-3
Editors: D.Acuña-Castroviejo, I.Rusanova, G.Escames © 2013 Nova Science Publishers, Inc.

Chapter 6

Melatonin and the Metabolic Syndrome

Eleonora S. Pagano, Pablo A. Scacchi Bernasconi, Roxana Reynoso, Pablo Scacchi and Daniel P. Cardinali*

[1]Departamento de Docencia e Investigación, Facultad de Ciencias Médicas,
Pontificia Universidad Católica Argentina,
Buenos Aires, Argentina

Abstract

Circadian disruption and sleep deprivation in contemporary "24/7 Society" lead to the predominance of pro-orexic and proinflammatory mechanisms that contribute to the high prevalence of obesity, diabetes and cardiovascular disease, all constituents of the metabolic syndrome (MS). Besides changes in life style, a successful therapy for MS requires a drug able to antagonize the trigger factors of MS and to correct the disturbed circadian rhythmicity observed in MS. This chapter deals with the analysis of the therapeutic validity of melatonin to fulfill that objective in MS. As an effective chronobiotic agent, melatonin can change the phase and the amplitude of the sleep/wake rhythm. In addition, it has cytoprotective and immunomodulatory properties that can be useful to prevent a number of MS sequelae including obesity, diabetes and cardiovascular disease. Melatonin prevents hyperadiposity in animal models of obesity and there is preliminary information that in low doses (2-5 mg/day) melatonin may curtail MS in humans. More recently, attention has been focused on the development of potent melatonin analogs with prolonged effects (ramelteon, agomelatine, tasimelteon). In clinical trials these analogs were employed in doses considerably higher than those usually employed for melatonin to treat insomnia and other sleep disorders, and as antidepressants. Clinical trials employing melatonin doses in the range of 50-100 mg/day are needed to assess its therapeutic value in MS.

Keywords: Metabolic syndrome; diabetes; obesity; melatonin; circadian rhythms; inflammation; free radicals

---

* E-mail: danielcardinali@fibertel.com.ar.

Introduction

Since the term "Metabolic Syndrome" (MS) was introduced by Gerry Reaven at the 1988 Banting Lecture [1] much attention has been paid on it. A search using the PubMed engine yielded a total number of 40,631 papers by the time this Chapter was written (October 2012). In contrast a concomitant search with the terms "melatonin" and "metabolic syndrome" only yielded 45 significant articles. Therefore our understanding of melatonin´s involvement in the metabolic syndrome has barely begun.

The MS is characterized by the presence of at least three of the following parameters: waist circumference >102 cm in males and >88 cm in females, triglycerides >150 mg/dl plasma, high density lipoproteins (HDL) <40 mg/dl plasma, blood pressure >130/85 mm Hg and fasting glucose >110 mg/dl [2]. MS and its related pathologies (obesity, diabetes and hypertension) constitute a true pandemia: it has 34 % prevalence on the worldwide population over 20 years, increasing with age and body mass index (BMI). Metabolic syndrome´s prevalence varied by race and ethnicity and the pattern is different for males and females.

Obesity and insulin resistance represent a problem of utmost clinical significance. Insulin-resistant states are characterized by the inability of insulin to induce proper signal transduction leading to defective glucose uptake in skeletal muscle tissue and impaired insulin-mediated effects. A high-fat diet, which contributes to insulin resistance, aggravates type 2 diabetes mellitus, stroke, and coronary artery disease and can feed back to influence the biological clock [3].

An obvious cause for the increasing prevalence of MS is the impending food availability while evolution has rather shaped humans for periods of food scarcity. Another important factor is sleep disturbance: evidence shows that we sleep on average 25% less than 40 years ago, with a 30% of adults reporting only 6 slept hours per night [4] a situation that may vary among Countries [5]. Thus, our current life style does no longer provide an environment for which we are adapted to. The increasing sleep debt and poorer sleep quality and a tendency to nocturnality allowed by artificial lighting and modern electronic devices they all define our current lifestyle, which causes the disruption of the sleep/wake cycle and other circadian rhythms [6].

It is thoroughly documented that circadian misalignment, as in the case of shift work, is associated with increased risk for obesity, diabetes and cardiovascular disease, which results from an inadequate adaptation to out of phase two major synchronizers, food and light exposure. Sleeping and eating at abnormal circadian times, chronically set up in shift work, and their consequences, defined the Shiftwork Maladaptation Syndrome [7]. Subjects exposed for 10 days to a laboratory protocol of a "28 h day" showed significant changes in circulating leptin (-17%), glucose (+6%) and insulin (+22%). They also completely reversed the daily cortisol rhythm and showed significantly increased mean arterial pressure (+3%), and reduced sleep efficiency (-20%) [8].

The association between circadian disruption and a higher risk of developing obesity and of type 2 diabetes has been demonstrated in a number of epidemiological studies. For example, in the Nurse Health Study (>70,000 participants), self-reported short (~5 h) and long duration of sleep (6- 9 h) was associated with symptomatic diabetes with a relative risk (odd ratio) of 1.345 for both short and long sleepers even after adjusting for confounding factors like diet or physical activity [9]. Also, in a Swedish study in which more than 2,000 people were followed for over 10 years, a short duration of sleep ($\leq$ 5 h) and difficulty in initiating and maintaining sleep were associated with higher incidence of diabetes in men even after adjusting for confounding factors like age, BMI, snoring, depression and hypertension [10]. In another study over 1000 outpatients, obese patients (BMI: 30-39 kg/m^2) reported a total sleep time per day 16 minutes lower than normal BMI subjects, with greater differences in extremely obese patients (BMI: 40-85 kg/m^2) [11]. Subjects who self-reported $\leq$ 6 h sleep were twice as likely to develop diabetes in the longitudinal Massachusetts Male Aging Study followed for more than 15 years. This elevated risk remained after adjusting for factors like age, waist circumference, smoking and education [12].

Obesity is a state of chronic oxidative stress, a major mechanism underlying the development of co-morbidities [13]. Oxidative stress is associated with several indexes of adiposity and a low antioxidant defense. Because reactive oxygen species (ROS) generation is a continuous and physiological phenomenon, cells possess efficient antioxidant systems that protect them from oxidative damage. These defense systems are thought to prevent free radicals from causing irreparable damage by reacting with lipids, proteins and nucleic acids. Inasmuch as melatonin has been demonstrated to be an effective chronobiotic (substance with the capacity to change the amplitude and timing of the biologic clock) and to have antioxidant [13], cytoprotective and immunomodulatory properties [14], a consideration of its possible role in the etiology of MS is directly relevant not only for providing new insights into the disease, but also for guiding the therapeutic use of melatoninergic agonists in the treatment of MS.

Circadian Organization and Obesity

Mammalian physiology and behavior follow daily variations or oscillations, defined as the circadian cycle (from the Latin "circa diem" about a day). The mammalian circadian timing system is ruled by a central pacemaker or rhythm generator located in the brain's suprachiasmatic nuclei (SCN). It also comprises peripheral oscillators located in almost every cell of the body [15]. A number of factors such as the light/dark cycle, food, ambient temperature and social cues can reset or phase shift the internal clock, and therefore they have been identified as synchronizers (or "Zeitgebers", a German term coined by Jürgen Aschof half-a-century ago) that can actually reset, or phase shift, the internal clock. Depending on when an organism is exposed to such an entraining agent, circadian rhythms can be advanced, delayed, or unshifted at all [15]. The circadian clock prepares individuals for predictable events such as food availability and sleep, and its disruption has strong metabolic consequences.

In an animal study aimed to determine whether nighttime light exposure ("light at night", LAN) had any effect on obesity, the effects of LAN on body mass were examined. Mice exposed to either bright or dim LAN have significantly increased body mass and reduced glucose tolerance related to mice kept in a standard light/dark cycle, even when total diary caloric intake was similar [16]. Dim light-exposed mice consumed 55.5% of their food during the light phase, as compared with 36.5% in controls. Restricting food consumption to the active phase in dim light mice prevented body mass gain. These results indicate that even low levels of LAN may disrupt the feeding timing and other metabolic signals, leading to excess weight gain. The central clock is daily synchronized to the environment by photic cues through the retina and transmitted to SCN neurons. In turn, the SCN influences circadian physiology and behavior via neuronal and humoral pathways, synchronizing local oscillators at their respective organs and tissues. Melatonin, cortisol and body temperature closely follow these daily oscillations. The SCN are not essential to run these periodic tissue changes because circadian clocks are self sustained, meaning that intrinsic oscillations for each cell can proceed with no need of an environmental signal. However, since the period is not exactly 24 h, they need to be daily synchronized to reset the system and prevent it to go out of phase by the SCN, or by food and temperature, if adequately trained, in order to independently run its own physiologic rhythm (see for revision [17]). In the last few years, there has been an intensive research on clock-controlled genes (CCG) in almost every human tissue: lymphocytes, skin, colon, brain tissue and adipose tissue, allowing a better understanding of their functions and regulations regarding the central clock.

The molecular basis for the rhythmicity of central and peripheral clocks is a negative feedback mechanism driven by the interaction of clock genes and their related proteins: *Clock* (circadian locomotor output cycles kaput), *Bmal1* (brain and muscle *Arnt*-like protein-1), *Per* (Period) *1, 2 y 3,* y *Cry* (Cryptochrome) *1 y 2* (see Figure 1).

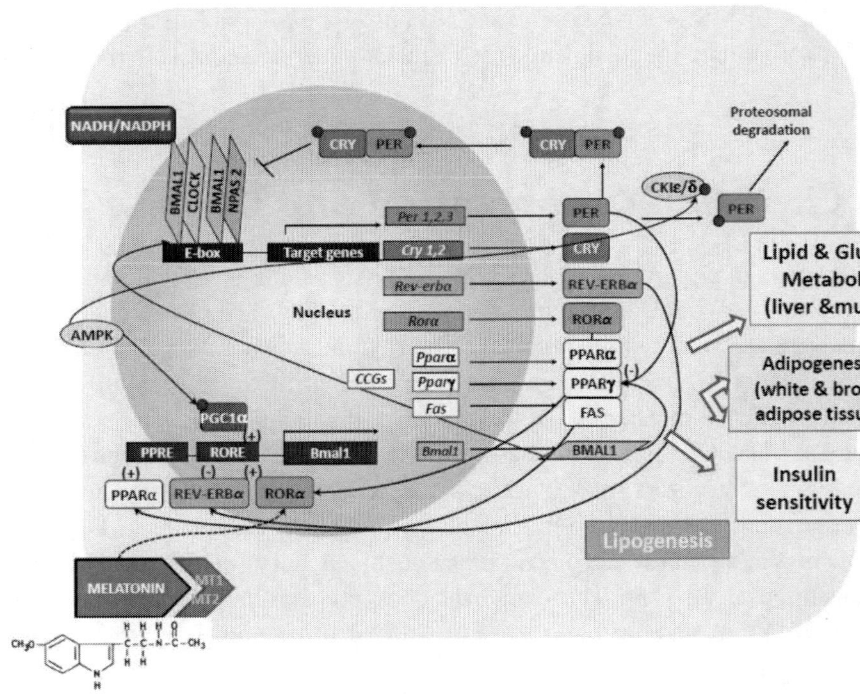

Figure 1. Clock genes, metabolism and obesity. Mammalian circadian clock is a negative feedback circuit of transcriptional and translational regulations. For details see text. PERs and CRYs phosphorylation (red circles) by CKIε/δ, (also regulated by AMPK) and concomitant PERs degradation close the circuit, defining circadian rhythmicity: BMAL1:CLOCK constitute the positive arm of the clock while PER:CRY, represent the negative one. Other genes like Rev-erbα (=NR1D1), Rorα, and particularly, Ppar and Pgc-1α, are involved in Bmal transcription. Some of these genes, Ppar, Fas, etc, are key regulators and/or players in metabolism and adipogenesis, underlining the circadian clock connection to obesity. Melatonin, via receptor and non-receptor mediated mechanisms, may regulate cellular clocks.

The protein heterodimer CLOCK: BMAL1 binds to E-box elements at the promoter region of *Per1, Per2, Per3, Cry1* and *Cry2,* inducing their transcription. Conversely, PER1-3 and CRY1-2 proteins heterodimerize in the cytoplasm and translocate to the nucleus where by interacting with the CLOCK: BMAL1 heterodimer, operate as negative regulators inhibiting their own transcription, thus stopping the cycle. PER phosphorylation by CKIε (casein kinase Iε), and CRY regulation by FBXL3, send them to proteolytic degradation, releasing CLOCK-BMAL1 to start a new cycle [18] (Figure 1). Through CCG and their downstream effectors, peripheral circadian clock components directly regulate many aspects of cell physiology, such as membrane trafficking, detoxification, nutrient metabolism, and the cell cycle [15].

Clock has a histone acetyltransferase intrinsic activity, and the deacetylase sirtuins (SIRT) counteract this function. SIRT are important regulator of aging, inflammation and metabolism. Since many other oscillating peripheral tissues transcripts encode proteins with central roles in the metabolism, it could be postulated a molecular link between energy balance, chromatin remodeling and hence epigenetics, and circadian physiology [17].

There is a large body of evidence that links feeding regimens and food components with the circadian system [19]. A high-fat diet (HFD) that contributes to insulin resistance, impaired glucose metabolism, and obesity, can feedback to influence the biological clock. Data from our Laboratory in a model of HFD obesity exemplify it (Figure 2).

In the adenohypophysis of control rats (fed with a 4% fat diet), *Clock* and *Bmal1* expression and *Per1* and *Per2* expression were in antiphase, *Clock* and *Bmal1* peaking during scotophase.

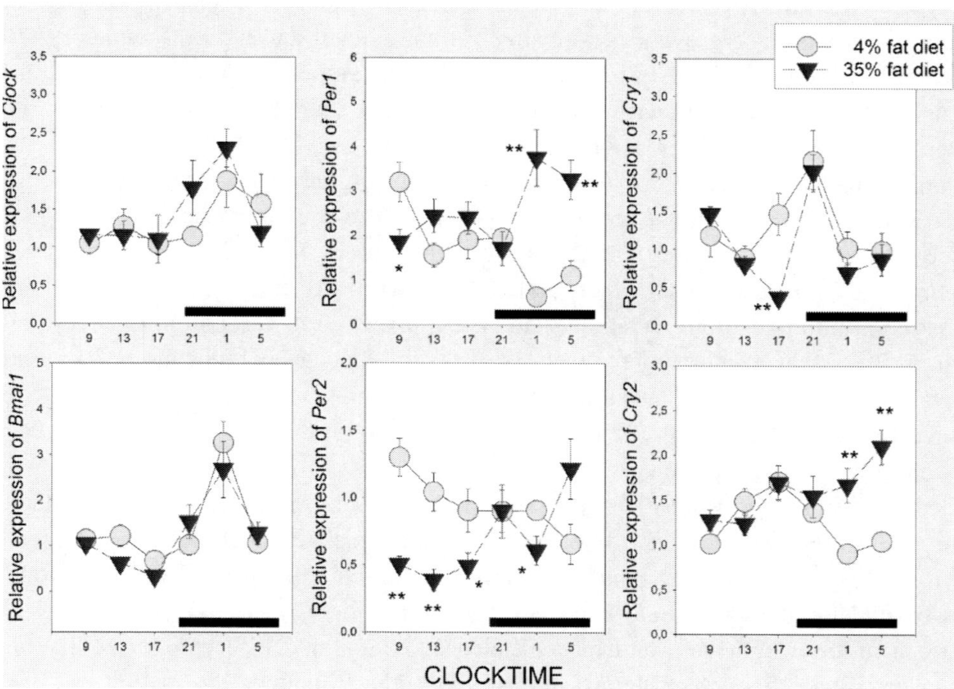

Figure 2. Circadian oscillating expression of clock genes is sensitive to a high fat diet. In this experiment rats were fed a 4% (control) or a 35% fat diet for 11 weeks. Wistar male rats groups (n=6-8) were killed by decapitation at six different time intervals through a 24 h cycle. Adenohypophysis was collected and RNA extracted. Shown are the means ± SEM of mRNA expression by Real Time PCR (**p<0.01, *p< 0.05 when compared to control rats in a Student´s t test) (data redrawn from [3]).

Maximal expression of *Cry1* and *Cry2* showed a phase delay of about 4 h as compared to *Per1-Per2*. Rats on a 35% fat diet exhibited a disrupted 24 h rhythmicity of *Per1*, *Per2*, *Cry1* and *Cry2* expression without affecting the diurnal oscillation of *Clock* or *Bmal*. *Per1* and *Per2* expression profile was almost inverted by the HFD (Figure 2). These results indicate that the inherent transcription, translation, and posttranslational modifications that give the clock its own natural rhythmicity are disrupted in obese rats.

The results of Figure 2 could also explain the reason why the circadian rhythmicity of many metabolism related hormones becomes disrupted during the MS and obesity development. A significant disruption on the rhythmicity of circulating prolactin, LH, TSH, testosterone, corticosterone, insulin, leptin, ghrelin, adiponectin, tumor necrosis factor- α (TNF-α), interleukin-1 and -6, and monocyte chemoattractant protein-1 could be identified in rats fed a 35% fat diet [20-22].

A decrease in amplitude of the 24 h rhythm in pineal melatonin content was also observed [20], underlining the significant effects that obesity has on circadian organization.

Melatonin Use in Experimental Models of MS/Obesity

Melatonin is a thoroughly conserved molecule present from unicells to higher vertebrates [23]. It affects a variety of functions such as sleep, seasonal reproduction, immunomodulation and circadian rhythmicity. In addition, when exogenously provided at pharmacological doses, melatonin inhibits tumor growth, presumably via antioxidant and anti-inflammatory effects, and acts as a chronobiotic, restoring the phase and the amplitude of circadian rhythmicity [23]. A number of studies indicate that melatonin has the ability to reduce obesity, type 2 diabetes, liver steatosis, hypertension and other features of MS [24,25]. Regarding glucose metabolism, melatonin treatment ameliorates the hyperglucemia in type 1 diabetic rats because it induces regeneration/ proliferation of β cells in the pancreas [26]. Pinealectomy, and the consequent circulating melatonin loss, results in marked hyperinsulinemia and triglyceride accumulation in the liver [27]. In line with this finding, long-term melatonin administration improves lipid metabolism in type 2 diabetic rats through normalizing insulin resistance [28]. Melatonin treatment ameliorates several diabetes complications, including the cardiovascular ones [29,30]: melatonin prevents experimental induced arrhythmias in the isolated rat heart [31] and it shows a cytoprotective effect at the early phase of a myocardial infarction [32].

Clearly, it is regarding to obesity where melatonin´s benefits can be of importance. A number of studies were addressed to assess whether melatonin could effectively reduce adiposity in obese rats. In a rat model of obesity, in which animals were fed with a HFD, 3 weeks of melatonin treatment (30 mg/kg) 1 h before lights out, induced almost a 50% decrease in body weight gain and feed efficiency. Although ineffective to modify plasma leptin, melatonin decreased circulating glucose and triglyceride levels [33].

Endogenous melatonin levels decrease with age, both in humans as in rats. Melatonin supplementation of middle-aged rats decreased body weight, visceral fat, plasma leptin and insulin to more youthful levels [34]. Middle-aged (10-month-old) rats fed on a liquid diet with high fat content achieved an 8% weight gain after 3 weeks. Animals receiving melatonin

(0.2 μg/ml) gained only a 4% body weight during the first 2 weeks and then stabilized [35]. Thus, melatonin reduced weight gain without affecting total food consumption and decreased plasma leptin levels within 3 wk-before decreasing plasma insulin. 8-week-long oral treatment of HFD-fed mice with melatonin significantly improved insulin sensitivity and glucose tolerance [36].

Rats on a 60% fructose diet develop MS after 4 or 6 weeks [37]. In these animals, serum insulin, triglyceride, total cholesterol, free fatty acids, uric acid, leptin and lipid peroxide concentrations, as well as hepatic triglyceride and cholesterol levels, increased. Relative intra-abdominal fat and liver weights also increased while serum HDL cholesterol and adiponectin concentrations decreased [37]. The 6-week high fructose feeding increased serum TNF-α and hepatic lipid peroxide concentrations and decreased hepatic reduced glutathione concentration (GSH) [38]. Daily intraperitoneal administration of melatonin (1 or 10 mg/kg body weight), starting at 4th week from the onset of fructose feeding, attenuated these changes at 6-wk in a dose dependent manner. Oral glucose tolerance tests in melatonin treated rats showed higher serum insulin response curve and normal serum glucose response curve than their control counterparts. These results indicate that melatonin improves metabolic syndrome induced by high fructose intake in rats [38].

It is known that diets incorporating fructose in drinking water at low concentrations (5% or less) for long periods, or concentrations of 10% fructose for short periods (up to 2 weeks), caused no change or even increase the tolerance to a glucose load [39]. In a recent experiment we assessed the effect of melatonin supplementation (2 mg/kg/day in the drinking water) at an early phase of the fructose-induced MS in rats (Figures 3 and 4). The expected increased tolerance to glucose overload was found as well as an increased systolic BP and augmented circulating levels of cholesterol. Melatonin was effective in normalizing abnormally elevated systolic BP and glucose tolerance as well as the abnormally high cholesterol levels (Figures 3 and 4). It is particularly promising to find therapeutic potential for melatonin at an early stage of the MS.

By studying a HFD model (35% fat) we also assessed melatonin´s ability to counteract these induced metabolic effects [22]. Animals were divided into three groups, two fed with a HFD and melatonin (2 mg/kg/day) or vehicle in drinking water for 11 weeks, and one fed normal diet (4% fat). The HFD disrupted normal 24 h patterns of circulating adiponectin, insulin and cholesterol.

Melatonin attenuated body weight increase, hyperglycemia and hyperinsulinemia, as well as the increase in mean plasma adiponectin, leptin, triglycerides and cholesterol levels [22]. Other animal models in which melatonin was effective to reduce obesity include the ovariectomized rat [40-42], the type 2 diabetic (OLETF) rat [28], HFD fed rabbits [43] and olanzapine-treated rats [44]. NEU-P11, a melatonin analog, also inhibited weight gain and ameliorated insulin sensitivity in HFD rats [45].

In a prediabetic rat model of diet-induced obesity (high caloric diet) 16 week melatonin treatment (4 mg/kg/day in the drinking water) reduced the metabolic sequelae and protected the heart against myocardial ischemia and reperfusion injury through activation of the reperfusion injury salvage kinases pathway (increased Akt and ERK activation, decreased p38 activation) [46]. Young male Zucker diabetic fatty rats which received melatonin (10 mg/kg/day in drinking water) for 6 weeks, reduced mean weight gain without affecting food intake, reduced triglyceride levels, elevated cholesterol-HDL and reduced cholesterol-low-density-lipoprotein (LDL) levels [47].

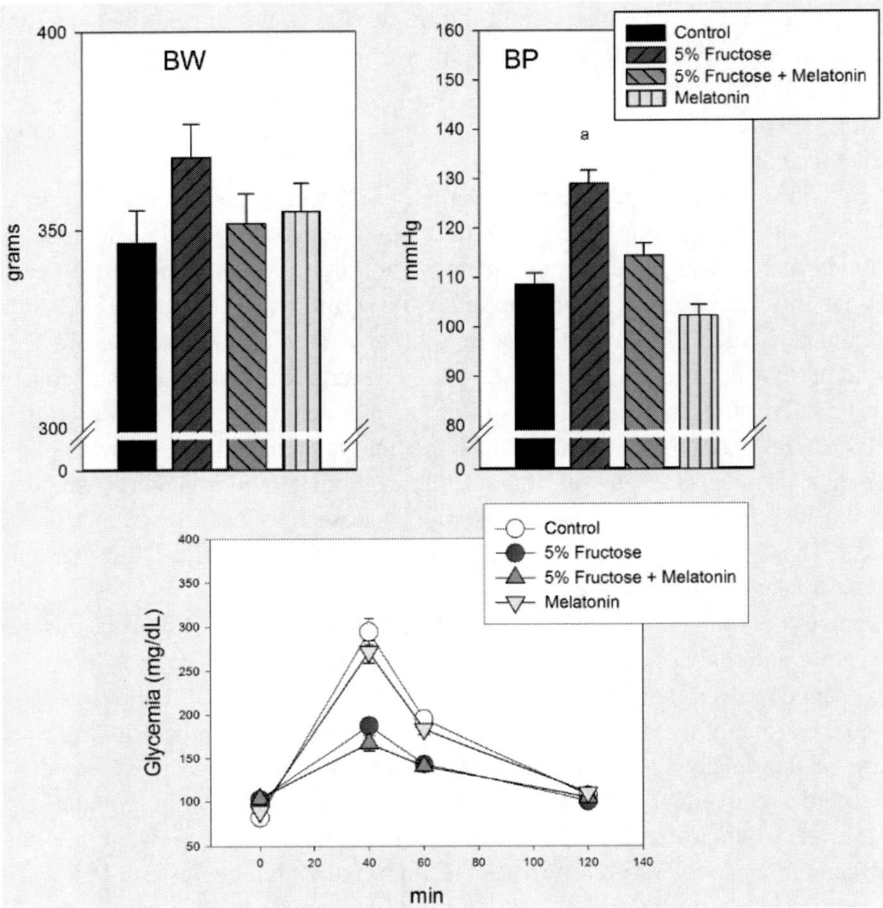

Figure 3. Effect of melatonin at an early phase of the MS produced by administering 5% fructose in the drinking water. Body weights (BW), systolic blood pressure (BP) and glucose tolerance were assessed at the time of sacrifice. Melatonin (25ug/ml) and fructose were given to the animals in the drinking water for 6 weeks. Groups of 6 rats were weighed and their BP was determined by a tail sphingometer. For the glucose tolerance test blood was collected from the tail tip at three different time intervals after glucose peritoneal injection. Shown are the means ± SEM. (a) $p < 0.01$ vs. all groups, one-way analysis of variance (ANOVA).

The reasons for melatonin´s effect on body weight in the absence of significant differences in food intake remain undefined. In seasonally active Siberian hamsters melatonin brought about an increase in the activity of the sympathetic nervous system innervating white fat thus increasing lipolysis [48]. At present, we do not know whether a similar mechanism exists in a nonseasonal species like the laboratory rat, or even in humans. Since all animal studies demonstrating effects of melatonin on metabolism have been conducted in nocturnal species, studies on melatonin effects on MS primate's models, like the rhesus monkey [49] would be very helpful. Melatonin may increase energy expenditure by brown adipose tissue [50]. Collectively, these results provide a strong support to melatonin´s counteracting effect on some of the disrupted features seen in diet-induced obesity in rats, in particular insulin resistance, dyslipidemia and overweight. Still, our knowledge is limited and further studies on this topic are needed.

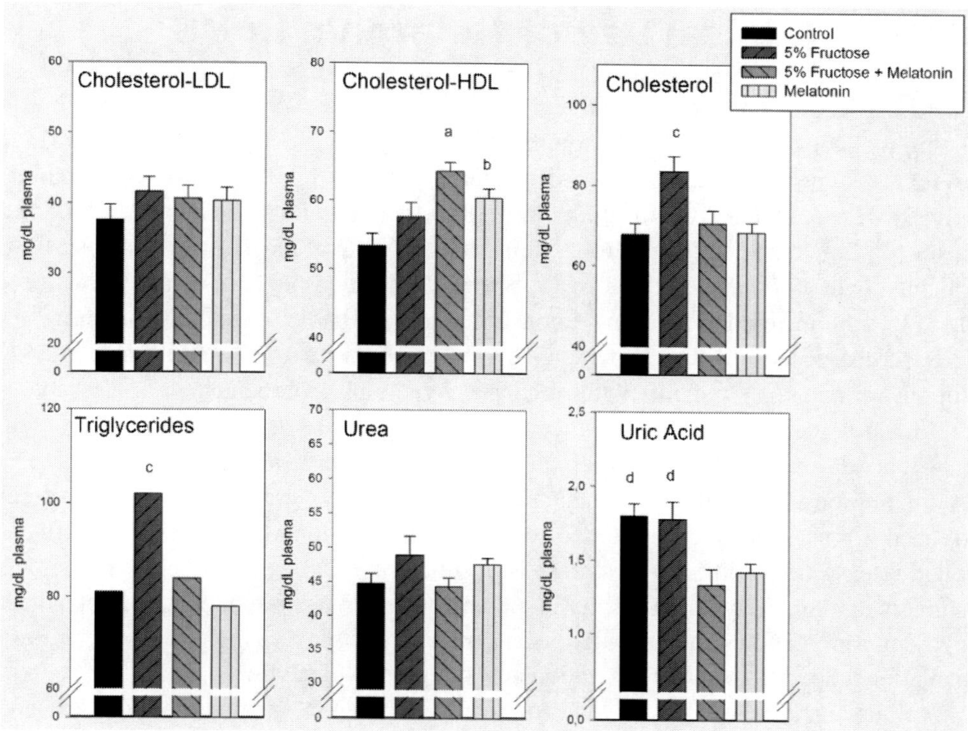

Figure 4. Effect of melatonin at an early phase of the MS produced by administering 5% fructose in the drinking water. The same rats used in the experiment shown in Figure 3 were killed by decapitation and blood was collected for the following determinations: total cholesterol, cholesterol-LDL, cholesterol-HDL, triglycerides, urea, and uric acid. Shown are the means ± SEM. (a) P< 0.01 vs. control, (b) P< 0.05 vs. control, (c) P< 0.01 vs. all groups, d P< 0.01, vs. melatonin, one-way ANOVA.

In view of the strong relationships found among food intake, weight gain and melatonin, some researchers have began to explore the molecular basis for it. It has been found that in murine Swiss 3T3-L1 preadipocytes melatonin functions as a negative regulator of adipogenesis, the process by which fibroblasts differentiate into functional adipocytes [51]. Melatonin would do so in part by inhibiting an essential transcription factor for this process, C/EBPβ. However, a contradicting study was published arguing that melatonin stimulates adipogenic differentiation by increasing C/EBPα and PPARγ expression, the two main transcription factors. Apparently, a classic mechanism involving a melatonin receptor would explain it, since it was counteracted by luzindole, a melatonin receptor antagonist [52].

Regarding melatonin effects on key metabolism regulating molecules, it was found that it increases leptin expression and potentiates insulin effects on epidydimal adipocytes [53]. In isolated adipocytes intermittently exposed to melatonin mimicking a circadian-like pattern insulin and melatonin jointly but neither alone, increase leptin expression by a 105%. Also dexamethasone proved to be synergic with melatonin by increasing leptin expression and release by a 75% [54]. In this model, during the "induced night" (+melatonin) Clock, Per-1 and FAS (fatty acid synthase) expression and leptin secretion was increased and lipolytic activity was reduced. However, information on the circadian profile of these metabolic genes is limited, and to assess it is becoming a priority task if we keep in mind that circadian disruption may be underlie emerging metabolic pathology that we are currently studying.

Clinical Use of Melatonin in MS

There are clinical results indicating that type 2 diabetic patients have low levels of circulating melatonin [55] with a concomitantly and expected melatonin membrane receptor mRNA expression upregulation [24]. Also, allelic variants for the melatonin receptor 1B (MTNR1B) were associated with fasting blood glucose level and/or the increased risk of type 2 diabetes [56-58]. These findings strongly bind melatonin to blood glucose homeostasis.

Patients with coronary artery disease show diminished melatonin secretion [59-62]. Remarkably, administered melatonin demonstrated to be capable of reducing nocturnal blood pressure in otherwise untreated hypertensive women [63], essential hypertensive men [64], nondipping women [65], patients with nocturnal hypertension [66] and in adolescents with type 1 diabetes mellitus [67,68]. A recent meta-analysis of randomized controlled trials indicates that add-on controlled-release melatonin to antihypertensive therapy is effective and safe in ameliorating nocturnal hypertension [69]. Accordingly, larger trials of longer duration would need to be conducted in order to determine the long-term beneficial effects of controlled-release melatonin in patients with nocturnal hypertension. As a pleiotropic molecule, melatonin may exert its antihypertensive and anti-remodeling effects offering cardiovascular protection in MS through its antioxidant and scavenging properties, preserving NO availability, specific receptor activation and sympathoplegic effects [3].

As well as in animal models, clinical studies have shown that melatonin provides benefits on lipid profiles. Melatonin treatment (1 mg/kg for 30 days) elevated cholesterol-HDL levels in peri- and postmenopausal women [70]. Several mechanisms can account for the hypolipidemic effects of melatonin, such as decrease in intestinal cholesterol absorption [71] or inhibition of cholesterol biosynthesis [72,73].

Catecholamine-induced hypercoagulability in acute stress contributing to thrombus growth after coronary plaque rupture was prevented by the administration of melatonin [74,75]. Platelet aggregation in vitro was inhibited by melatonin via a time-dependent, dose-response effect [76-79]. In light of the herein results, melatonin may have a protective effect in reducing the atherothrombotic risk in MS.

A recent open-label study which included 33 healthy volunteers and 30 MS patients treated with melatonin was carried out [80]. Patients with MS (not responding to a 3-month lifestyle modification) had significantly higher B values and total cholesterol, cholesterol LDL, triglycerides, systolic and diastolic blood pressure, glycemia, fibrinogen, and erythrocyte thiobarbituric acid-reactive substrate (TBARs) levels when compared to controls.

They also had lower levels of cholesterol HDL levels and reduced activities of catalase, glutathione peroxidase and superoxide dismutase in erythrocytes. Melatonin (5-mg/day/2 hr before bedtime/2 months) decreased significantly hypertension and improved the serum lipid profile and the antioxidative status [80]. Collectively, the above discussed results suggest that melatonin therapy may be of benefit for patients with MS, particularly with arterial hypertension. Undoubtedly, more studies are needed in order to assess a melatonin proper doses/ treatment duration/administration time relationship in MS patients. Information from PubMed indicates that there are a few ongoing clinical trials involving melatonin and MS and/or related pathologies (Table 1).

Table 1. Clinical trials related to MS involving melatonin (Source: PubMed)

Clinical Trial	Status	Condition	Drug	Sponsor	Outcome measure
Melatonin and the Metabolic	Recruiting	Metabolic	Melatonin Placebo	Emory University	Metabolic components
Melatonin Metabolism Abnormality in Patients With Schizophrenia or Schizoaffective Disorder Treated With Olanzapine	Recruiting	Schizophrenia; Schizoaffective Disorder; Bipolar Disorder; Obesity; Metabolic Syndrome	Olanzapin Melatonin	Seattle Institute for Biomedical and Clinical Research; Eli Lilly and Company	Nocturnal melatonin production, assay of urinary 6-sulfatoxymelatonin (aMT6s) adjusted for creatinine; Metabolic indices including weight, waist and hip measurements, and metabolic tests
Effects of Metformin and Oral Hormonal Contraceptive in Adolescents With Polycystic Ovary Syndrome	Recruiting	Polycystic Ovary Syndrome	Metmorfin Placebo	Federal University of São Paulo	Serum melatonin; hormonal and metabolic measurements, clinical assessment
Melatonin and Adiponectin in Hypertensive Kidney Transplant	Completed	Hypertension; Kidney Transplant		Sheba Medical Center	
Myo-inositol	Recruiting	Perimenopause	Myo-mel Placebo	AGUNCO Obstetrics and Gynecology Centre	
Effects of Melatonin and Oxygen Consumption and Choroidal Blood Flow	Completed	Vasospastic Syndrome	Melatonin Placebo	University Hospital, Basel, Switzerland	Choroidal blood flow; oxygen consumption; Co2 production; skin temperature; rectal temperature; blood pressure; eye tension
Melatonin for Prevention of Metabolic	Recruiting	Schizophrenia; Schizophreniform Disorder; Brief Psychotic Disorder; Substance Induced Psychosis	Melatonin Placebo	Guilan University of Medical Sciences	At week 4 and 8: Weight; Triglyceride; HDL; LDL; Total Cholesterol; Fasting blood sugar; blood pressure; body mass index (BMI) waist to hip ratio; Positive and negative syndrome scale (PANSS) also at week 8; Insulin at week 8; Number of adverse events at the end of the study in each group; Changes from baseline in HOMA-IR values at week 8

Chronobiologic Therapy in MS

Daily rhythms affecting most components of the cardiovascular system, such as heart rate, blood pressure, platelet and endothelial function, have been epidemiologically reported to be disturbed, particularly with a morning peak of cardiovascular incidents, such as ischemic stroke, myocardial infarction, sudden cardiac death and ventricular arrhythmias [81,82].

Incidentally, this is the moment in which the augmented endogenous melatonin levels at night have come back to basal values. Recent studies have established mechanistic links between time-of-day-dependent oscillations in myocardial metabolism and the autonomous cardiomyocyte circadian clock, which regulates myocardial glucose uptake, glycolysis/ hexosamine biosynthetic pathway, and pyruvate oxidation, as well as glycogen, triglyceride, and protein turnover [83].

Circadian clocks within individual cardiovascular cells confer the advantage of anticipation of the onset of neurohumoral stimuli before and increased energetic demand during the wake period.

As in many diseases, particularly those related to MS, hypertension, cardiovascular disease, obesity, diabetes, etc., the cumulative evidence supports the hypothesis that many of us sustain: metabolic rhythms attenuation and/or disruption contribute to the etiology of the disease.

Diabetes mellitus, a major risk factor for the development of heart disease and/or MS in human beings, is associated with a phase shift in the cardiac circadian clock [83]. Actually, metformin, a commonly-used antidiabetic drug, exerts differential effects on CCG in different target tissues, with phase advances in the liver and phase delays in the muscle (in clock and metabolic genes and/or protein expression). It does so by activating AMPK, inhibiting acetyl CoA carboxylase, the rate limiting enzyme in fatty acid synthesis, and activating liver casein kinase I α (CKIα) and muscle CKIε, known modulators of the positive loop of the circadian clock [84].

Therefore, a combined strategy of melatonin and bright light administration to augment the circadian amplitude and synchronize endogenous rhythms seems to be promising in MS. However, to our knowledge, there is currently no study involving bright light + melatonin in MS. Regarding the bright light effect only, when 25 overweight and obese subjects were assigned to 6 weeks of moderate exercise with or without bright light treatment, body weight and BMI decreased significantly with exercise regardless whether they were in the light or non-light treatment group [85].

With exercise, body fat decreased significantly only in the light treatment group. Mood scores improved significantly with exercise in the light group, but there were no significant changes regarding sleep.

So this preliminary study is the first to show that addition of bright light treatment plus a 6-week moderate exercise program can modify body composition by significantly reducing body fat. This is of particular importance, because visceral fat has been implicated as a major factor in the development of MS.

Conclusion

Melatonin can provide an innovative strategy in MS by combining its effects on circadian rhythmicity with its cytoprotective properties. Melatonin protects against several comorbidities of MS, including diabetes and concomitant oxyradical-mediated damage, inflammation, microvascular disease and atherothrombotic risk. At an early stage of MS treatment, a non pharmacological approach as lifestyle modification, a low-fat diet, and physical exercise are commonly recommended. Patients who are refractory to these changes are treated with drugs (hypotensive, lipid-lowering, antidiabetic drugs) that may have significant side effects.

Melatonin has a high safety profile and it reduces the toxicity of many pharmaceutical agents. In addition, it is usually remarkably well tolerated e.g. very high doses (300 mg melatonin/day) were given orally for up to 2 years to amyotrophic lateral sclerosis patients and found to be safe [86].

As melatonin is a short-lived molecule having a limited duration of action (half-life 0.54–0.67 h), analogs with a high affinity for melatonin receptors and a longer duration of action have been synthesized with a potential therapeutic efficacy to treat circadian disorders [87]. To what extent the new melatoninergic agents approved by the US Food and Drug Administration or the European Medicines Agency (ramelteon, agomelatine) or those who are in the process of being approved (tasimelteon) share the protective activity of melatonin in MS remains to be defined. A recent study indicates that ramelteon given in drinking water (8 mg/kg/day) for 8 weeks to spontaneously hypertensive Wistar-Kyoto male rats significantly attenuated age-associated increase of systolic blood pressure and age-associated body weight gain [88]. In view of the higher binding affinities, longest half-life and relative higher potencies of the different melatonin agonists, studies using 2 or 3 mg/day of melatonin are probably unsuitable to give appropriate comparison of the effects of the natural compound. Hence, clinical trials employing melatonin doses in the range of 50–100 mg/day are warranted before the relative merits of the melatonin analogs versus melatonin can be settled [87].

Acknowledgment

Studies in authors´ laboratories were supported by grants from the Agencia Nacional de Promoción Científica y Tecnológica, Argentina (PICT 2007-01045) and the University of Buenos Aires (M048). DPC is a Professor Emeritus, University of Buenos Aires. DPC, PS and ESP are Research Career Awardees from the Argentine Research Council (CONICET).

References

[1] Reaven GM: Banting lecture 1988. Role of insulin resistance in human disease. *Diabetes,* 1988;37:1595-1607.

[2] Reiter RJ, Tan DX, Korkmaz A, Ma S: Obesity and metabolic syndrome: Association with chronodisruption, sleep deprivation, and melatonin suppression. *Ann. Med.,* 2011; 44:564-577.

[3] Cardinali DP, Cano P, Jimenez-Ortega V, Esquifino AI: Melatonin and the metabolic syndrome: physiopathologic and therapeutical implications. *Neuroendocrinology,* 2011;93:133-142.

[4] National Sleep Foundation: Sleep in America Poll 2003,Washington, DC, USA, National Sleep Foundation, 2003.

[5] Bin YS, Marshall NS, Glozier NS: Secular changes in sleep duration among Australian adults, 1992-2006. *Med. J. Aust.,* 2011;195:670-672.

[6] Bixler E: Sleep and society: an epidemiological perspective. *Sleep Med.* 2009;10 Suppl 1:S3-S6.

[7] LaDou J: Health effects of shift work. West J Med 1982;137:525-530.

[8] Scheer FA, Hilton MF, Mantzoros CS, Shea SA: Adverse metabolic and cardiovascular consequences of circadian misalignment. *Proc. Natl. Acad. Sci. U S A,* 2009;106:4453-4458.

[9] Ayas NT, White DP, Al Delaimy WK, Manson JE, Stampfer MJ, Speizer FE, Patel S, Hu FB: A prospective study of self-reported sleep duration and incident diabetes in women. *Diabetes Care*, 2003;26:380-384.

[10] Mallon L, Broman JE, Hetta J: High incidence of diabetes in men with sleep complaints or short sleep duration: a 12-year follow-up study of a middle-aged population. *Diabetes Care,* 2005;28:2762-2767.

[11] Vorona RD, Winn MP, Babineau TW, Eng BP, Feldman HR, Ware JC: Overweight and obese patients in a primary care population report less sleep than patients with a normal body mass index. *Arch. Intern. Med.,* 2005;165:25-30.

[12] Yaggi HK, Araujo AB, McKinlay JB: Sleep duration as a risk factor for the development of type 2 diabetes. *Diabetes Care*, 2006;29:657-661.

[13] Vincent HK, Innes KE, Vincent KR: Oxidative stress and potential interventions to reduce oxidative stress in overweight and obesity. *Diabetes Obes. Metab.,* 2007;9:813-839.

[14] Sanchez-Barcelo EJ, Mediavilla MD, Tan DX, Reiter RJ: clinical uses of melatonin: evaluation of human trials. *Curr. Med. Chem.,* 2010; 17: 2070 -2095.

[15] Dibner C, Schibler U, Albrecht U: The mammalian circadian timing system: organization and coordination of central and peripheral clocks. *Annu. Rev. Physiol.,* 2010;72:517-549.

[16] Fonken LK, Workman JL, Walton JC, Weil ZM, Morris JS, Haim A, Nelson RJ: Light at night increases body mass by shifting the time of food intake. *Proc. Natl. Acad. Sci. U S A,* 2010;107:18664-18669.

[17] Bellet MM, Sassone-Corsi P: Mammalian circadian clock and metabolism - the epigenetic link. *J. Cell Sci.,* 2010;123:3837-3848.

[18] Gimble JM, Sutton GM, Bunnell BA, Ptitsyn AA, Floyd ZE: Prospective influences of circadian clocks in adipose tissue and metabolism. *Nat. Rev. Endocrinol.,* 2011;7:98-107.

[19] Froy O: The relationship between nutrition and circadian rhythms in mammals. *Front Neuroendocrinol.,* 2007;28:61-71.

[20] Cano P, Jimenez-Ortega V, Larrad A, Toso CF, Cardinali DP, Esquifino AI: Effect of a high-fat diet on 24-h pattern of circulating levels of prolactin, luteinizing hormone, testosterone, corticosterone, thyroid-stimulating hormone and glucose, and pineal melatonin content, in rats. *Endocrine,* 2008; 33:118-125.

[21] Cano P, Cardinali DP, Ríos-Lugo MP, Fernández-Mateos MP, Reyes MP, Esquifino AI: Effect of a high-fat diet on 24-hour pattern of circulating adipocytokines in rats. *Obesity*, 2009;117:1866-1871.
[22] Rios-Lugo MJ, Cano P, Jimenez-Ortega V, Fernández-Mateos MP, Scacchi PA, Cardinali DP, Esquifino AI: Melatonin effect on plasma adiponectin, leptin, insulin, glucose, triglycerides and cholesterol in normal and high fat-fed rats. *J. Pineal Res.,* 2010;49:342-348.
[23] Hardeland R, Cardinali DP, Srinivasan V, Spence DW, Brown GM, Pandi-Perumal SR: Melatonin - a pleiotropic, orchestrating regulator molecule. *Progr. Neurobiol.,* 2011;93:350-384.
[24] Peschke E, Stumpf I, Bazwinsky I, Litvak L, Dralle H, Muhlbauer E: Melatonin and type 2 diabetes - a possible link? *J. Pineal Res.,* 2007; 42: 350-358.
[25] Peschke E, Muhlbauer E: New evidence for a role of melatonin in glucose regulation. *Best Pract. Res. Clin. Endocrinol. Metab.,* 2010; 24: 829-841.
[26] Kanter M, Uysal H, Karaca T, Sagmanligil HO: Depression of glucose levels and partial restoration of pancreatic beta-cell damage by melatonin in streptozotocin-induced diabetic rats. *Arch. Toxicol.,* 2006; 80: 362-369.
[27] Nishida S, Sato R, Murai I, Nakagawa S: Effect of pinealectomy on plasma levels of insulin and leptin and on hepatic lipids in type 2 diabetic rats. *J. Pineal Res.,* 2003; 35: 251-256.
[28] Nishida S, Segawa T, Murai I, Nakagawa S: Long-term melatonin administration reduces hyperinsulinemia and improves the altered fatty-acid compositions in type 2 diabetic rats via the restoration of Delta-5 desaturase activity. *J. Pineal Res.,* 2002;32:26-33.
[29] Paskaloglu K, Sener G, Ayangolu-Dulger G: Melatonin treatment protects against diabetes-induced functional and biochemical changes in rat aorta and corpus cavernosum. *Eur. J. Pharmacol.,* 2004; 499: 345-354.
[30] Reyes-Toso CF, Linares LM, Ricci CR, Obaya-Naredo D, Pinto JE, Rodriguez RR, Cardinali DP: Melatonin restores endothelium-dependent relaxation in aortic rings of pancreatectomized rats. *J. Pineal Res.,* 2005; 39: 386-391.
[31] Tan DX, Manchester LC, Reiter RJ, Qi W, Kim SJ, El Sokkary GH: Ischemia /reperfusion-induced arrhythmias in the isolated rat heart: prevention by melatonin. *J. Pineal Res.,* 1998;25:184-191.
[32] Castagnino HE, Lago N, Centrella JM, Calligaris SD, Farina S, Sarchi MI, Cardinali DP: Cytoprotection by melatonin and growth hormone in early rat myocardial infarction as revealed by Feulgen DNA staining. *Neuro. Endocrinol. Lett.,* 2002;23:391-395.
[33] Prunet-Marcassus B, Desbazeille M, Bros A, Louche K, Delagrange P, Renard P, Casteilla L, Penicaud L: Melatonin reduces body weight gain in Sprague Dawley rats with diet-induced obesity. *Endocrinology,* 2003; 144: 5347-5352.
[34] Wolden-Hanson T, Mitton DR, McCants RL, Yellon SM, Wilkinson CW, Matsumoto AM, Rasmussen DD: Daily melatonin administration to middle-aged male rats suppresses body weight, intraabdominal adiposity, and plasma leptin and insulin independent of food intake and total body fat. *Endocrinology,* 2000; 141: 487-497.
[35] Puchalski SS, Green JN, Rasmussen DD: Melatonin effect on rat body weight regulation in response to high-fat diet at middle age. *Endocrine,* 2003; 21: 163-167.

[36] Sartori C, Dessen P, Mathieu C, Monney A, Bloch J, Nicod P, Scherrer U, Duplain H: Melatonin improves glucose homeostasis and endothelial vascular function in high-fat diet-fed insulin-resistant mice. *Endocrinology,* 2009;150:5311-5317.

[37] Tran LT, Yuen VG, McNeill JH: The fructose-fed rat: a review on the mechanisms of fructose-induced insulin resistance and hypertension. *Mol. Cell Biochem.,* 2009;332:145-159.

[38] Kitagawa A, Ohta Y, Ohashi K: Melatonin improves metabolic syndrome induced by high fructose intake in rats. *J. Pineal Res.,* 2012; 52: 403-413.

[39] Roglans N, Sanguino E, Peris C, Alegret M, Vazquez M, Adzet T, Diaz C, Hernandez G, Laguna JC, Sanchez RM: Atorvastatin treatment induced peroxisome proliferator-activated receptor alpha expression and decreased plasma nonesterified fatty acids and liver triglyceride in fructose-fed rats. *J. Pharmacol. Exp. Ther.,* 2002; 302: 232-239.

[40] Ciortea R, Costin N, Braicu I, Haragas D, Hudacsko A, Bondor C, Mihu D, Mihu CM: Effect of melatonin on intra-abdominal fat in correlation with endometrial proliferation in ovariectomized rats. *Anticancer Res.,* 2011; 31: 2637-2643.

[41] Ladizesky MG, Boggio V, Albornoz LE, Castrillón P, Mautalen CA, Cardinali DP: Melatonin increases oestradiol-induced bone formation in ovariectomized rats. *J. Pineal Res.,* 2003; 34: 143-151.

[42] Sanchez-Mateos S, Alonso-Gonzalez C, Gonzalez A, Martinez-Campa CM, Mediavilla MD, Cos S, Sanchez-Barcelo EJ: Melatonin and estradiol effects on food intake, body weight, and leptin in ovariectomized rats. *Maturitas,* 2007;58:91-101.

[43] Hussein MR, Ahmed OG, Hassan AF, Ahmed MA: Intake of melatonin is associated with amelioration of physiological changes, both metabolic and morphological pathologies associated with obesity: an animal model. *Int. J. Exp. Pathol.,* 2007;88: 19-29.

[44] Raskind MA, Burke BL, Crites NJ, Tapp AM, Rasmussen DD: Olanzapine-induced weight gain and increased visceral adiposity is blocked by melatonin replacement therapy in rats. *Neuropsychopharmacology,* 2007; 32: 284-288.

[45] She M, Deng X, Guo Z, Laudon M, Hu Z, Liao D, Hu X, Luo Y, Shen Q, Su Z, Yin W: NEU-P11, a novel melatonin agonist, inhibits weight gain and improves insulin sensitivity in high-fat/high-sucrose-fed rats. *Pharmacol. Res.,* 2009; 59: 248-253.

[46] Nduhirabandi F, Du Toit EF, Blackhurst D, Marais D, Lochner A: Chronic melatonin consumption prevents obesity-related metabolic abnormalities and protects the heart against myocardial ischemia and reperfusion injury in a prediabetic model of diet-induced obesity. *J. Pineal Res.,* 2010.

[47] Agil A, Navarro-Alarcon M, Ruiz R, Abuhamadah S, El Mir MY, Vazquez GF: Beneficial effects of melatonin on obesity and lipid profile in young Zucker diabetic fatty rats. *J. Pineal Res*., 2011;50:207-212.

[48] Bartness TJ, Demas GE, Song CK: Seasonal changes in adiposity: the roles of the photoperiod, melatonin and other hormones, and sympathetic nervous system. *Exp. Biol. Med.,* (Maywood) 2002; 227: 363-376.

[49] Bremer AA, Stanhope KL, Graham JL, Cummings BP, Wang W, Saville BR, Havel PJ: Fructose-fed rhesus monkeys: a nonhuman primate model of insulin resistance, metabolic syndrome, and type 2 diabetes. *Clin. Transl. Sci.,* 2011;4:243-252.

[50] Tan DX, Manchester LC, Fuentes-Broto L, Paredes SD, Reiter RJ: Significance and application of melatonin in the regulation of brown adipose tissue metabolism: relation to human obesity. *Obes. Rev.,* 2010; 12: 167-188.

[51] Alonso-Vale MI, Andreotti S, Mukai PY, Borges-Silva CN, Peres SB, Cipolla-Neto J, Lima FB: Melatonin and the circadian entrainment of metabolic and hormonal activities in primary isolated adipocytes. *J. Pineal Res.* 2008;45:422-429.

[52] Gonzalez A, Alvarez-Garcia V, Martinez-Campa C, Alonso-Gonzalez C, Cos S: Melatonin promotes differentiation of 3T3-L1 fibroblasts. *J. Pineal Res.,* 2012; 52:12-20.

[53] Alonso-Vale MI, Andreotti S, Peres SB, Anhe GF, das NB-S, Neto JC, Lima FB: Melatonin enhances leptin expression by rat adipocytes in the presence of insulin. *Am. J. Physiol. Endocrinol. Metab.,* 2005; 288: E805-E812.

[54] Alonso-Vale MI, Andreotti S, Borges-Silva CN, Mukai PY, Cipolla-Neto J, Lima FB: Intermittent and rhythmic exposure to melatonin in primary cultured adipocytes enhances the insulin and dexamethasone effects on leptin expression. *J. Pineal Res.,* 2006;41:28-34.

[55] Tutuncu NB, Batur MK, Yildirir A, Tutuncu T, Deger A, Koray Z, Erbas B, Kabakci G, Aksoyek S, Erbas T: Melatonin levels decrease in type 2 diabetic patients with cardiac autonomic neuropathy. *J. Pineal Res.,* 2005; 39: 43-49.

[56] Dietrich K, Birkmeier S, Schleinitz D, Breitfeld J, Enigk B, Muller I, Bottcher Y, Lindner T, Stumvoll M, Tonjes A, Kovacs P: Association and evolutionary studies of the melatonin receptor 1B gene (MTNR1B) in the self-contained population of Sorbs from Germany. *Diabet. Med.,* 2011; 28:1373-1380.

[57] Kim JY, Cheong HS, Park BL, Baik SH, Park S, Lee SW, Kim MH, Chung JH, Choi JS, Kim MY, Yang JH, Cho DH, Shin HD, Kim SH: Melatonin receptor 1 B polymorphisms associated with the risk of gestational diabetes mellitus. *BMC Med. Genet.,* 2011;12:82.

[58] Prokopenko I, Langenberg C, Florez JC, Saxena R, Soranzo N, Thorleifsson G, Loos RJ, Manning AK, Jackson AU, Aulchenko Y, Potter SC, Erdos MR, Sanna S, Hottenga JJ, Wheeler E, Kaakinen M, Lyssenko V, Chen WM, Ahmadi K, Beckmann JS, Bergman RN, Bochud M, Bonnycastle LL, Buchanan TA, Cao A, Cervino A, Coin L, Collins FS, Crisponi L, de Geus EJ, Dehghan A, Deloukas P, Doney AS, Elliott P, Freimer N, Gateva V, Herder C, Hofman A, Hughes TE, Hunt S, Illig T, Inouye M, Isomaa B, Johnson T, Kong A, Krestyaninova M, Kuusisto J, Laakso M, Lim N, Lindblad U, Lindgren CM, McCann OT, Mohlke KL, Morris AD, Naitza S, Orru M, Palmer CN, Pouta A, Randall J, Rathmann W, Saramies J, Scheet P, Scott LJ, Scuteri A, Sharp S, Sijbrands E, Smit JH, Song K, Steinthorsdottir V, Stringham HM, Tuomi T, Tuomilehto J, Uitterlinden AG, Voight BF, Waterworth D, Wichmann HE, Willemsen G, Witteman JC, Yuan X, Zhao JH, Zeggini E, Schlessinger D, Sandhu M, Boomsma DI, Uda M, Spector TD, Penninx BW, Altshuler D, Vollenweider P, Jarvelin MR, Lakatta E, Waeber G, Fox CS, Peltonen L, Groop LC, Mooser V, Cupples LA, Thorsteinsdottir U, Boehnke M, Barroso I, Van Duijn C, Dupuis J, Watanabe RM, Stefansson K, McCarthy MI, Wareham NJ, Meigs JB, Abecasis GR: Variants in MTNR1B influence fasting glucose levels. *Nat. Genet.,* 2009; 41: 77-81.

[59] Dominguez-Rodriguez A, Abreu-Gonzalez P, Garcia MJ, Sanchez J, Marrero F, Armas-Trujillo D: Decreased nocturnal melatonin levels during acute myocardial infarction. *J. Pineal Res.,* 2002; 33: 248-252.

[60] Girotti L, Lago M, Yanovsky O, Carbajales J, Elizari M, Brusco LI, Cardinali DP: Low urinary 6-sulphatoxymelatonin levels in patients with coronary artery disease. *J. Pineal Research.,* 2000;29:138-142.

[61] Sakotnik A, Liebmann PM, Stoschitzky K, Lercher P, Schauenstein K, Klein W, Eber B: Decreased melatonin synthesis in patients with coronary artery disease. *Eur. Heart J.,* 1999; 20: 1314-1317.

[62] Yaprak M, Altun A, Vardar A, Aktoz M, Ciftci S, Ozbay G: Decreased nocturnal synthesis of melatonin in patients with coronary artery disease. *Int. J. Cardiol.,* 2003;89:103-107.

[63] Cagnacci A, Cannoletta M, Renzi A, Baldassari F, Arangino S, Volpe A: Prolonged melatonin administration decreases nocturnal blood pressure in women. *Am. J. Hypertens.,* 2005;18:1614-1618.

[64] Scheer FA, Van Montfrans GA, Van Someren EJ, Mairuhu G, Buijs RM: Daily nighttime melatonin reduces blood pressure in male patients with essential hypertension. *Hypertension,* 2004;43:192-197.

[65] Jonas M, Garfinkel D, Zisapel N, Laudon M, Grossman E: Impaired nocturnal melatonin secretion in non-dipper hypertensive patients. *Blood Press.,* 2003;12:19-24.

[66] Grossman E, Laudon M, Yalcin R, Zengil H, Peleg E, Sharabi Y, Kamari Y, Shen-Orr Z, Zisapel N: Melatonin reduces night blood pressure in patients with nocturnal hypertension. *Am. J. Med.,* 2006; 119: 898-902.

[67] Cavallo A, Daniels SR, Dolan LM, Bean JA, Khoury JC: Blood pressure-lowering effect of melatonin in type 1 diabetes. *J. Pineal Res.,* 2004; 36: 262-266.

[68] Cavallo A, Daniels SR, Dolan LM, Khoury JC, Bean JA: Blood pressure response to melatonin in type 1 diabetes. *Pediatr. Diabetes,* 2004; 5: 26-31.

[69] Grossman E, Laudon M, Zisapel N: Effect of melatonin on nocturnal blood pressure: meta-analysis of randomized controlled trials. *Vasc. Health Risk Manag.*, 2011;7:577-584.

[70] Tamura H, Nakamura Y, Narimatsu A, Yamagata Y, Takasaki A, Reiter RJ, Sugino N: Melatonin treatment in peri- and postmenopausal women elevates serum high-density lipoprotein cholesterol levels without influencing total cholesterol levels. *J. Pineal Res.,* 2008; ;45:101-105.

[71] Hussain SA: Effect of melatonin on cholesterol absorption in rats. *J. Pineal Res.,* 2007;42:267-271.

[72] Muller-Wieland D, Behnke B, Koopmann K, Krone W: Melatonin inhibits LDL receptor activity and cholesterol synthesis in freshly isolated human mononuclear leukocytes. *Biochem. Biophys. Res. Commun.*, 1994; 203: 416-421.

[73] Esquifino A, Agrasal C, Velazquez E, Villanua MA, Cardinali DP: Effect of melatonin on serum cholesterol and phospholipid levels, and on prolactin, thyroid-stimulating hormone and thyroid hormone levels, in hyperprolactinemic rats. *Life Sci.,* 1997; 61: 1051-1058.

[74] Wirtz PH, Bartschi C, Spillmann M, Ehlert U, von Kanel R: Effect of oral melatonin on the procoagulant response to acute psychosocial stress in healthy men: a randomized placebo-controlled study. *J. Pineal Res.,* 2008; 44: 358-365.

[75] Wirtz PH, Spillmann M, Bartschi C, Ehlert U, von Kanel R: Oral melatonin reduces blood coagulation activity: a placebo-controlled study in healthy young men. *J. Pineal Res.,* 2008;44:127-133.
[76] Del Zar MM, Martinuzzo M, Cardinali DP, Carreras LO, Vacas MI: Diurnal variation in melatonin effect on adenosine triphosphate and serotonin release by human platelets. *Acta Endocrinologica,* 1990; 123: 453-458.
[77] Martinuzzo M, Del Zar MM, Cardinali DP, Carreras LO, Vacas MI: Melatonin effect on arachidonic acid metabolism to cyclooxygenase derivatives in human platelets. *J. Pineal Res.,* 1991; 11: 111-115.
[78] Vacas MI, Del Zar MM, Martinuzzo M, Cardinali DP: Binding sites for ^{3}H-melatonin in human platelets. *J. Pineal Res.,* 1992; 13: 60-65.
[79] Vacas MI, Del Zar MM, Martinuzzo M, Falcon C, Carreras LO, Cardinali DP: Inhibition of human platelet aggregation and thromboxane B2 production by melatonin. Correlation with plasma melatonin levels. *J. Pineal Res.,* 1991;11:135-139.
[80] Kozirog M, Poliwczak AR, Duchnowicz P, Koter-Michalak M, Sikora J, Broncel M: Melatonin treatment improves blood pressure, lipid profile, and parameters of oxidative stress in patients with metabolic syndrome. *J. Pineal Res.,* 2011;50:261-266.
[81] Dominguez-Rodriguez A, Abreu-Gonzalez P, Sanchez-Sanchez JJ, Kaski JC, Reiter RJ: Melatonin and circadian biology in human cardiovascular disease. *J. Pineal Res.,* 2010;49:14-22.
[82] Ruger M, Scheer FA: Effects of circadian disruption on the cardiometabolic system. *Rev. Endocr. Metab. Disord.,* 2009; 10: 245-260.
[83] Chatham JC, Young ME: Regulation of myocardial metabolism by the cardiomyocyte circadian clock. *J. Mol. Cell Cardiol.,* 2012.
[84] Barnea M, Haviv L, Gutman R, Chapnik N, Madar Z, Froy O: Metformin affects the circadian clock and metabolic rhythms in a tissue-specific manner. *Biochim. Biophys. Acta,* 2012;1822:1796-1806.
[85] Dunai A, Novak M, Chung SA, Kayumov L, Keszei A, Levitan R, Shapiro CM: Moderate exercise and bright light treatment in overweight and obese individuals. *Obesity,* (Silver Spring) 2007; 15: 1749-1757.
[86] Weishaupt JH, Bartels C, Polking E, Dietrich J, Rohde G, Poeggeler B, Mertens N, Sperling S, Bohn M, Huther G, Schneider A, Bach A, Siren AL, Hardeland R, Bahr M, Nave KA, Ehrenreich H: Reduced oxidative damage in ALS by high-dose enteral melatonin treatment. *J. Pineal Res.,* 2006; 41: 313-323.
[87] Cardinali DP, Srinivasan V, Brzezinski A, Brown GM: Melatonin and its analogs in insomnia and depression. *J. Pineal Res.,* 2012;52:365-375.
[88] Oxenkrug GF, Summergrad P: Ramelteon attenuates age-associated hypertension and weight gain in spontaneously hypertensive rats. *Ann. N Y Acad. Sci.,* 2010; 1199 : 114-120.

In: New Developments in Melatonin Research ISBN: 978-1-62618-843-3
Editors: D.Acuña-Castroviejo, I.Rusanova, G.Escames © 2013 Nova Science Publishers, Inc.

Chapter 7

Melatonin and Their Protective Role on Oxidative Cell Damage: Interplay between Oxidative Stress and Tumorigenesis

Luiz Gustavo de Almeida Chuffa, Beatriz Aparecida Fioruci and Fábio Rodrigues Ferreira Seiva[2]
[1]Department of Anatomy, IBB/UNESP,
Univ Estadual Paulista, SP, Brazil
[2]Department of Chemistry and Biochemistry, IBB/UNESP, Brazil
Univ Estadual Paulista, SP, Brazil

Abstract

Melatonin, an indolamine produced by pineal gland at night, has been implicated in the treatment of many dysfunctions including oxidative disorders, apoptosis, and cancer. It is indisputable that melatonin represents an important molecule used for antioxidant therapies at cellular levels, preventing subsequent changes that results in cell damage. Melatonin is a very potent free radical scavenger, reactive species which can be extremely deleterious to macromolecules into the cells. Direct antioxidant properties of melatonin have been shown both in vitro and in vivo. Alternatively, melatonin also stimulates several antioxidant activities, protecting the cells from oxidative stress. Thus, to focus on the antioxidant effects of melatonin, several experimental and clinical studies have been carried in an attempt to assess the activity of melatonin towards radical-induced damage. The cell oxidation is one of the main causes leading to tumorigenic process. Recently, a wide range of studies has focused attention on the positive correlation between major cell signaling-induced cancer, such as the MAP kinase and PI3K/Akt pathways, and the increasing oxygen/nitrogen species formation. Particularly, melatonin has a dual effect on intracellular redox state regarding its antiproliferative action and its cytotoxic effect directly to cancer cells. As far as we could investigate, there is no compiled data regarding melatonin, oxidative stress and cancer studies which we believe to be extremely important for the hormone divulgation and to encourage further researches. This chapter briefly presents a review of the melatonin metabolism (biosynthesis, distribution, cellular responsiveness, and degradation), followed by an introductory topic to the free radicals world, broaching the main mechanisms in which they participate, and their consequences. The next topics include the extensively studied relations between free radicals and cancer development (addressing some specific and aggressive cancer types), focusing on standard and alternative treatment methodologies.

Introduction

Melatonin: Biosynthesis, Distribution, Cellular responsiveness and degradation.

Biosynthesis

Melatonin, also known as N-acetyl-5-methoxytryptamine, is an endogenous indoleamine produced by pineal gland at night. Among other important functions, melatonin plays an essential role in the regulation of sleep-wake cycle by directly controlling the circadian rhythms and, consequently the bodily functions and activities. Thus, daily and seasonal rhythms of changing melatonin are quite informative for time of day and time of year, serving as a bioclock or a physiological pacemaker in vertebrates [1].

The first precursor of melatonin biosynthesis is the amino acid tryptophan, in which after several enzymatic steps including hydroxylation, decarboxylation, N-acetylation and O-methylation, the melatonin is formed. During melatonin synthesis, two important enzymes are required; the arylalkylamine N-acetyltransferase (AA-NAT) and the hydroxyindole O-methyltransferase (HIOMT). Over the past years, AA-NAT was considered the rate-limiting enzyme during melatonin synthesis, because its activity is synchronized with the circadian rhythm at pineal gland level [2, 3]. More recently, direct or indirect evidences have pointed HIOMT as a rate-limiting enzyme for melatonin synthesis [4]. In pinealocytes, β-adrenergic receptors activate G-protein subunits which, in turn, stimulate adenylate cyclase activity. When activated, both α_1-adrenergic and β-adrenergic receptors cause elevation in Ca^{+2} activity, and consecutively the activation of prostaglandins and protein kinase C (PKC) [5]. Ultimately, protein kinase up-regulates nuclear CREB gene, responsible for driving the production of N-acetyltransferase [6].

Distribution and Cellular Responsiveness

Melatonin was believed to be only synthetized by the pineal gland. Nowadays, it is well recognized a variety of extrapineal tissues and organs capable of producing melatonin. These include retina, lens, ciliary body, skin, brain regions, thymus, bone marrow, gut, ovary, testicle, placenta and lymphocytes [7]. Although extrapineal melatonin is largely produced, it appears not to contribute in the regulation of circadian rhythm (no function as a chemical signal of light/dark cycle). In contrast, surgical removal of pineal gland, or even chemical pinealectomy, caused a severe reduction in melatonin levels [8]. Tan et al. [9] stated that extrapineal melatonin is locally consumed by the surrounding tissues as a protective mechanism against oxidative damage, since it has antioxidant and anti-inflammatory properties [10].

Table 1. Representation of the well-known melatonin receptors (MT1, MT2 and MT3) and their activities in nervous system and other peripheral tissues and cells

Tissues/cells	*Melatonin Receptors*		
	MT1	MT2	MT3
Hypothalamus	+	+	–
Pituitary	+	–	–
Suprachiasmatic nucleus	–	–	–
Retina	–	+	+
Vasoconstriction/dilatation	+	+	–
Insulin/leptin secretion	+	–	–
Immune cells	+	+	+
Adrenal cortex	+	–	–
Testes	+	–	–
Ovary	+	–	–

Positive and negative signal (+/-) indicates presence or absence of the melatonin receptor subtype, respectively, in the specific tissues/cells.

MT1: melatonin receptor-subtype 1; MT2: melatonin receptor-subtype 2; MT3: melatonin receptor-subtype 3.

In addition, extrapineal melatonin might be bound to melatonin-binding proteins for both inhibition and storage. Differential interactions between melatonin and its receptors was facilitated after the discovery of the radioligand 2-[$_{125}$I]-iodomelatonin [11]. The physiological actions of melatonin are mediated via two G-protein-coupled MT(1) and MT(2) receptors, with low picomolar (MT1) and low nanomolar (MT2) affinities, respectively [12]. MT3, formerly known as Melc, is a non-mammalian melatonin receptor similar to human enzyme quinone reductase [13]. These receptors present unique molecular and pharmacological characteristics [14, 15]. MT1 and MT2 receptors are consisted of 350 and 362 amino acids, respectively, and they have glycosylation sites in N-terminus for protein kinase C (PKC) and protein kinase A (PKA) phosphorylation [16]. Also, MT1 and MT2 share a NRY motif in intracellular loop II of G protein-coupled receptor, which is involved in trafficking and cell signaling [17].

Taken overall, the tissues expressing both MT1 and MT2 proteins include suprachiasmatic nucleus, pars tuberalis, arteries, retina, pancreas, kidney, adrenal, testis and immune cells. Table 1 summarizes the action sites of the three melatonin receptors (MT1, MT2 and MT3) already described in different tissues and cells.

Melatonin: Metabolism and Degradation

Melatonin is metabolized in the liver, where it is first hydroxylated at the C6 position by cytochrome P450 mono-oxygenases, (isoenzymes CYP1A2, CYP1A1, and to a lesser extent CYP1B1) and then conjugated with sulfate to be excreted as 6-sulfatoxymelatonin [18].

Moreover, melatonin can be metabolized by a non-enzymatic process in all cells, and curiously at extracellular level, by several free radicals and other oxidants. It is converted into cyclic-3-hydroxy melatonin when directly scavenges 2 hydroxyl radicals. The so called N1-acetyl-N2-formyl-5-methoxykynuramine (AFMK) has been investigated as one of melatonin's metabolites. AFMK seems to be the central metabolite derived from melatonin oxidation in non-hepatic tissues [19]. Importantly, the kynurenic pathway of melatonin derivatives includes a series of possible free radical scavengers following the sequence: melatonin → cyclic 3-hydroxymelatonin → AFMK → AMK (N-acetyl-5-methoxykynuramine).

Oxidative Stress: A Brief Overview

The maintenance of the cell "redox state" homeostasis is extremely necessary in order to enable the life. In all living organisms, oxidative stress results from intensive metabolic reactions that utilize oxygen, and because of that, represents a disturbance in the equilibrium of pro-oxidant/antioxidant status.

The exceeding ROS (reactive oxygen species) can lead to irreversible damage in cellular lipids (lipid peroxidation), protein (protein oxidation), DNA (DNA oxidation), thereby affecting their normal function. Oxidative stress has gained focus in an attempt to explain a number of human diseases including cancer and related malignancies, chronic inflammation, metabolic diseases and the ageing process.

Free radicals can be defined as molecules or fragments that contain one or more unpaired electrons on its atomic orbitals [20]. A lack of electron(s) usually promotes its instability and gives a considerable degree of reactivity to these radicals. ROS as well as reactive nitrogen species (RNS) are products of cellular metabolism. Both ROS and RNS play a dual role having deleterious and beneficial effects on organic systems [21]. Beneficial effects include physiological roles in response to anoxia against infectious agent, during activation of cell signaling systems, and at low concentration to induce mitogenic responses.

The reactive radicals derived from oxygen molecule that can be formed into the cells include peroxyl (ROO•), superoxide anion (O_2•−), hydroxyl (•OH), hydrogen peroxide (H_2O_2), alkoxyl (LO•) radicals and others [21]. For radicals derived from nitrogen molecule, NO• is a small molecule that contains unpaired electron on the *y* orbital. NO• is formed in biological tissues by specific nitric oxide synthases (NOS), which converts arginine into citrulline. Generally, nitric oxide and superoxide anion react to produce a very powerful oxidative molecule, the peroxynitrite anion (ONOO−), which can cause DNA fragmentation and lipid oxidation [22].

The hydroxyl radical (•OH), is a neutral form of the hydroxide ion, and has a high capacity of reactivity, making it a very dangerous radical presenting a short half-life of approximately 10^{-9} s [23]. •OH reacts to its local formation and is maintained within a strict physiological interval.

Free Radicals and Melatonin

Melatonin has shown unquestionable effects on reducing lipid peroxidation and DNA degradation. Regarding to DNA oxidation, a dual effect of melatonin scavenging free radicals and/or activating DNA reparation enzymes is recognized [24].

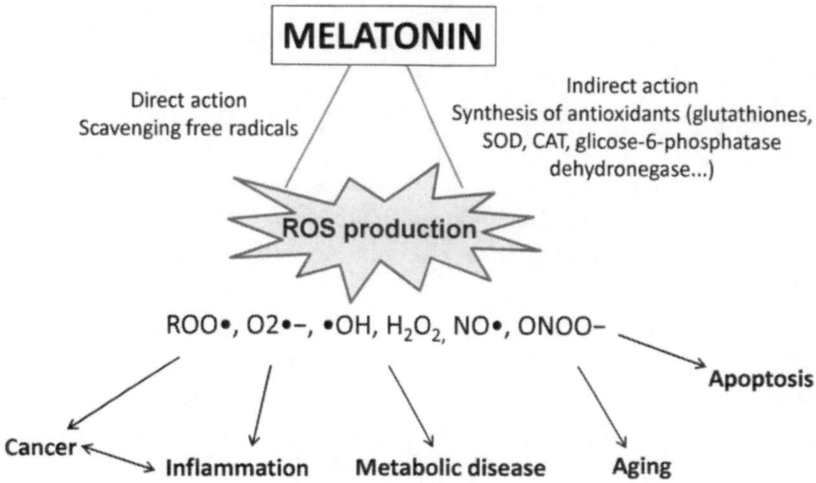

Figure 1. Melatonin' actions as natural antioxidant on ROS generation and potential applications in some human diseases. SOD: superoxide dismutase, CAT: catalase, ROS: reactive oxygen species, ROO•: lipid hydroperoxide, O2•–: superoxide anion, •OH: hydroxyl radical, H_2O_2: hydrogen peroxide, NO•: nitric oxide, ONOO–: nitrite peroxide.

This property confers to melatonin an advantage compared to other antioxidants in which their action is limited to the solubility partitioning between extra- and intra-cellular compartments. Melatonin is therefore highly dependent on its lipidic and aqueous phases.

Several indole derivatives similar to melatonin, such as 5-hydroxytryptophol, 5-hydroxytryptophan, 5-methoxytryptophol, pinoline (6-methoxy-1,2,3,4-tetrahydro-beta-carboline), 5-methoxytryptamine, and tryptoline (1,2,3,4-tetrahydro-beta-carboline) also exert their antioxidant activity [25, 26]. The powerful role of melatonin in preventing cell damage arising from reactive oxygen species is undisputable. Melatonin promote its direct effect by neutralizing hydroxyl radicals, hydrogen peroxide, hypochlorus acid, superoxide anion radical, singlet oxygen and others [26-30], see Figure 1.

Furthermore, it has been documented that melatonin stimulates both activities and expressions of antioxidant enzymes, i.e., superoxide dismutase, catalase, glutathione peroxidase, glutathione reductase, glucose-6-phosphate dehydrogenase, the high activity in which represent the main source of NADPH production, an essential substrate for glutathione reductase activity (Figure 1). It stimulates the glutathione production by cells [27, 31] when activating the γ-glutamylcysteine synthase, an enzyme responsible for glutathione synthesis, and also promotes the conversion of oxidized glutathione (GSSG) into its reduced form

(GSH) by glutathione reductase. Conversely, melatonin also inhibits the activity of pro-oxidant enzymes such as nitric oxide synthase and aminolevulinate synthase [32]

Additionally, N-acetylserotonin, a direct precursor of melatonin, has shown a stronger antioxidant capacity than melatonin in an experimental condition [33].

Cancer, Free radicals and Melatonin

Clinical investigations have reported that circulating melatonin is depressed in patients with primary tumors including both endocrine-dependent (endometrial, mammary, and prostate cancer) and endocrine-independent tumors (gastric, lung, and colorectal cancer). This reduction is most pronounced in patients with advanced primary tumors in which a clear negative correlation with tumor-size and volume exists [34]. Melatonin is pointed to be an oncostatic agent since it has direct effect on cell proliferation and cytokine secretion [35, 36] In animals bearing carcinogen-induced tumors, melatonin therapy was efficient in reducing the number, size and incidence of tumors while increases tumor latency. It has been recognized that melatonin may inhibits the proliferation rate of tumor cells by acting on cell cycle regulation [35, 37], interaction with sex steroid-dependent tissue [36], and mainly via its antioxidant capacity as free-radical scavenger [38]. The human organism is well supported with immune and non-immune anticarcinogenic strategies for cancer. Many studies have implicated oxidative stress as participating in initiation, promotion, and progression of tumor [39]. Also, free radicals generated after carcinogen exposure or by metabolic changes may cause instability or damage on DNA structure, uncontrolled growth of tumor cells, resistance to chemotherapy, cell invasion and metastasis [40, 41].

The antineoplastic activity of melatonin has been extensively studied in both *in vivo* and *in vitro* models of carcinogenesis [41-43]. Besides acting as a free radical scavenger *per se*, melatonin exerts its effects by altering gene expression at physiological level and through immunomodulatory and anti-apoptotic effects [7]. Melatonin can modulate several estrogen-regulated proteins, inhibits the estrogen receptor (ER) gene activities, and arrests the metastatic potential of the cells [44]. Cellular mechanisms have been proposed to mediate the oncostatic effects of melatonin. One of them is related to suppression of linoleic acid uptake and consequently the conversion into 13-hydroxyoctadecadienoic acid, which strongly activates EGFR/MAPK mitogenic signaling [7]. Melatonin also exerts their oncostatic effects through stimulation of monocytes, macrophages, lymphocytes, and natural killer cells [45], enhancing mainly the production of IL-1, IL-6, TNF-α, and IL-12 by monocytes [46] and IL-2, IL-6, and IFN-γ from human mononuclear cells [47].

In tumor cells, melatonin is able to stimulate ROS formation [48], making them undergo apoptosis [49]. To date, this mechanism remains controversial since some authors claim that melatonin prevent apoptosis of tumor cells in vitro and in vivo [50, 51]. In addition, melatonin has been shown to induce apoptotic cell death through ROS generation in many cancer cells including human myeloid HL60, Jurkat, Molt-4 tumor cells [52], human colorectal cancer cells and lymphoma cells [53, 54]. In mice, daily melatonin reduces the weight and size of S-91 melanoma tumors, and inhibits "in vitro" cell proliferation. This properties was attributed to the increases in both catalase and glutathione peroxidase activities [55]. Despite melatonin has an attenuating effect on ROS production, its action in some tumor cells is completely opposite. The presence of ROS in cancer cells means that tumors are resistant under mild oxidative stress compared to normal cells, and this condition may potentially be explored therapeutically by drugs or agents that augment ROS levels or weaken their antioxidant defenses by cells. Thus, the melatonin treatment reduces effectively the antioxidant defenses depleting glutathione systems [56]. In accordance to Bejarano et al. melatonin disrupted mitochondrial function causing elevation of intracellular ROS [50]. The increased ROS appears to be one of the main effects to evoke apoptosis in cancer cells. Also, a persistent elevation of ROS and consecutive oxidative stress present in cancer cells may lead to oncogenic mutation by successive damages on DNA. This can result in mutant gene products that reduce the effectiveness of chemotherapeutic agents, mainly molecular targeted therapies [57].

Surprisingly, melatonin treatment enhances the viability of normal cells by increasing intracellular GSH concentrations at low pharmacological levels (1 μM – 10 nM), but in contrast, it can serve as pro-oxidant at high levels (1 – 0.1 mM) in human liver cancer and leukaemia [52, 58].

Signaling Pathways for Carcinogenesis, ROS and Melatonin

There are several potential consequences eliciting ROS-induced DNA damages that may result in mutagenic and genetic alterations linked to carcinogenesis initiation and cancer development. These genetic changes include those related to constitutively major signaling pathways, such as PI3K/Akt and MAP kinase pathways. Previous studies have showed that ROS, especially H_2O_2, can activate the MAP kinase signaling leading to consequent cellular proliferation [59, 60], Figure 2.

Furthermore, ROS can activate the cytosolic nuclear factor-κB (NFκB) in many cases [61], see Figure 2. It has been investigated how ROS can interact or cooperate with these genetic disturbances as a result of the MAP kinase and PI3K/Akt alterations, such as mutations in BRAF, Ras, PTEN, and PIK3CA, during promotion and progression of cancer pathogenesis [62;63]. In models of squamous cell carcinoma, the complex ROS/mTORC1 caused downregulation in both p21 and p27 levels, and also damaged DNA, indicating that inhibition of p21 and p27 might facilitate G1/S transition of cell cycle possibly leading to error-prone DNA replication [64].

More recently, NADPH oxidase inhibitors, which are responsible for attenuating ROS formation, have shown correlation with reduction of COX-2 expression, and ERK/JNK-AP1 pathways ameliorating bladder cancer cell development [65]. Environmental carcinogens, such as 4-(methylnitrosamino)-1-(3-pyridyl)-1-butanone (NNK), is able to elevate ROS, leading to Raf-independent ERK activation and subsequent induction of cell proliferation and DNA damage [66]. Melatonin has been useful for the treatment of immune diseases and cancer, as it reduces inflammatory injuries by blocking transcription factors and NFκB [67], thus reducing further ROS formation within the cells (Figure 2). In the same context, melatonin seems to inhibit the activation of inducible NO synthase (iNOS) and cyclooxygenase 2 (COX-2) both activated in chronic inflammation-related disorders [68], Figure 2. Melatonin decreases Sphingosine kinase 1 (SPHK1) activity, and suppressed phospho-Akt and vascular endothelial growth factor (VEGF) production in prostate cancer cells during hypoxia. Consistently, melatonin inhibits ROS generation in these cells under hypoxia [69]. There is compelling data showing the suppressive effects of melatonin on tumorigenesis [52, 70, 71], and the efficiency of melatonin treatment has been documented in patients with advanced cancer stages. A randomized controlled trial was conducted by Mills et al. (2005) in more than 620 different solid tumors considering its effects at 1 year survival. In this context, melatonin was able to reduce the risk of death after 1 year without any other adverse effect [72]. Also, a study involving women with metastatic breast cancer progressed in response to tamoxifen has proved that melatonin may promote tumor regression when given orally at doses of 20 mg/day, in the evening hours [73]. Melatonin at pharmacological levels (10(-3) m) induced apoptosis and suppressed cell proliferation in breast cancer.

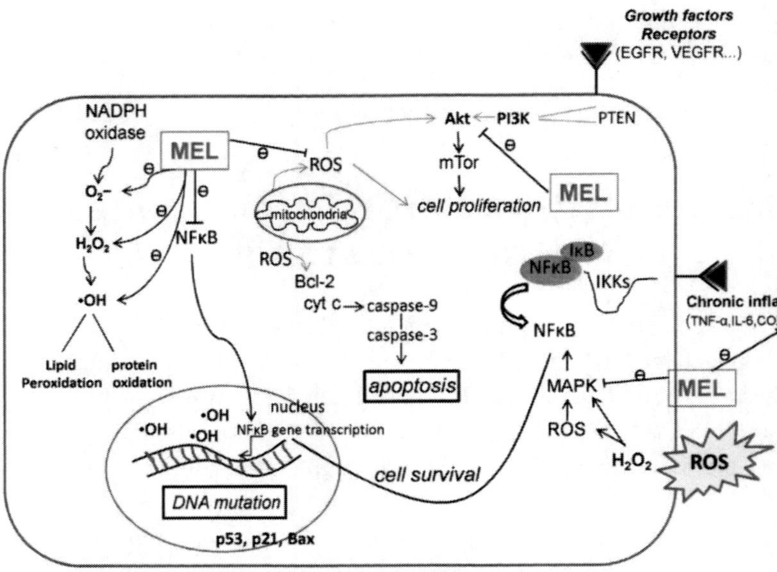

Figure 2. Differential signaling mechanisms by which the cell is activated depends on several molecular factors. Growth factors binding to their receptors may stimulate PI3K/Akt and mTOR pathways causing cell proliferation. The complex NADPH oxidase is the main source for ROS generation, where final •OH can be translocated into the nucleus damaging DNA structures and proteins related to tumor suppression, such as p53, p21, and Bax. Furthermore, mediators of cancer-linked chronic inflammation activates IKK complex, thus leading Iκβ to phosphorylation and consecutive liberation of NFκβ to regulate nuclear gene transcription (cell survival). ROS, especially H_2O_2, was seen to activate NFκβ via direct effect on MAPK pathways. Notably, an intense ROS production during mitochondria metabolism can undergo cellular apoptosis after sequestration of Bcl-2-like anti-apoptotic factor, allowing cyt c to activate the cascade of caspases. Importantly, melatonin exerts fundamental influence on these signaling pathways against cell damage and cell cycle deregulation. Melatonin directly neutralizes different ROS arising from external or internal part of the cell. Melatonin can reduces cancer-related inflammatory injuries by blocking NFκβ further reducing ROS formation, and it can also inhibit both MAPK and PI3K/Akt signaling, and the activity of many inflammatory mediators (iNOS, COX-2, IL-6, and TNF-α). MAPK: mitogen-activated protein kinase; NFκβ: nuclear factor-κβ; Iκβ: NFκβ transcription factor inhibitor; IKK: Iκβ kinase, mTOR: mammalian target of rapamycin; PTEN: phosphatase and tensin homolog (tumor suppressor gene); p53-p21,Bax: tumor suppressor proteins; ROS: reactive oxygen species; TNF-α: tumoral necrosis factor; IL-6: interleukin 6; COX 2: cyclooxygenase 2; iNOS: inducible nitric oxide synthase; EGFR: epidermal growth factor receptor; VEGFR: vascular endothelial growth factor receptor; O_2^-: superoxide anion; •OH: hydroxyl radical; H_2O_2: hydrogen peroxide; MEL: melatonin; ϴ: inhibitory action by melatonin.

The reduction of proliferation rate was accompanied by inhibition of COX-2 expression and prostaglandin E(2) production, and NFκB signaling. Moreover, melatonin blocked phosphorylation of PI3K, Akt, PRAS40, and GSK-3 proteins, thereby inactivating the PI3K/Akt pathway.

Furthermore, melatonin induced Apaf-1 expression, and stimulated caspase-3 and caspase-9 activities, leading to activation of the classical Apaf1-dependent apoptotic pathway [74].

Breast Cancer, ROS and Melatonin

Breast cancer is one of the most frequently leading causes of death among women aged 40 to 55 years [75]. The numerous risk factors are age, hormonal imbalance, genetic characteristics, augment in estradiol/ER-α ratio, ionizing radiation-related oxidative damages, and others [76]. Recently, studies have hypothesized that the increased risks for breast cancer involving night shift work (night workers, nurses, flight attendants) is due to high bright light-exposure, and consequent inhibition of melatonin secretion [77-80]. Notably, Cohen et al. suggested that a possible decline of melatonin production by pineal gland could promote hyperestrogenism, a highly relevant condition for developing breast cancer [81].

Melatonin treatment has antiproliferative and oncostatic actions to breast cancer, since it functions as antagonist of estradiol-induced cell proliferation and invasion [71]. At low concentrations, melatonin increases expression of p53, p21 and reduces the binding of estradiol-ER-α-calmodulin complex to DNA, besides the activity of aromatase. In breast cancer bearing-animal, melatonin was able to increase activities of catalase, glutathione peroxidase, and superoxide dismutase while cause a reduction of malondialdehyde, NO levels and NO synthase [82]. Lee et al. (2012) have provided aberrant DNA methylation in human breast cancer cell lines, and melatonin treatment led to down-regulation in oncogenic genes (EGR3 and POU4F2/Brn-3b), and up-regulation of tumor suppressor gene GPC3 suggesting a potential mechanism of its anticancer effects [83]. Also, the clinical utility of melatonin depends on their properties as an excellent adjuvant associated with drugs currently used for breast cancer prevention (antiaromatases and antiestrogens). In addition, the antioxidant actions of melatonin represent a suitable strategy to reduce oxidative damage arising from chemotherapy, especially radiotherapy and anthracyclines treatment [84]. Briefly, melatonin can prevent or inhibit the development of breast cancer.

Prostate Cancer, ROS and Melatonin

Prostate cancer is a common malignancy among men and the second leading cause of death in USA [85]. The risk factors are associated with aging, ethnical factors, hormone disturbances, dietary components, and family history [86]. There are several molecular targets that have been implicated as survival booster for prostate cancer, such as Bcl-2 and COX-2 overexpression, increased ROS formation, altered androgen receptor signaling, mutation of p53, elevation in expression of inhibitor apoptosis protein (IAP), NFκB, and AP-1 [87, 88].

Generally, patients with prostate cancer exhibit a lower level of melatonin than those age-matched controls, and furthermore, melatonin reduces the cell growth of hormone-dependent and -refractory human prostate cancer [89]. A recent study showed that melatonin treatment almost doubles the total GSH content in LNCaP and PC3 *in vitro* cells [88]. Also, pre-incubation with melatonin prevented significantly the toxicity by chemotherapeutic agents. More importantly, after depleting GSH content by chemotherapy, the PC3 cells had increased DNA fragmentation during c-radiation treatment, and melatonin prevented completely this condition. In prostate cancer, melatonin inhibited the DNA binding to NFκB via MT(1) receptor-induced PKA and PKC stimulation, and upregulated p27(kip1) transcription consequently causing cell antiproliferation. Notably, MT1-mediated inhibition of activated NFκB provides a novel mechanism for melatonin treatment in prostate cancer chemoprevention and chemotherapy [90].

Colorectal Cancer, ROS and Melatonin

Patients with colorectal carcinoma exhibit a great amplitude of melatonin peak and elevation in nocturnal plasma melatonin [91]. Consistently, the high concentrations of melatonin in the colon enhance the capacity of scavenging free radicals generated from intense cellular metabolism, and stimulate the immune response. Melatonin plays a protective role against the invasiveness and advanced stages of colorectal carcinoma whose pathogenesis involves damages due high levels of reactive oxygen metabolites. The actions of melatonin as scavenger of free radicals were experimentally demonstrated in models of colitis and ulcers [92, 93] where instillation of melatonin significantly decreased lipid peroxidation and the appearance of nitrotyrosine (Cuzzocrea et al. 2001), a biomarker of nitrosative stress, in colonic mucosa. These effects were linked to a direct scavenging of peroxynitrite molecules [94].

Previous studies confirmed that administration of melatonin ameliorates colitis through downregulation of the enzymes iNOS and COX-2 [95, 96], as well as reducing PGE2 and NO content [96]. In addition, short-term melatonin successfully reduces the myeloperoxidase (MPO) activity and attenuates the TNF-α production, both positively influenced by the development of colitis [97].

Liver Cancer, ROS and Melatonin

Hepatocellular carcinoma (HCC) is the most frequent form of liver cancer and chronic infection with hepatitis C virus associated with alcoholism is the main risk factor for developing HCC [98]. An increased production of ROS has been documented both in humans and animal model of liver disease [99, 100]. These early events enhance the progression of the disease by a build-up of DNA oxidative damage in patients with cirrhosis and chronic hepatitis [101, 102]. Cardin et al. found that in hepatocellular carcinoma, the high miR-92 expression is positively correlated with telomerase activity, 8-hydroxydeoxyguanosine (8-OHdG) levels, and Bad/Bax mRNA expression [103].

Dewa et al. have demonstrated that ROS production linked to increased level of DNA oxidation, as well as lipid and protein oxidation, might be involved in the liver cancer-promoting mechanism [104]. In many cancer types, including liver cancer, ROS interact with NF-κB signaling, and the transcription of NF-κB-dependent genes stimulates ROS in the cell.

In this context, transforming cells can use ROS signals to induce cell proliferation and tumor progression. Notably, exacerbated ROS production beyond a considerable threshold makes cancer cells undergo apoptosis. Thus, melatonin-like therapeutic agents that either promote ROS generation or reduce the antioxidant defenses in cancer cells represent the potential to kill these cells with little damage on normal cells [105]. Nishimura et al. have been reported "in vitro" that melatonin may also prevent HCC by decreasing NADPH-dependent ROS formation in hepatic microsomes [106].

Pancreas Cancer, ROS and Melatonin

Pancreatic cancer is the fourth most common cause of death in the USA [107]. Recent reports have indicated that general phytochemicals targeting ROS metabolism may selectively kill the tumor cells when ROS generation reach a toxic threshold. In order to better understanding this aggressive cancer type, several molecular inhibitors of tumor growth has been extensively studied (COX-2 and tyrosine kinase inhibitors, farnesyl transferase and matrix metalloproteinase (MMPs) inhibitors [108].

Lipid peroxidation (LPO) is associated with the promotion of pancreatic cancer [109]. Melatonin reduced lipid peroxidation (LPO) in pancreatic cancer-bearing animal, and after 24 weeks of administration, LPO levels returned to those of control animals [110]. In a model of pancreatic carcinogenesis, a significant depletion of GSH, catalase, SOD and GSH-Px were found, and conversely, melatonin treatment recovered the whole antioxidant status. Although a strong relationship exists between oxidative stress and cancer, additional studies will help to clarify more precisely the antioxidant action of melatonin underlying anti-tumoral mechanisms in pancreatic cancer [110].

Conclusion

Oxygen is indispensable for obtaining energy during the aerobic process, and the natural metabolism enables the cell to generate ROS. Overproduction of ROS is thought to play detrimental effects in the development of several cancer types mainly through the induction of oxidative DNA damage or by altering the cell cycle regulation. Some drug therapies have reached antitumor effects via ROS-dependent activation of apoptotic cell death, suggesting the ROS as an antitumor strategy. Melatonin treatment has drawn attention serving as direct scavenger of free radicals or stimulating a number of antioxidant defenses in health cells. Otherwise, melatonin can promote exacerbated ROS productions leading to cancer cell death. Administration of melatonin has shown not only a promising role on the inhibition of numerous cancer pathways by its oncostatic properties, but also improvements in quality of life and functional status in patients suffering from aggressive cancers, such as breast, prostate, colorectal, liver, and pancreas cancer. Briefly, melatonin may be useful into the integrative aspects of cancer therapy either as a unique agent or in combination with other standard therapies.

References

[1] Reiter R.J. The melatonin rhythm: both a clock and a calendar. *Experientia*, 1993 Aug 15;49(8):654-64.

[2] Foulkes N.S, Borjigin J, Snyder S.H, Sassone-Corsi P. Rhythmic transcription: the molecular basis of circadian melatonin synthesis. *Trends Neurosci.,* 1997 Oct;20(10):487-92.

[3] Karolczak M, Korf H.W, Stehle J.H. The rhythm and blues of gene expression in the rodent pineal gland. *Endocrine,* 2005 Jul;27(2):89-100.

[4] Ribelayga C, Pevet P, Simonneaux V. HIOMT drives the photoperiodic changes in the amplitude of the melatonin peak of the Siberian hamster. *Am. J. Physiol. Regul. Integr. Comp. Physiol.,* 2000 May;278(5):R1339-R1345.

[5] Krause D.N, Dubocovich M.L. Regulatory sites in the melatonin system of mammals. *Trends Neurosci.,* 1990 Nov;13(11):464-70.

[6] Klein D.C. Photoneural regulation of the mammalian pineal gland. *Ciba. Found. Symp.,* 1985;117:38-56.

[7] Srinivasan V, Spence D.W, Pandi-Perumal S.R, Trakht I, Cardinali D.P. Therapeutic actions of melatonin in cancer: possible mechanisms. *Integr. Cancer Ther.*, 2008 Sep;7(3):189-203.

[8] Vakkuri O, Rintamaki H, Leppaluoto J. Plasma and tissue concentrations of melatonin after midnight light exposure and pinealectomy in the pigeon 4. *J. Endocrinol.,* 1985 May;105(2):263-8.

[9] Tan D.X, Manchester L.C, Terron M.P, Flores L.J, Tamura H, Reiter R.J. Melatonin as a naturally occurring co-substrate of quinone reductase-2, the putative MT3 melatonin membrane receptor: hypothesis and significance. *J. Pineal. Res.,* 2007 Nov;43(4): 317-20.

[10] Rodriguez C, Mayo J.C, Sainz R.M, Antolin I, Herrera F, Martin V, et al. Regulation of antioxidant enzymes: a significant role for melatonin. *J. Pineal. Res.,* 2004 Jan;36(1):1-9.

[11] Dubocovich M.L, Takahashi J.S. Use of 2-[125I]iodomelatonin to characterize melatonin binding sites in chicken retina. *Proc. Natl. Acad. Sci. USA,* 1987 Jun;84(11):3916-20.

[12] Dubocovich M.L. Melatonin receptors: are there multiple subtypes?. *Trends Pharmacol. Sci.,* 1995 Feb;16(2):50-6.

[13] Nosjean O, Ferro M, Coge F, Beauverger P, Henlin J.M, Lefoulon F, et al. Identification of the melatonin-binding site MT3 as the quinone reductase 2. *J. Biol. Chem.,* 2000 Oct 6;275(40):31311-7.

[14] Dubocovich M.L, Masana M.I, Iacob S, Sauri D.M. Melatonin receptor antagonists that differentiate between the human Mel1a and Mel1b recombinant subtypes are used to assess the pharmacological profile of the rabbit retina ML1 presynaptic heteroreceptor. *Naunyn. Schmiedebergs Arch. Pharmacol.,* 1997 Mar;355(3):365-75.

[15] Reppert S.M, Weaver D.R, Godson C. Melatonin receptors step into the light: cloning and classification of subtypes. *Trends Pharmacol. Sci.,* 1996 Mar;17(3):100-2.

[16] Ferguson S.S. Evolving concepts in G protein-coupled receptor endocytosis: the role in receptor desensitization and signaling9. *Pharmacol. Rev.,* 2001 Mar;53(1):1-24.

[17] Nelson C.S, Ikeda M, Gompf H.S, Robinson M.L, Fuchs N.K, Yoshioka T, et al. Regulation of melatonin 1a receptor signaling and trafficking by asparagine-124. *Mol. Endocrinol.*, 2001 Aug;15(8):1306-17.

[18] Claustrat B, Brun J, Chazot G. The basic physiology and pathophysiology of melatonin. Sleep Med Rev 2005 Feb;9(1):11-24.

[19] Hardeland R. Antioxidative protection by melatonin: multiplicity of mechanisms from radical detoxification to radical avoidance. *Endocrine.*, 2005 Jul;27(2):119-30.

[20] Halliwell B, Zhao K, Whiteman M. Nitric oxide and peroxynitrite. The ugly, the uglier and the not so good: a personal view of recent controversies. *Free Radic. Res.*, 1999 Dec;31(6):651-69.

[21] Valko M, Rhodes C.J, Moncol J, Izakovic M, Mazur M. Free radicals, metals and antioxidants in oxidative stress-induced cancer. *Chem. Biol. Interact., 2006* Mar 10;160(1):1-40.

[22] Carr A.C, McCall M.R, Frei B. Oxidation of LDL by myeloperoxidase and reactive nitrogen species: reaction pathways and antioxidant protection. *Arterioscler. Thromb. Vasc. Biol.*, 2000 Jul;20(7):1716-23.

[23] Pastor N, Weinstein H, Jamison E, Brenowitz M. A detailed interpretation of OH radical footprints in a TBP-DNA complex reveals the role of dynamics in the mechanism of sequence-specific binding. *J. Mol. Biol.*, 2000 Nov 17;304(1):55-68.

[24] Vijayalaxmi, Reiter R.J, Herman T.S, Meltz M.L. Melatonin reduces gamma radiation-induced primary DNA damage in human blood lymphocytes. *Mutat. Res.*, 1998 Feb 2;397(2):203-8.

[25] Keithahn C, Lerchl A. 5-hydroxytryptophan is a more potent in vitro hydroxyl radical scavenger than melatonin or vitamin C. *J. Pineal. Res.*, 2005 Jan;38(1):62-6.

[26] Millan-Plano S, Piedrafita E, Miana-Mena F.J, Fuentes-Broto L, Martinez-Ballarin E, Lopez-Pingarron L, et al. Melatonin and structurally-related compounds protect synaptosomal membranes from free radical damage. *Int. J. Mol. Sci.*, 2010;11(1): 312-28.

[27] Chuffa L.G, Amorim J.P, Teixeira G.R, Mendes L.O, Fioruci B.A, Pinheiro P.F, et al. Long-term melatonin treatment reduces ovarian mass and enhances tissue antioxidant defenses during ovulation in the rat. *Braz. J. Med. Biol. Res.*, 2011 Mar;44(3):217-23.

[28] Chuffa L.G, Amorim J.P, Teixeira G.R, Mendes L.O, Fioruci B.A, Pinheiro PF, et al. Long-term exogenous melatonin treatment modulates overall feed efficiency and protects ovarian tissue against injuries caused by ethanol-induced oxidative stress in adult UChB rats. *Alcohol. Clin. Exp. Res.*, 2011 Aug;35(8):1498-508.

[29] Stasica P, Ulanski P, Rosiak J.M. Melatonin as a hydroxyl radical scavenger. *J. Pineal. Res.*, 1998 Aug;25(1):65-6.

[30] Ximenes V.F, Silva S.O, Rodrigues M.R, Catalani L.H, Maghzal G.J, Kettle A.J, et al. Superoxide-dependent oxidation of melatonin by myeloperoxidase 5. *J. Biol. Chem.*, 2005 Nov 18;280(46):38160-9.

[31] Winiarska K, Fraczyk T, Malinska D, Drozak J, Bryla J. Melatonin attenuates diabetes-induced oxidative stress in rabbits. *J. Pineal. Res.*, 2006 Mar;40(2):168-76.

[32] Pozo D, Reiter R.J, Calvo J.R, Guerrero J.M. Inhibition of cerebellar nitric oxide synthase and cyclic GMP production by melatonin via complex formation with calmodulin. *J. Cell Biochem.*, 1997 Jun 1;65(3):430-42.

[33] Stuss M, Wiktorska J.A, Sewerynek E. N-acetylserotonin reduces lipopolysaccharide-induced lipid peroxidation in vitro more effectively than melatonin. *Neuro Endocrinol. Lett.,* 2010;31(4):489-96.

[34] Bartsch C, Bartsch H. Melatonin in cancer patients and in tumor-bearing animals. *Adv. Exp. Med. Biol.,* 1999;467:247-64.

[35] Feletou M, Vanhoutte PM. Endothelial dysfunction: a multifaceted disorder (The Wiggers Award Lecture). *Am. J. Physiol. Heart Circ. Physiol.,* 2006 Sep;291(3):H985-1002.

[36] Kilic E, Kilic U, Reiter R.J, Bassetti C.L, Hermann D.M. Prophylactic use of melatonin protects against focal cerebral ischemia in mice: role of endothelin converting enzyme-1. *J. Pineal. Res.,* 2004 Nov;37(4):247-51.

[37] Maestroni G.J. The immunotherapeutic potential of melatonin. *Expert Opin. Investig. Drugs,* 2001 Mar;10(3):467-76.

[38] Carrillo-Vico A, Guerrero J.M, Lardone PJ, Reiter R.J. A review of the multiple actions of melatonin on the immune system. *Endocrine,* 2005 Jul;27(2):189-200.

[39] Klaunig J.E, Xu Y, Isenberg J.S, Bachowski S, Kolaja K.L, Jiang J, et al. The role of oxidative stress in chemical carcinogenesis. *Environ. Health Perspect.,* 1998 Feb;106 Suppl 1:289-95.

[40] Jakobisiak M, Lasek W, Golab J. Natural mechanisms protecting against cancer. *Immunol. Lett.,* 2003 Dec 15;90(2-3):103-22.

[41] Karbownik M, Lewinski A, Reiter R.J. Anticarcinogenic actions of melatonin which involve antioxidative processes: comparison with other antioxidants. *Int. J. Biochem. Cell Biol.,* 2001 Aug;33(8):735-53.

[42] Blask D.E, Sauer L.A, Dauchy R.T, Holowachuk E.W, Ruhoff MS. New insights into melatonin regulation of cancer growth. *Adv. Exp. Med. Biol.,* 1999;460:337-43.

[43] Karasek M, Pawlikowski M. Antiproliferative effects of melatonin and CGP 52608. *Biol. Signals Recept.,* 1999 Jan;8(1-2):75-8.

[44] Srinivasan V, Pandi-Perumal S.R, Trahkt I, Spence DW, Poeggeler B, Hardeland R, et al. Melatonin and melatonergic drugs on sleep: possible mechanisms of action. *Int. J. Neurosci.,* 2009;119(6):821-46.

[45] Martins E Jr, Fernandes L.C, Bartol I, Cipolla-Neto J, Costa Rosa L.F. The effect of melatonin chronic treatment upon macrophage and lymphocyte metabolism and function in Walker-256 tumour-bearing rats. *J. Neuroimmunol.,* 1998 Feb;82(1):81-9.

[46] Morrey K.M, McLachlan J.A, Serkin C.D, Bakouche O. Activation of human monocytes by the pineal hormone melatonin. *J. Immunol.,* 1994 Sep 15;153(6): 2671-80.

[47] Garcia-Maurino S, Gonzalez-Haba M.G, Calvo J.R, Rafii-El-Idrissi M, Sanchez-Margalet V, Goberna R, et al. Melatonin enhances IL-2, IL-6, and IFN-gamma production by human circulating CD4+ cells: a possible nuclear receptor-mediated mechanism involving T helper type 1 lymphocytes and monocytes. *J. Immunol.,* 1997 Jul 15;159(2):574-81.

[48] Pirozhok I, Meye A, Hakenberg O.W, Fuessel S, Wirth M.P. Serotonin and melatonin do not play a prominent role in the growth of prostate cancer cell lines. *Urol. Int.,* 2010;84(4):452-60.

[49] Pawlikowski M, Winczyk K, Karasek M. Oncostatic action of melatonin: facts and question marks. *Neuro Endocrinol. Lett.,* 2002 Apr;23 Suppl 1:24-9.

[50] Bejarano I, Espino J, Marchena A.M, Barriga C, Paredes S.D, Rodriguez AB, et al. Melatonin enhances hydrogen peroxide-induced apoptosis in human promyelocytic leukaemia HL-60 cells. *Mol. Cell Biochem.,* 2011 Jul;353(1-2):167-76.

[51] Espino J, Bejarano I, Ortiz A, Lozano G.M, Garcia J.F, Pariente J.A, et al. Melatonin as a potential tool against oxidative damage and apoptosis in ejaculated human spermatozoa. *Fertil. Steril.,* 2010 Oct;94(5):1915-7.

[52] Buyukavci M, Ozdemir O, Buck S, Stout M, Ravindranath Y, Savasan S. Melatonin cytotoxicity in human leukemia cells: relation with its pro-oxidant effect. *Fundam. Clin. Pharmacol.,* 2006 Feb;20(1):73-9.

[53] Paternoster L, Radogna F, Accorsi A, Cristina A.M, Gualandi G, Ghibelli L. Melatonin as a modulator of apoptosis in B-lymphoma cells. *Ann. NY Acad. Sci.,* 2009 Aug;1171:345-9.

[54] Wenzel U, Nickel A, Daniel H. Melatonin potentiates flavone-induced apoptosis in human colon cancer cells by increasing the level of glycolytic end products. *Int. J. Cancer,* 2005 Aug 20;116(2):236-42.

[55] Kadekaro AL, Andrade L.N, Floeter-Winter L.M, Rollag M.D, Virador V, Vieira W, et al. MT-1 melatonin receptor expression increases the antiproliferative effect of melatonin on S-91 murine melanoma cells. *J. Pineal. Res.,* 2004 Apr;36(3):204-11.

[56] Albertini M.C, Radogna F, Accorsi A, Uguccioni F, Paternoster L, Cerella C, et al. Intracellular pro-oxidant activity of melatonin deprives U937 cells of reduced glutathione without affecting glutathione peroxidase activity. *Ann. NY Acad. Sci.,* 2006 Dec;1091:10-6.

[57] Wondrak G.T. Redox-directed cancer therapeutics: molecular mechanisms and opportunities. *Antioxid. Redox. Signal.,* 2009 Dec;11(12):3013-69.

[58] Osseni R.A, Rat P, Bogdan A, Warnet J.M, Touitou Y. Evidence of prooxidant and antioxidant action of melatonin on human liver cell line HepG2. *Life Sci.,* 2000 Dec 15;68(4):387-99.

[59] Aikawa R, Komuro I, Yamazaki T, Zou Y, Kudoh S, Tanaka M, et al. Oxidative stress activates extracellular signal-regulated kinases through Src and Ras in cultured cardiac myocytes of neonatal rats. *J. Clin. Invest.,* 1997 Oct 1;100(7):1813-21.

[60] Guyton K.Z, Gorospe M, Kensler T.W, Holbrook N.J. Mitogen-activated protein kinase (MAPK) activation by butylated hydroxytoluene hydroperoxide: implications for cellular survival and tumor promotion. *Cancer Res.,* 1996 Aug 1;56(15):3480-5.

[61] Durackova Z. Some current insights into oxidative stress. *Physiol. Res.,* 2010;59(4):459-69.

[62] Xing M. BRAF mutation in papillary thyroid cancer: pathogenic role, molecular bases, and clinical implications. *Endocr. Rev.,* 2007 Dec;28(7):742-62.

[63] Xing M. Genetic alterations in the phosphatidylinositol-3 kinase/Akt pathway in thyroid cancer. *Thyroid.,* 2010 Jul;20(7):697-706.

[64] Ji W.T, Yang S.R, Chen J.Y, Cheng Y.P, Lee Y.R, Chiang M.K, et al. Arecoline downregulates levels of p21 and p27 through the reactive oxygen species/mTOR complex 1 pathway and may contribute to oral squamous cell carcinoma. *Cancer Sci.,* 2012 Jul;103(7):1221-9.

[65] Chen C.C, Cheng Y.Y, Chen S.C, Tuan Y.F, Chen Y.J, Chen C.Y, et al. Cyclooxygenase-2 expression is up-regulated by 2-aminobiphenyl in a ROS and

MAPK-dependent signaling pathway in a bladder cancer cell line. *Chem. Res. Toxicol.,* 2012 Mar 19;25(3):695-705.

[66] Rathore K, Wang H.C. Green tea catechin extract in intervention of chronic breast cell carcinogenesis induced by environmental carcinogens. *Mol. Carcinog.,* 2012 Mar;51(3):280-9.

[67] Li J.H, Yu J.P, Yu H.G, Xu X.M, Yu L.L, Liu J, et al. Melatonin reduces inflammatory injury through inhibiting NF-kappaB activation in rats with colitis. *Mediators Inflamm.,* 2005 Aug 31;2005(4):185-93.

[68] Deng W.G, Tang S.T, Tseng H.P, Wu K.K. Melatonin suppresses macrophage cyclooxygenase-2 and inducible nitric oxide synthase expression by inhibiting p52 acetylation and binding. *Blood,* 2006 Jul 15;108(2):518-24.

[69] Cho S.Y, Lee H.J, Jeong S.J, Lee H.J, Kim H.S, Chen C.Y, et al. Sphingosine kinase 1 pathway is involved in melatonin-induced HIF-1alpha inactivation in hypoxic PC-3 prostate cancer cells. *J. Pineal. Res.,* 2011 Aug;51(1):87-93.

[70] Anisimov V.N, Popovich I.G, Zabezhinski M.A, Anisimov S.V, Vesnushkin G.M, Vinogradova I.A. Melatonin as antioxidant, geroprotector and anticarcinogen. *Biochim. Biophys. Acta.,* 2006 May;1757(5-6):573-89.

[71] Cos S, Blask D.E, Lemus-Wilson A, Hill A.B. Effects of melatonin on the cell cycle kinetics and "estrogen-rescue" of MCF-7 human breast cancer cells in culture. *J. Pineal. Res.,* 1991 Jan;10(1):36-42.

[72] Mills E, Wu P, Seely D, Guyatt G. Melatonin in the treatment of cancer: a systematic review of randomized controlled trials and meta-analysis. *J. Pineal. Res.,* 2005 Nov;39(4):360-6.

[73] Lissoni P, Barni S, Meregalli S, Fossati V, Cazzaniga M, Esposti D, et al. Modulation of cancer endocrine therapy by melatonin: a phase II study of tamoxifen plus melatonin in metastatic breast cancer patients progressing under tamoxifen alone. *Br. J. Cancer,*1995 Apr;71(4):854-6.

[74] Wang Y.M, Jin B.Z, Ai F, Duan C.H, Lu Y.Z, Dong T.F, et al. The efficacy and safety of melatonin in concurrent chemotherapy or radiotherapy for solid tumors: a meta-analysis of randomized controlled trials. Cancer *Chemother Pharmacol.,* 2012 May;69(5):1213-20.

[75] Parkin D.M. International variation. *Oncogene,* 2004 Aug 23;23(38):6329-40.

[76] Key T.J, Verkasalo P.K, Banks E. Epidemiology of breast cancer. *Lancet,* Oncol 2001 Mar;2(3):133-40.

[77] Lie J.A, Kjaerheim K. Cancer risk among female nurses: a literature review. *Eur. J. Cancer Prev.,* 2003 Dec;12(6):517-26.

[78] Pinheiro S.P, Schernhammer E.S, Tworoger S.S, Michels K.B. A prospective study on habitual duration of sleep and incidence of breast cancer in a large cohort of women. *Cancer Res.,* 2006 May 15;66(10):5521-5.

[79] Rafnsson V, Tulinius H, Jonasson J.G, Hrafnkelsson J. Risk of breast cancer in female flight attendants: a population-based study (Iceland). *Cancer Causes Control.,* 2001 Feb;12(2):95-101.

[80] Schernhammer E.S, Kroenke C.H, Laden F, Hankinson S.E. Night work and risk of breast cancer. *Epidemiology,* 2006 Jan;17(1):108-11.

[81] Cohen M, Lippman M, Chabner B. Role of pineal gland in aetiology and treatment of breast cancer. *Lancet,* 1978 Oct 14;2(8094):814-6.

[82] Moselhy SS, A.l mslmani M.A. Chemopreventive effect of lycopene alone or with melatonin against the genesis of oxidative stress and mammary tumors induced by 7,12 dimethyl(a)benzanthracene in sprague dawely female rats. *Mol. Cell Biochem.,* 2008 Dec;319(1-2):175-80.

[83] Lee S.E, Kim S.J, Yoon H.J, Yu S.Y, Yang H, Jeong S.I, et al. Genome-wide profiling in melatonin-exposed human breast cancer cell lines identifies differentially methylated genes involved in the anticancer effect of melatonin. *J. Pineal. Res.,* 2012 Jun 27.

[84] Sanchez-Barcelo E.J, Mediavilla M.D, Alonso-Gonzalez C, Reiter R.J. Melatonin uses in oncology: breast cancer prevention and reduction of the side effects of chemotherapy and radiation. *Expert. Opin. Investig. Drugs,* 2012 Jun;21(6):819-31.

[85] Jemal A, Murray T, Ward E, Samuels A, Tiwari R.C, Ghafoor A, et al. Cancer statistics, 2005. *CA Cancer J. Clin.,* 2005 Jan;55(1):10-30.

[86] Ross R.K, Pike M.C, Coetzee G.A, Reichardt J.K, Yu M.C, Feigelson H, et al. Androgen metabolism and prostate cancer: establishing a model of genetic susceptibility. *Cancer Res.,* 1998 Oct 15;58(20):4497-504.

[87] Krajewska M, Krajewski S, Banares S, Huang X, Turner B, Bubendorf L, et al. Elevated expression of inhibitor of apoptosis proteins in prostate cancer. *Clin. Cancer Res.,* 2003 Oct 15;9(13):4914-25.

[88] Sainz R.M, Reiter R.J, Tan D.X, Roldan F, Natarajan M, Quiros I, et al. Critical role of glutathione in melatonin enhancement of tumor necrosis factor and ionizing radiation-induced apoptosis in prostate cancer cells in vitro. *J. Pineal. Res.,* 2008 Oct;45(3):258-70.

[89] Sainz R.M, Mayo JC, Tan D.X, Leon J, Manchester L, Reiter R.J. Melatonin reduces prostate cancer cell growth leading to neuroendocrine differentiation via a receptor and PKA independent mechanism. *Prostate,* 2005 Apr 1;63(1):29-43.

[90] Shiu S.Y, Leung W.Y, Tam C.W, Liu V.W, Yao K.M. Melatonin MT(1) receptor-induced transcriptional up-regulation of p27(Kip1) in prostate cancer antiproliferation is mediated via inhibition of constitutively active nuclear factor kappa B (NF-kappaB): potential implications on prostate cancer chemoprevention and therapy. *J. Pineal. Res.,* 2012 Jun 20.

[91] Vician M, Zeman M, Herichova I, Jurani M, Blazicek P, Matis P. Melatonin content in plasma and large intestine of patients with colorectal carcinoma before and after surgery. *J. Pineal. Res.,* 1999 Oct;27(3):164-9.

[92] Ganguly K, Sharma A.V, Reiter R.J, Swarnakar S. Melatonin promotes angiogenesis during protection and healing of indomethacin-induced gastric ulcer: role of matrix metaloproteinase-2. *J. Pineal. Res.,* 2010 Sep;49(2):130-40.

[93] Pentney P.T, Bubenik G.A. Melatonin reduces the severity of dextran-induced colitis in mice. *J. Pineal. Res.,* 1995 Aug;19(1):31-9.

[94] Cuzzocrea S, Zingarelli B, Costantino G, Caputi A.P. Protective effect of melatonin in a non-septic shock model induced by zymosan in the rat. *J. Pineal. Res.,* 1998 Aug;25(1):24-33.

[95] Cuzzocrea S, Mazzon E, Serraino I, Lepore V, Terranova ML, Ciccolo A, et al. Melatonin reduces dinitrobenzene sulfonic acid-induced colitis. *J. Pineal. Res.,* 2001 Jan;30(1):1-12.

[96] Dong W.G, Mei Q, Yu J.P, Xu J.M, Xiang L, Xu Y. Effects of melatonin on the expression of iNOS and COX-2 in rat models of colitis. *World J. Gastroenterol.,* 2003 Jun;9(6):1307-11.

[97] Marquez E, Sanchez-Fidalgo S, Calvo J.R, la de Lastra C.A, Motilva V. Acutely administered melatonin is beneficial while chronic melatonin treatment aggravates the evolution of TNBS-induced colitis. *J. Pineal. Res.,* 2006 Jan;40(1):48-55.

[98] Kuske L, Mensen A, Mullhaupt B, Negro F, Semela D, Moradpour D, et al. Characteristics of patients with chronic hepatitis C who develop hepatocellular carcinoma. *Swiss Med. Wkly,* 2012;142:w13651.

[99] Sasaki Y. Does oxidative stress participate in the development of hepatocellular carcinoma?. *J. Gastroenterol.,* 2006 Dec;41(12):1135-48.

[100] Tsai WL, Chung RT. Viral hepatocarcinogenesis. *Oncogene,* 2010 Apr 22;29(16):2309-24.

[101] Farinati F, Cardin R, Bortolami M, Burra P, Russo F.P, Rugge M, et al. Hepatitis C virus: from oxygen free radicals to hepatocellular carcinoma. *J. Viral. Hepat.,* 2007 Dec;14(12):821-9.

[102] Fujita N, Horiike S, Sugimoto R, Tanaka H, Iwasa M, Kobayashi Y, et al. Hepatic oxidative DNA damage correlates with iron overload in chronic hepatitis C patients. *Free Radic. Biol. Med.,* 2007 Feb 1;42(3):353-62.

[103] Romilda C, Marika P, Alessandro S, Enrico L, Marina B, Andromachi K, et al. Oxidative DNA damage correlates with cell immortalization and mir-92 expression in hepatocellular carcinoma. *BMC Cancer,* 2012;12:177.

[104] Dewa Y, Nishimura J, Muguruma M, Jin M, Kawai M, Saegusa Y, et al. Involvement of oxidative stress in hepatocellular tumor-promoting activity of oxfendazole in rats. *Arch. Toxicol.,* 2009 May;83(5):503-11.

[105] Fang J, Nakamura H, Iyer A.K. Tumor-targeted induction of oxystress for cancer therapy. *J. Drug. Target.,* 2007 Aug;15(7-8):475-86.

[106] Nishimura J, Saegusa Y, Dewa Y, Jin M, Kawai M, Kemmochi S, et al. Antioxidant enzymatically modified isoquercitrin or melatonin supplementation reduces oxidative stress-mediated hepatocellular tumor promotion of oxfendazole in rats. *Arch. Toxicol.,* 2010 Feb;84(2):143-53.

[107] Tummala P, Junaidi O, Agarwal B. Imaging of pancreatic cancer: An overview. *J. Gastrointest. Oncol.,* 2011 Sep;2(3):168-74.

[108] Pino S.M, Xiong H.Q, McConkey D, Abbruzzese JL. Novel therapies for pancreatic adenocarcinoma. *Curr. Gastroenterol. Rep.,* 2004 Apr;6(2):119-25.

[109] Wenger FA, Kilian M, Jacobi C.A, Mautsch I, Peter F.J, Guski H, et al. Effects of octreotide on liver metastasis and intrametastatic lipid peroxidation in experimental pancreatic cancer. *Oncology,* 2001;60(3):282-8.

[110] Ruiz-Rabelo J.F, Vazquez R, Perea M.D, Cruz A, Gonzalez R, Romero A, et al. Beneficial properties of melatonin in an experimental model of pancreatic cancer. *J. Pineal. Res.,* 2007 Oct;43(3):270-5.

In: New Developments in Melatonin Research ISBN: 978-1-62618-843-3
Editors: D.Acuña-Castroviejo, I.Rusanova, G.Escames © 2013 Nova Science Publishers, Inc.

Chapter 8

The Importance of Melatonin in Ovaries of Higher Mammals

Or Friedman, Raoul Orvieto, Benjamin Fisch and Ronit Abir*

Infertility and IVF Unit, Beilinson Women Hospital, Rabin Medical Center, Petach Tikvah and Sackler School of Medicine, Tel Aviv University, Tel Aviv, and Infertility and IVF Unit, Department of Obstetrics and Gynecology, Barzilai Medical Center, Ashkelon and Faculty of Health science, Ben Gurion University of the Negev, Beer Sheva, Israel

Abstract

Melatonin is an endogenous mediator of photoperiod information and a molecular component of the circadian time-keeping system. In seasonal animals, melatonin synchronizes annual breeding via natural photoperiod signals. In humans, menstruation related psychopathologies have been linked to light and darkness and thereby, to melatonin. Melatonin acts on the ovary via the brain-hypothalamus-pituitary pathway and through its ovarian receptors. It is not only retained from the blood circulation, but also produced in the ovary; indeed levels of melatonin are higher in follicular fluid (correlated with follicular growth) than in serum. Melatonin regulates the expression of gonadotropin releasing hormone (GnRH) and receptor (GnRHR), which promotes the maintenance of corpus luteus in pregnancy, and the release of follicle stimulating hormone (FSH) and luteinzing hormone (LH), influencing their effect on follicular growth, ovulation, luteinization. Melatonin also alters steioroidogenesis in various mammals including humans, in a species-dependent manner. Additionally melatonin exerts antioxidant activity, protecting the ovulating oocyte from free radical damage and abolishing H2O2 inhibition on progesterone production. Accordingly it is apparently involved in various

* Corresponding author: Ronit Abir, Ph.D, Infertility and IVF Unit, Beilinson's Women Hospital, Rabin Medical Center, Petach Tikva, 49100, Israel, Fax: 972 3 9376608; Email: ronita@clalit.org.il.

infertility conditions with oxidative stress, such as PCOS and endometriosis. Melatonin holds promise in the treatment of luteal phase defects and as a supplement to the *in vitro* maturation culture medium of germinal-vesicle-stage oocytes. Melatonin also holds promise in the preservation/restoration of fertility in cancer patients and may also protect ovarian follicles against radio/chemotherapy damage. Further clinical studies are needed to increase our understanding of the reproductive role of melatonin in higher mammals which may open new horizons for ovarian infertility management.

Introduction

I. Melatonin and Its Receptors

Melatonin (N-acetyl-5-methoxytryptamine) is a small, lipophylic molecule derived from the amino acid tryptophan. Tryptophan is transformed into 5-hydroxytryptophan by the mitochondrial enzyme tryptophan-5-hydroxylase [1]. 5-Hydroxytryptophan is, in turn, decarboxylated to serotonin by the cytoplasmic enzyme decarboxylase [2]. Another cytoplasmic enzyme called serotonin-acetyltransferase (NAT), transforms serotonin to N-acetyl serotonin [3]. The final step in the pathway is the conversion of N-acetylserotonin by acetylserotonin O-methyltransferase (ASMT) to melatonin [3]. ASMT has been reported to be the rate-limiting enzyme in melatonin's biosynthesis [4] instead of NAT [5].

Melatonin serves as an endogenous mediator of photoperiodic information and a molecular component of the circadian time keeping system [6]. Its synthesis and secretion fluctuate in a circadian rhythm that is entrained to a 24 h light/dark cycle. Melatonin is activated by several mechanisms [7]. The first involves melatonin binding to its receptors in the plasma membrane MT1 (or Mel_{1a} or MTNR1A) and MT2 (or Mel_{1b} or MTNR1B) [8]. The genes encoding the melatonin receptors are historically referred to as melatonin receptor 1A (*MTNR1A*) and melatonin receptor 1B (*MTNRIB)*, respectively. MT1 and MT2 are found in a wide variety of tissues with different expression profiles [9]. Studies have shown all cloned melatonin receptors bind 2-[1251]-melatonin and melatonin at picomolar affinity (KD 25-160pM). The receptors are coupled to cyclic adenylate cyclate (cAMP) inhibition via pertussis-toxin-sensitive G-proteins [10]. Both MT1 and MT2 have pathways that inhibit forskolin-stimulated cAMP formation [11], and melatonin coupling to these receptors leads to the inhibition of cyclic guanosine monophosphate (cGMP) [12].

Melatonin apparently acts as a natural ligand for the three-member retinoid-related orphan nuclear hormone receptor family (RZR/ROR): RZR/ROR α is expressed in various organs; RZR β is specific to the brain and retina [13]; and ROR γ is preferentially expressed in human skeletal muscle cDNA [14].

The immunomodulatory effects and possibly also a portion of the circadian effects are partially mediated through melatonin activation of nuclear receptors that repress 5-lipoxygenase mRNA expression in human B cell lines [15]. In addition, melatonin may be activated by binding to intracellular proteins such as calmodulin, which participates in second messenger signal transduction; this directly antagonizes calmodulin binding to Ca+2 [16]. Finally, melatonin has important antioxidative effects, which have been extensively investigated in various pathological conditions associated with free radicals and related reactants, such as ischemia/reperfusion, inflammation, ionizing radiation, and mitochondrial toxins [17-19].

In this chapter we will discuss mainly the importance of melatonin in ovaries of high mammals. Studies in rodents are included only in so far as they have implications for higher mammals.

II. Relevant Aspects of Human Oogenesis and Folliculogenesis

The *in vivo* development of female germ cells and ovarian follicles is discussed here in brief, focusing on topics essential for the understanding of later sections [20].

The female is born with a complete pool of germ cells (oocytes). Their number declines gradually from birth to menopause [21]. The number of germ cells in the fetal ovary peaks at about seven million in mid-pregnancy, and then drops dramatically during the third trimester [20]. Meiotic division usually commences gradually in the third month of gestation, and the diplothen stage is achieved within weeks. The nucleus during the primary oocyte stage of oogenesis, termed the gereminal vesicle (GV) is round and large. Just before birth, the oocytes are arrested at the diplothen stage of the prophase of the first meiotic division. They have completed genetic recombination and do not undergo any additional nuclear maturation until puberty, when menstrual cycles are initiated.

Most of the follicles in the human ovary are primordial follicles (30-50 μm in diameter) with a single flat somatic-granulosa cell (GC) layer surrounding the oocyte. Their growth regulation is not hormonal, and the exact factors that stimulate their development are unknown. Primordial follicles are activated when their GC become cuboidal, and they are then termed primary follicles (50-80 μm in diameter). Primary follicles develop to secondary follicles (80 μm -0.2 mm in diameter) characterized by an increased proliferation rate of the GC and consequent formation of a multilaminar layer. A definitive theca layer is created from the stroma cells surrounding the secondary follicle. Steroid hormones are synthesized through complex interactions between the GC and theca cells. During the secondary follicular stage, the oocyte starts to grow, and a glycoprotein coat, the zona pellucida (ZP), forms between the oocyte and the innermost layer of the GCs. The final follicular stage consists of development of antral follicles (early antral follicle: 0.2-0.4 mm in diameter) containing a fluid-filled cavity within several layers of cuboidal GC; the innermost layers surrounding the oocytes are termed cumulus cells. Cumulus cells play very important roles in oocyte growth and maturation, supply nutrients [22] and/or messenger molecules for oocyte development [23], and mediate hormonal effects on oocytes [24]. Cumulus cell expansion is considered an important marker for oocyte maturation.

At puberty, the hypothalamic gonadotropin releasing hormone (GnRH) is secreted in pulsate discharges and stimulates the normal production of the pituitary gonadotropins, namely, follicle stimulating hormone (FSH) and luteinizing hormone (LH) [25, 26]. GnRH is also considered as a luteolytic factor that can directly increase granulosa cell apoptosis [27, 28]. FSH levels rise in the first half of the menstrual cycle before ovulation, inducing follicular development and growth from secondary stages (the follicular phase) [20]. The new formation of LH receptors, induced by FSH, is an obligatory step in the differentiation and maturation of the GC and is essential for the initiation of luteinization [29]. A primordial follicle reaches the ovulatory antral size (18-20 mm in diameter) within six to nine months [30].

Ovulation occurs at the mid menstrual cycle and is stimulated by a drastic increase in baseline LH levels (LH surge) [26]. The ovulation mechanism has been compared with an inflammatory reaction [31] involving also reactive oxygen species (ROS) [32]. ROS inhibit progesterone production by luteal cells, thereby potentially damaging GC undergoing luteinization [33].

This action is mediated by steroidogenic enzyme inhibition and cholesterol transport to the mitochondria by intracellular carrier proteins [33, 34]. In addition, ROS disrupt the plasma membrane of luteal cells by way of lipid peroxidation and via the modulating effect of cytochrome P450 enzyme activity [32, 35-39].

The follicle copes with excessive ROS with antioxidant enzymes, such as superoxide dismutase, glutathione peroxidase, and catalase, and nonenzymatic antioxidants such as vitamin E, vitamin C, and glutathione [32, 38, 39]. The balance between ROS and antioxidants within the follicle is apparently important for luteinizing GC function during ovulation.

The first meiotic division is completed, with the extrusion of the first polar body enclosed between the oocyte and the ZP, forming a mature oocyte [26, 39]. The ovarian site from which ovulation occurs, develops into a progesterone-secreting gland, the corpus luteum. The remaining days until the end of the cycle are termed the luteal phase.

Effect of Light and Darkness on Ovarian Function

Melatonin functions in the reproductive system of higher mammals, such as sheep, goats, pigs, cows, buffalos and humans [40-42]. The mechanism for synchronizing breeding in seasonal animals involves the interpretation of natural environmental signals, the duration of exposure to daylight (photoperiod) and melatonin activity. The precise nature of this mechanism remains unclear. Two explanations have been offered using studies of sheep models, both of which are based on three assumptions: there is no specific signal that stops reproductive activity; the shortening day (i.e., longer duration of melatonin activity) after the summer solstice sustains breeding; and an endogenous circannual rhythm prevails to stop cycling [43].

The more accepted "duration" model posits that the endogenous circannual reproductive rhythm is synchronized to natural photoperiodic changes via corresponding changes in the level of secretion of endogenous melatonin. The alternative "phase coincidence" model, based on the external coincidence model of Pittendrigh and Minis (1964), posits that the endogenous circadian pacemaker phase is sensitive to light and darkness (i.e.: melatonin), and the timing of reproductive activity depends on the coincidence in time of the circadian rhythm sensitive to a certain level of melatonin secreted [44]. The phase coincidence model is not necessarily contingent on the existence of an endogenous circannual reproduction rhythm, but the lack of an appropriate marker makes it is difficult to examine this parameter experimentally.

Studies in highly seasonal animals, such as Romney Marsh sheep, yielded varying melatonin secretion patterns under natural conditions [45]. In the shorter days of autumn and winter, this sensitive phase occurs within the natural darkness of the longer night, and as such, may provide the short-day signal that directly induces a reproductive response. However, it is also possible that signal stopping ovarian activity is the recoincidence of light with the sensitive phase of the circadian pacemaker following the end of winter. This notion is supported by findings that exogenous melatonin can block the effect of light, but only when coincident with the circadian pacemaker phase [46], and that breeding can be driven by exogenous melatonin even in the presence of a conflicting photoperiod [47]. Thus, endogenous melatonin may be more important than darkness per se.

In humans, the high follicular phase levels of melatonin in winter have been suggested to inhibit serum LH [48]. Accordingly, exposure to bright light was found to significantly increase levels of prolactin, LH, FSH and the number of ovulatory cycles [49].

Interestingly, psychopathologies linked to menstruation may be connected with light and darkness; specifically, depression-associated menstrual disorders [50], and depressive symptoms specific to the luteal phase and pregnancy [51]. Bright light therapy has been shown to improve these depressive symptoms, perhaps owing to an increase in melatonin in response to the bright light itself [49].

Melatonin's Effect on the Ovary via the Hypothalamic-Hypophysial Axis

Melatonin probably acts on the ovary via the brain and pituitary [42], by regulating the aftereffects of gonadotropin release on hypothalamic monoamine and GnRH [40], and possibly on cAMP and Ca 2+ dependent intracellular mechanisms in the hypophysis [41]. In rats and probably also humans, melatonin inhibits LH secretion from the hypophysis [52], and regulates LH receptor (LHR), GnRH and GnRH receptor (GnRHR), probably through mitogen-activated protein kinase pathway [53].

Moreover, melatonin's direct administration upregulated LH mRNA receptor expression, enhanced human chrorionic gonadotropin (hCG) stimulated progesterone secretion. By binding to the their ovarian receptors, the gondotropins effect steroidogenesis and gametogenesis [29]; thus, differences in melatonin –stimulated levels of FSH receptor (FSHR) and LHR influence the effect of gonadotropins on follicular growth, ovulation, and luteinization [54, 55]. Accordingly, the administration of exogenous melatonin and progesterone to women induced LH secretion, blocked ovulation, and increased the in luteal-phase progesterone without affecting FSH or inhibiting estradiol [56].

Direct Effects of Melatonin in the Ovary

Accumulating evidence suggest that melatonin has also a direct effect on ovarian cells [57, 58], through MT1 and MT2, which are expressed in human ovaries and granulosa cells [59, 60]. These findings were supported by studies in which *MTNR1A* gene expression was identified in bovine oocytes and their cumulus cells, *MTNR1B* gene expression, in oocytes [61]. Melatonin was found in human preovulatory follicular fluid at concentrations three fold higher than in serum [62, 63]. Although evidnence shows follicular fluid melatonin is derived from the blood circulation [62-64], melatonin is probably also synthesized in the human ovary [65], as suggested by kinetic analyses showing that the Michaelis constant (Km) for ovarian substrates of melatonin synthesizing enzymes NAT and hydoryindole-O-methyltransferase (HIOMT) was similar to those of the pineal gland. Furthermore, a study in cows detected ASMT expression in both oocytes and cumulus cells [61].

The LH/hCG ratio is an important rescue factor in corpus luteum maintenance in early pregnancy. In addition, GnRH is a direct inhibitor of human granulosa-luteal cells [66], and may play an important role in corpus luteum regression, as indicated by the increase in GnRH and its receptor mRNA during spontaneous luteinization *in vitro* [28]; thus GnRH downregulation may reflect the corpus luteum state. The high levels of melatonin in the follicular fluid [67] and the presence of its binding sites in the granulosa-luteal cells [60], suggest that melatonin directly modulates steroidogenesis and possibly luteolysis via its ovarian receptors [67, 68]. The administration of melatonin to human granulosa lutelal cells regulated LH mRNA receptor expression [53], enhanced human chorionic gonadotropin (hCG) production, stimulated progesterone secretion, and inhibited GnRH and GnRHR expression [28].

However, the direct effect of melatonin on female sex-steroid production remains controversial. Some reports showed no or even negative effects of melatonin on progesterone production in growing and luteinized granulosa cells from pigs, cattle and humans [62, 69-73], whereas others reported melatonin-stimulated secretion in monkeys and humans [53, 73-76]. One study found melatonin failed to stimulate estradiol secretion after culturing antral porcine follicles [77]; however, others noted that melatonin stimulated estradiol secretion in cultured porcine GC [72], but not in ovine GC [78]. These discrepancies may be explained by differences in cell type tested (theca or GC), experimental model used (cell or follicle culture), species tested, and dose and duration of treatment [79-81].

Indirect Effect of Melatonin on the Ovary via Its Antioxidant Activity

Besides melatonin effects via the hypothalamic-pituitary axis and its ovarian MT1 and MT2 receptors, melatonin may exert an indirect effect on folliculogenesis. Follicular atresia, ovulation, oocyte maturation and corpus luteum formation have its broad free- radical scavenging and antioxidant and antiapoptotic activity [82-84]. Owing to their small size and highly lipophylic properties [18], melatonin molecules cross all cell membranes and easily reach subcellular compartments, including mitochondria and nuclei, where it accumulates at high concentrations [85].

Acting as a free radical scavenger and broad-spectrum antioxidant, it then prevents lipid peroxidation [82, 83], protein, and DNA damage [84]. In particular, melatonin preserves optimal mitochondrial function and homeostasis by reducing and preventing oxidative stress, thereby curtailing subsequent apoptotic events and cell death [86-88].

Human melatonin's follicular concentration increases with follicular growth [70]. Thus, its antioxidant activity during ovulation protects human oocytes from free radical damage. Melatonin also abolishes the inhibitory effect of H2O2 on progesterone production by luteinized GC [89], stimulating the potential of luteinizing ROS damage to progesterone production in the ovulating follicle.

Melatonin in Female Infertility

Melatonin and Luteal Phase Defects

Luteal phase defects have been implicated as a cause of infertility and spontaneous miscarriage [89]. Findings of significantly elevated serum lipid peroxidase levels in patients with luteal phase defects compared to women with normal luteal function [90], suggested that in some cases, luteal phase defects might be a result of oxidative stress. Therefore, melatonin supplementation may serve as useful treatment in this setting [89].

Clinical *in vitro* Oocyte Maturation and Poor Oocyte Quality

Melatonin may enhance the *in vitro* maturation of oocytes, either via its action on the ovarian receptors or its direct and indirect antioxidant activities [61]. Specifically, as an antioxidant melatonin might protect cumulus cells against apoptosis [75, 91,92], or enhance their expansion [91]. Experimental studies have shown that melatonin supplementation to the culture medium of GV-stage oocytes promoted cumulus cell expansion in pigs and cows [61, 91], and increased nuclear maturation in cows, pigs [91, 93] and buffalos [94]. To the best of our knowledge similar experiments have not been performed with immature human oocytes.

However, melatonin has been used to treat infertility due to poor oocyte quality in women [95]. The rationale of this approach is based on findings that increasing the melatonin concentration in follicular fluid seems to reduce lipid peroxidation and consequent damage to oocyte DNA [94, 95].

Endometriosis

Endometriosis is a chronic inflammatory disease that is characterized by implantation and growth of endometrial tissue outside the uterine cavity [96]. It is progressive and recurrent in nature, affecting an estimated 21%-44% of infertile patients. It has also been identified in 4%-22% of fertile women [96, 96, 97]. Manifestations include chronic pelvic pain, progressive dysmenorrheal, dyspareunia and infertility. The cause in unknown. It is believed to be multifactorial and associated with general peritoneal cavity inflammatory response. Studies suggest that during menstruation, endometrial fragments reach the fallopian tubes and the peritoneal cavity in a retrograde manner, implant on the serosal surfaces of the peritoneal cavity, and undergo progressive proliferation and bleeding each successive menstrual cycle. Oxidative stress inducers at these sites, may include erythrocytes, apoptotic endometrial cells, and undigested endometrial cells in the menstrual effluent [98].

ROS are involved in the local inflammatory process and pathophysiology of endometriosis with localized pelvic inflammatory reaction [99]. The increase in peritoneal fluid volume together with activated macrophages induces oxidative stress, lipid peroxide formation, inducible nitric oxide synthase activity, and the production of nitric oxide and other by-products of apolipoprotein and peroxide interactions. In addition, ROS lead to increased levels of cytokines, growth factors, prostaglandins, free iron, free heme and other proinflammatory mediators, and their increased deposition is at a close proximity to the peritoneal endometriotic implants [98].

Melatonin was shown to induce a regression in endometriosis in mice (100). Specifically, its administration arrested lipid peroxidation and protein oxidation, downregulated the activity and expression of pro-matrix metallopeptidase 9 (MMP-9), a marker of endometriosis progression and severity, and increased tissue inhibitors of metalloproteinase (TIMP-1), another endometriosis marker. Intraperitoneal melatonin administration to a rat model of endometriosis suggested that melatonin might prevent endometriosis and induce its regression via MMP regulation [101]. Others using a similar model, noted a significant reduction in explant volume which they attributed to melatonin's antioxidant, anti-inflamatory, and immunomodulatory effects [102]. Melatonin also significantly decreased explant levels of cyclooxygenase-2 positive cells and malondialdehyde, a lipid peroxidation product and marker of free-radical-induced tissue changes, while elevating levels of superoxide dismutase and catalase.

Polycystic Ovarian Syndrome (PCOS)

PCOS is a common endocrine disorder that causes female infertility due to anovulation, and decreased oocyte and embryo quality [103]. Other clinical features include hyperandrogenism, hyperinsulinemia, insulin resistance, hirsutism, and obesity. PCOS is characterized by ROS generation from mononuclear cells, an increase in serum lipid peroxidation products, protein oxidation, and follicular DNA damage [104, 105]. The oxidative stress may be responsible for poor oocyte quality and damage.

There is an increase in malondialdehyde in the follicular fluid, which was used as a marker of free radical-induced tissue damage [106], and in apoptotic/damaged GC because of lipid peroxidation [107]. Levels of urinary 6-sulfatoxymelatonin, the major enzymatic metabolite of melatonin, are increased as well [108]. The hormone leptin has also been related to PCOS. Leptin is produced mainly in adipose tissue [109]. Levels are high in serum and follicular fluid in obese women [109, 110]. In rat models of PCOS, daily melatonin administration to rats reduced body weight, intraabdominal adiposity, and serum/plasma leptin levels [111], whereas pinealectomy increased leptin [112]. The mechanism whereby decreased melatonin levels interact with increased leptin levels in PCOS is still unclear. Interestingly, one study of patients with PCOS reported high concentrations of melatonin in serum and low concentrations in ovarian follicles [80].

Various studies are investigating the connection between PCOS and single-nucleotide polymorphisms (SNPs) [113]. A clinical and phenotypic overlap exists between PCOS and type 2 diabetes mellitus (T2DM) [114]. The *MTNR1B* gene, located on human chromosome 11q21-q22, is also a candidate gene marker for T2DM. Studies suggest that disturbance in circadian rhythmicity may affect metabolic control and increase the risk of diabetes [76]. Specifically, the distribution of the genotypes and allelic frequencies of rs1083093, could lead to functional and activity changes of melatonin, as well as melatonin deficiency. These were found to be significantly higher in women with PCOS than in the sex-and age-matched general population [115, 116]. A higher frequency in GG and GC genotypes were observed in a Chinese PCOS population [115]. Therefore, there seems a connection between melatonin's signaling pathway and PCOS [115, 116].

Premature Ovarian Failure (POF)

POF is defined by sex steroid deficiency, elevated gonadotropins and amenorrhea in women less than 40 years old [117]. It can be due to a genetically predetermined reduction in the number of ovarian follicles at birth or to accelerated follicular depletion (atresia), or follicular dysfunction [118], mostly consequent to radiotherapy or chemotherapy [119, 120]. Autoimmune mechanisms are probably involved in pathogenesis of up to 30% of cases [30]. These include also ovarian autoantibodies against GC, theca cells, and against the ZP [121-123].

In patients with cancer who undergo radiotherapy, ovarian damage is usually attributable to direct pelvic irradiation, although scattered radiation can be harmful as well [119, 124]. The depletion of primordial follicles is dose-dependant [125]. The mechanism underlying the effect of direct radiation is a disruption of sensitive cellular molecules; the indirect effects of ionizing radiation occur through interactions with cellular water molecules, resulting in the production of highly reactive free radicals, such as the hydroxyl radical (OH). Studies have shown that free radicals are responsible to 60%-70% of the tissue, cellular and DNA damage [124, 125].

Exogenous melatonin has been shown to inhibit radiation-induced follicular atresia in mice [125, 126]. At the cellular level, melatonin may directly protect against chromosome damage by interacting with OH, thereby converting it to an intermediate, low-toxic, indolyl (melatonyl) radical that melatonin subsequently scavenges [125, 127]. Indolyl, in turn, scavenges a second OH to generate cyclic 3-hydroxy melatonin. Melatonin can also indirectly alter the final amount of chromosomal damage by activating oxidative repair enzymes, and it may exert a receptor-mediated protective effect. Studies in mice and rats have found melatonin to be highly effective in protecting against ionizing radiation [128, 129]. Additionally, pretreatment with melatonin reduced plasma and erythrocyte malondialdehyde levels in rats with oxidative damage from total body irradiation [130]. However, this effect did not extend to conditions in which melatonin was administered after radiation [128]; that is melatonin had to be present inside the cell for it to be effective.

Oxidative stress also plays an important role in chemotherapy-induced cytotoxicity and gonadotoxicity. Some chemotherapeutic medications are known to generate mitochondrial ROS, including alkylating agents (e.g., cyclophosphamide, ifosfamide), platinum agents (e.g., cisplatin), antitumour antibiotics (e.g., doxorubicin, dounorubicin, bleomycin). Findings in patients with cancer and rats [131], melatonin administration together with different chemotherapeutic agents reduced several side effects, such as thrombocytopenia. Considering its protective-antioxidant effect in this setting [18, 132], melatonin may be useful for protecting follicles and oocytes from free-radical damage also in patients undergoing chemotherapy.

It may also be true for autoimmune ovarian POF. In mice, melatonin had a direct protecting effect against ovarian failure caused by antiovarian antibodies [132, 133]. Melatonin restored oocyte meiotic maturation and survival by its anti-inflammatory and antiapoptotic effects.

Fertility Restoration

Cryopreservation of ovarian tissue containing immature ovarian follicles is a major option for fertility preservation; in many cases the only alternative [134]. So far, the autologous transplantation of cryopreserved–thawed ovarian tissue has resulted in about 30 live births [135-137].

However, too-slow graft revascularization after transplantation can lead to substantial follicular loss due to ischemia [20, 138]. Therefore, methods to improve and hasten graft vascularization are needed, particularly treatments with a minimal potential for dangerous side effects, so that they can eventually be applied in autotransplantation for fertility restoration in women.

Melatonin might play a beneficial role in fertility preservation/restoration in young female patients with cancer. Besides its preventive action against free-radical damage, melatonin reduces Bcl2 expression and caspase-3 activity [139], thereby reducing the apoptotic mitochondrial pathawy. It also seems to be devoid of dangerous side effects.

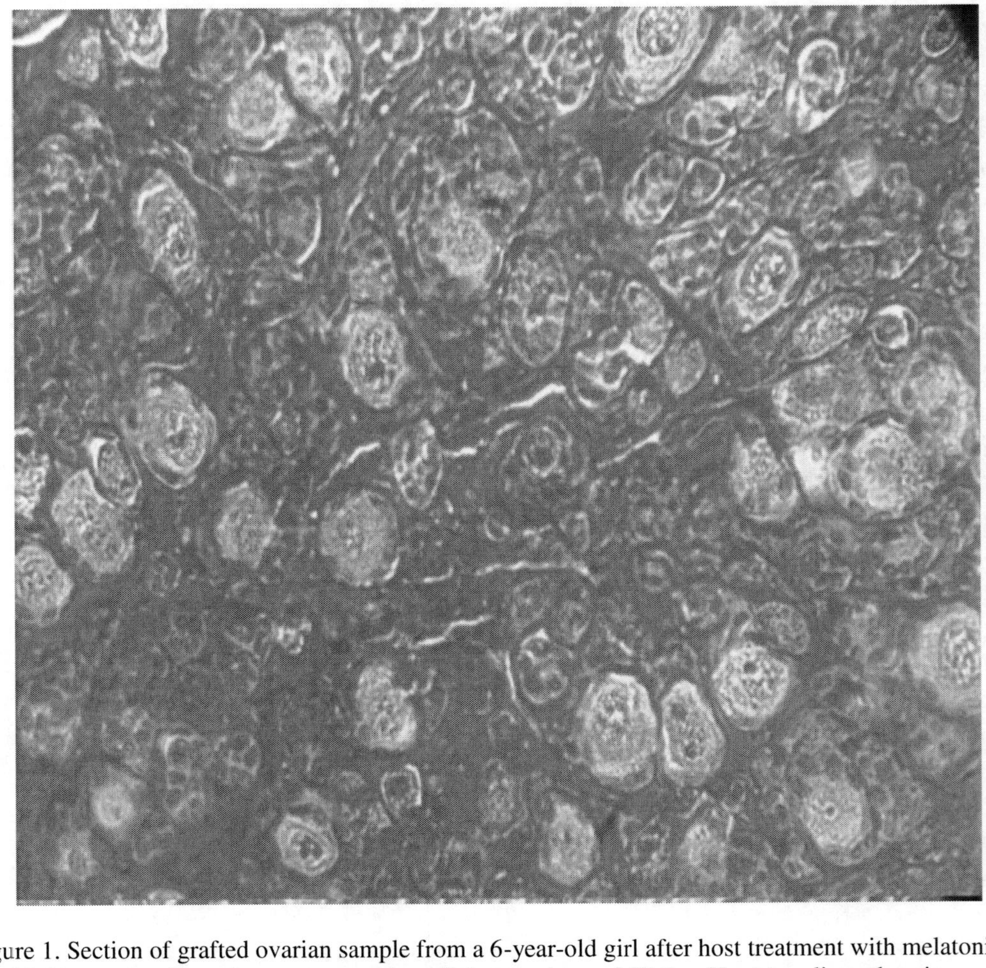

Figure 1. Section of grafted ovarian sample from a 6-year-old girl after host treatment with melatonin in the drinking water. Note the numerous primordial and primary follicles. Hematoxylin and eosin, original magnification x400.

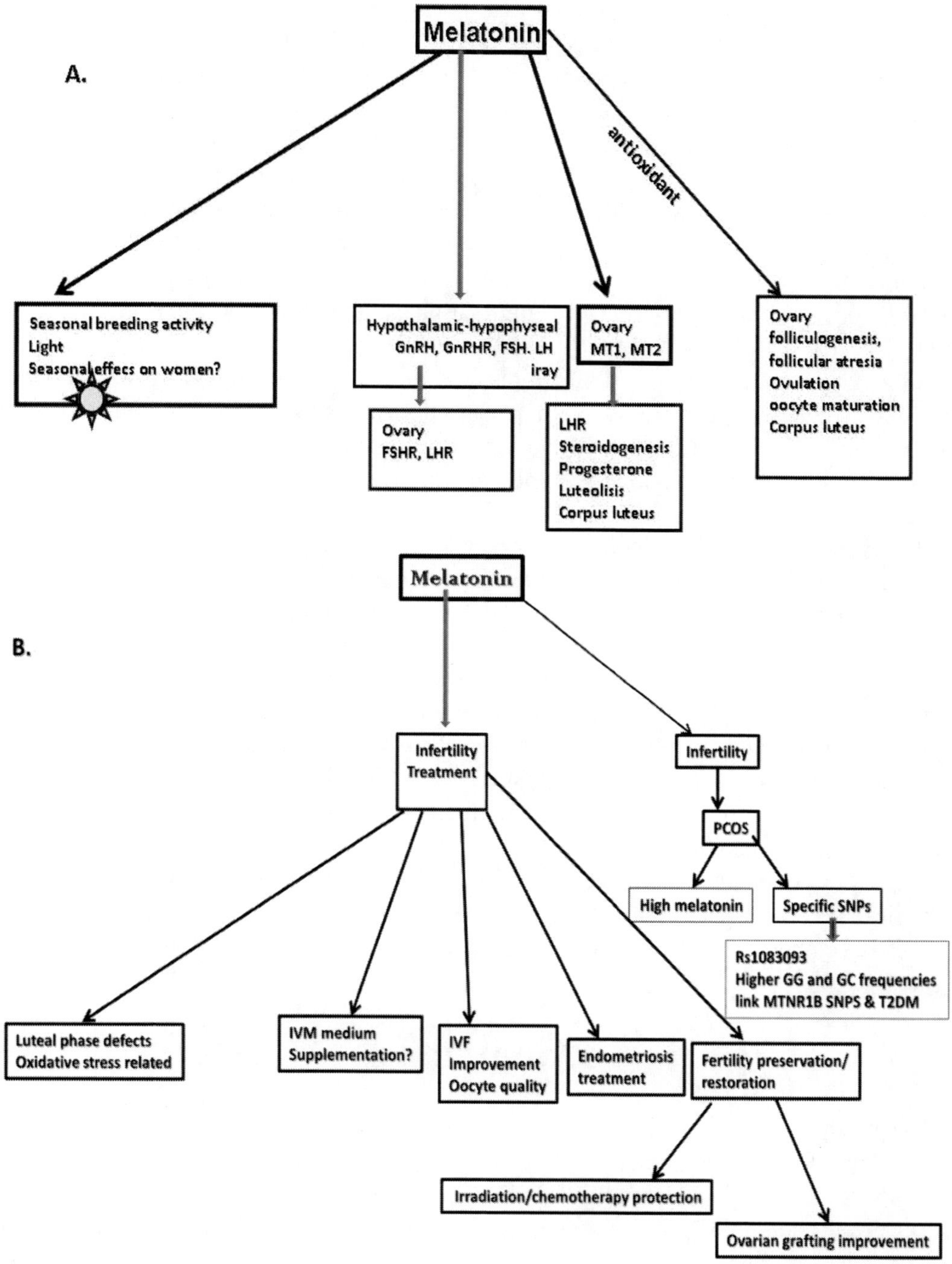

Figure 2. A. Normal effects of melatonin in the ovary of higher mammals. *Note*: GnRH=gonadotropin realizing hormone, GnRHR= gonadotropin realizing hormone receptor, FSH=follicle stimulating hormone, FSHR=follicle stimulating hormone receptor, LH=luteinizing hormone, LHR=luteinizing hormone receptor, MT1=melatonin receptor 1, MT2=melatonin receptor 2.
B. Effects of melatonin in putative fertility treatment and PCOS. *Note*: IVM=*in vitro* maturation; IVF=*in vitro* fertilization, PCOS=polycystic ovarian syndrome, SNPs=single nucleotide polymorphisms, MTNR1B=melatonin receptor 1B, T2DM=type 2 diabetes mellitus.

There are already studies suggesting that melatonin may be a key player in improving future ovarian reimplantation techniques in women [134, 139-141].

In the initial experiments, immunodeficient mice engrafted with ovarian tissue can serve as useful models for examining graft survival [134, 138, 142]. Melatonin treatment to murine hosts engrafted with vitrified-warmed ovaries from mice improved follicular survival and development, cumulus–oocyte complex quality, ovarian size, with homogenous distribution of granulosa and stroma cells [140]. Others reported a reduction in necrosis of ovarian graft tissue in rat hosts injected with melatonin shortly before grafting [141]. Moreover, the addition of melatonin to the drinking water of immunodeficient mice engrafted with frozen-thawed human ovarian tissue prevented graft shrinkage and reduced cellular graft apoptosis (Figure 1).

Although ovarian transplantation has resulted in live births [137], it carries the risk of reintroducing malignancies [20, 142, 143]. This drawback could be overcome by embryo transfer after *in vitro* fertilization of oocytes from primordial follicles matured *in vitro*. Therefore, researchers are seeking methods to improve techniques of culturing primordial follicles.

However, uncertainties regarding the signals that prompt the initial activation of the primordial follicles continue to hinder the development of a successful culture system. Melatonin may be involved in this process, by regulating follicular development via its ovarian receptors and antioxidant activity, and modulating the production of growth factors that support follicular development. A recent study showed that addition of a combination of melatonin with FSH to the culture medium of goat preantral follicles increased follicular and oocyte diameters and resulted in viable follicles with normal ultrastructure [144]. Furthermore, melatonin was shown to stimulate the production of factors such as insulin-like growth factor-I, which is involved in GC proliferation, steroidogenesis and *in vitro* follicular growth in rats, cows and humans.

There is evidence that melatonin functions through multiple receptors, and also as a direct free radical scavenger, suggesting melatonin's involvement in ovarian physiology including follicular development, ovulation, oocyte maturation, and luteal function (Figure 2).

Conclusion

The mechanism for synchronizing the annual timing of breeding in seasonal animals involves the interpretation of natural environmental signals, commonly photoperiod via the pineal hormone melatonin. Highly seasonal animals exhibited varying melatonin secretion patterns under natural conditions. In women, there are high follicular phase melatonin levels in winter that have been suggested to inhibit serum LH, and bright light exposure might increase prolactin, LH, FSH and the number of ovulatory cycles. In addition, menstrual-associated psychopathologies might be linked with light and darkness; specifically, depression-associated menstrual disorders and luteal phase and pregnancy depressive symptoms.

In addition, melatonin abnormalities seem to be involved in infertility pathologies such as PCOS and endometriosis. Melatonin is a potentially safe promising putative fertility medication and might open new horizons in infertility management, as it improves oocyte quality, increases fertilization rates and reduces follicular fluid oxidative damage. Melatonin might also have roles in improving fertility preservation and restoration both in ovarian protection against radiation and chemotherapy and by improving outcomes of ovarian grafting.

Further knowledge of the effect of melatonin in the ovaries of higher animal mammalian species will contribute to our understanding of its importance in humans. Melatonin could become an important medication for improving ovarian function and its use might open new approaches to the management of various ovarian fertility problems. For the use of melatonin in infertility, clinical trials should be conducted in future years.

References

[1] Lovenberg W, Jequier E, Sjoerdsma A. Tryptophan hydroxylation: measurement in pineal gland, brainstem, and carcinoid tumor. *Science,* 1967 Jan 13;155(3759):217-9.

[2] Lovenberg W, Weissbach H, Udenfriend S. Aromatic L-amino acid decarboxylase. *J. Biol. Chem.,* 1962 Jan;237:89-93.

[3] Wurtman RJ, Axelrod J. The Pineal Gland. Sci Am 1965 Jul;213:50-60.

[4] Liu T, Borjigin J. N-acetyltransferase is not the rate-limiting enzyme of melatonin synthesis at night. *J. Pineal. Res.,* 2005 Aug;39(1):91-6.

[5] Klein DC, Weller JL. Indole metabolism in the pineal gland: a circadian rhythm in N-acetyltransferase. *Science,* 1970 Sep 11;169(3950):1093-5.

[6] Claustrat B, Brun J, Chazot G. The basic physiology and pathophysiology of melatonin. Sleep Med Rev 2005 Feb;9(1):11-24.

[7] Macchi M.M, Bruce J.N. Human pineal physiology and functional significance of melatonin. *Front Neuroendocrinol.,* 2004 Sep;25(3-4):177-95.

[8] Dubocovich M.L, Rivera-Bermudez M.A, Gerdin M.J, Masana M.I. Molecular pharmacology, regulation and function of mammalian melatonin receptors. *Front Biosci.,* 2003 Sep 1;8:d1093-d1108.

[9] Delagrange P, Atkinson J, Boutin JA, Casteilla L, Lesieur D, Misslin R, et al. Therapeutic perspectives for melatonin agonists and antagonists. *J. Neuroendocrinol.,* 2003 Apr;15(4):442-8.

[10] New D.C, Tsim ST, Wong Y.H. G protein-linked effector and second messenger systems involved in melatonin *signal transduction. Neurosignals,* 2003 Mar;12(2):59-70.

[11] Reppert S.M, Weaver D.R, Godson C. Melatonin receptors step into the light: cloning and classification of subtypes. *Trends Pharmacol. Sci.,* 1996 Mar;17(3):100-2.

[12] Petit L, Lacroix I, de CP, Strosberg A.D, Jockers R. Differential signaling of human Mel1a and Mel1b melatonin receptors through the cyclic guanosine 3'-5'-monophosphate pathway. *Biochem. Pharmacol.,* 1999 Aug 15;58(4):633-9.

[13] Missbach M, Jagher B, Sigg I, Nayeri S, Carlberg C, Wiesenberg I. Thiazolidine diones, specific ligands of the nuclear receptor retinoid Z receptor/retinoid acid receptor-related orphan receptor alpha with potent antiarthritic activity. *J. Biol. Chem.,* 1996 Jun 7;271(23):13515-22.

[14] Hirose T, Smith R.J, Jetten A.M. ROR gamma: the third member of ROR/RZR orphan receptor subfamily that is highly expressed in skeletal muscle. *Biochem. Biophys. Res. Commun.,* 1994 Dec 30;205(3):1976-83.

[15] Steinhilber D, Brungs M, Werz O, Wiesenberg I, Danielsson C, Kahlen JP, et al. The nuclear receptor for melatonin represses 5-lipoxygenase gene expression in human B lymphocytes. *J. Biol. Chem.,* 1995 Mar 31;270(13):7037-40.

[16] Pozo D, Reiter RJ, Calvo JR, Guerrero J.M. Inhibition of cerebellar nitric oxide synthase and cyclic GMP production by melatonin via complex formation with calmodulin. *J. Cell Biochem.,* 1997 Jun 1;65(3):430-42.

[17] Allegra M, Reiter R.J, Tan D.X, Gentile C, Tesoriere L, Livrea M.A. The chemistry of melatonin's interaction with reactive species. *J. Pineal. Res.,* 2003 Jan;34(1):1-10.

[18] Reiter R.J, Manchester L.C, Tan D.X. Melatonin in walnuts: influence on levels of melatonin and total antioxidant capacity of blood. *Nutrition,* 2005 Sep;21(9):920-4.

[19] Tan D.X, Hardeland R, Manchester L.C, Poeggeler B, Lopez-Burillo S, Mayo JC, et al. Mechanistic and comparative studies of melatonin and classic antioxidants in terms of their interactions with the ABTS cation radical. *J. Pineal. Res.,* 2003 May;34(4):249-59.

[20] Feigin E, Abir R, Fisch B, Kravarusic D, Steinberg R, Nitke S, et al. Laparoscopic ovarian tissue preservation in young patients at risk for ovarian failure as a result of chemotherapy/irradiation for primary malignancy. *J. Pediatr. Surg.,* 2007 May;42(5):862-4.

[21] Kaipia A, Hsueh AJ. Regulation of ovarian follicle atresia. *Annu. Rev. Physiol.,* 1997;59:349-63.

[22] Eppig J.J. The relationship between cumulus cell-oocyte coupling, oocyte meiotic maturation, and cumulus expansion. *Dev. Biol.,* 1982 Jan;89(1):268-72.

[23] Buccione R, Schroeder A.C, Eppig J.J. Interactions between somatic cells and germ cells throughout mammalian oogenesis. *Biol. Reprod.,* 1990 Oct;43(4):543-7.

[24] Zuelke K.A, Brackett B.G. Luteinizing hormone-enhanced in vitro maturation of bovine oocytes with and without protein supplementation. *Biol. Reprod.,* 1990 Nov;43(5):784-7.

[25] Chen L, Wert S.E, Hendrix E.M, Russell P.T, Cannon M, Larsen W.J. Hyaluronic acid synthesis and gap junction endocytosis are necessary for normal expansion of the cumulus mass. *Mol. Reprod. Dev.,* 1990 Jul;26(3):236-47.

[26] Speroff L. The effect of aging on fertility. *Curr. Opin. Obstet. Gynecol.,* 1994 Apr;6(2):115-20.

[27] Adashi E.Y, Resnick C.E, Svoboda M.E, Van Wyk J.J. Somatomedin-C synergizes with follicle-stimulating hormone in the acquisition of progestin biosynthetic capacity by cultured rat granulosa cells. *Endocrinology,* 1985 Jun;116(6):2135-42.

[28] Nathwani P.S, Kang S.K, Cheng K.W, Choi K.C, Leung P.C. Regulation of gonadotropin-releasing hormone and its receptor gene expression by 17beta-estradiol in cultured human granulosa-luteal cells. *Endocrinology,* 2000 May;141(5):1754-63.

[29] Hillier S.G, Smyth C.D, Whitelaw P.F, Miro F, Howles C.M. Gonadotrophin control of follicular function. *Horm. Res.,* 1995;43(5):216-23.

[30] Conway G.S. Clinical manifestations of genetic defects affecting gonadotrophins and their receptors. *Clin. Endocrinol.,* (Oxf) 1996 Dec;45(6):657-63.

[31] Richards J.S, Russell D.L, Ochsner S, Espey L.L. Ovulation: new dimensions and new regulators of the inflammatory-like response. *Annu. Rev. Physiol.,* 2002;64:69-92.
[32] Agarwal A, Nandipati K.C, Sharma R.K, Zippe C.D, Raina R. Role of oxidative stress in the pathophysiological mechanism of erectile dysfunction. *J. Androl.,* 2006 May;27(3):335-47.
[33] Behrman H.R, Kodaman P.H, Preston S.L, Gao S. Oxidative stress and the ovary. *J. Soc. Gynecol. Investig.,* 2001 Jan;8(1 Suppl Proceedings):S40-S42.
[34] Behrman H.R, Aten R.F. Evidence that hydrogen peroxide blocks hormone-sensitive cholesterol transport into mitochondria of rat luteal cells. *Endocrinology,* 1991 Jun;128(6):2958-66.
[35] Carlson J.C, Sawada M, Boone D.L, Stauffer JM. Stimulation of progesterone secretion in dispersed cells of rat corpora lutea by antioxidants. *Steroids,* 1995 Mar;60(3):272-6.
[36] Gatzuli E, Aten R.F, Behrman H.R. Inhibition of gonadotropin action and progesterone synthesis by xanthine oxidase in rat luteal cells. *Endocrinology,* 1991 May;128(5):2253-8.
[37] Vega M, Carrasco I, Castillo T, Troncoso J.L, Videla L.A, Devoto L. Functional luteolysis in response to hydrogen peroxide in human luteal cells. *J. Endocrinol.,* 1995 Oct;147(1):177-82.
[38] Al-Gubory K.H, Bolifraud P, Germain G, Nicole A, Ceballos-Picot I. Antioxidant enzymatic defence systems in sheep corpus luteum throughout pregnancy. *Reproduction,* 2004 Dec;128(6):767-74.
[39] Goud A.P, Goud P.T, Diamond M.P, Gonik B, Abu-Soud H.M. Reactive oxygen species and oocyte aging: role of superoxide, hydrogen peroxide, and hypochlorous acid. *Free Radic. Biol. Med.,* 2008 Apr 1;44(7):1295-304.
[40] Reiter R.J. The pineal and its hormones in the control of reproduction in mammals. *Endocr. Rev.,* 1980;1(2):109-31.
[41] Vanecek J. Melatonin inhibits increase of intracellular calcium and cyclic AMP in neonatal rat pituitary via independent pathways. *Mol. Cell Endocrinol.,* 1995 Feb;107(2):149-53.
[42] Vanecek J. Cellular mechanisms of melatonin action. *Physiol. Rev.,* 1998 Jul;78(3):687-721.
[43] Barrell G.K, Moenter S.M, Caraty A, Karsch F.J. Seasonal changes of gonadotropin-releasing hormone secretion in the ewe. *Biol. Reprod.,* 1992 Jun;46(6):1130-5.
[44] Guerin M.V, Matthews C.D. Alterations of estrous activity in the ewe by circadian-based manipulation of the endogenous pacemaker. *J. Biol. Rhythms,* 1998 Feb;13(1):60-9.
[45] Matthews C.D, Guerin M.V, Napier A.J. Is a critical interval of the circadian pacemaker at dusk responsive to light and melatonin responsible for the timing of estrus in the Romney Marsh ewe?. *J. Biol. Rhythms,* 1995 Dec;10(4):308-18.
[46] Guerin M.V, Deed J.R, Matthews C.D. The coincidence of light and melatonin with a specific phase of the circadian pacemaker is important for the timing of seasonal breeding in the ewe. *J. Biol. Rhythms,* 2000 Dec;15(6):514-23.
[47] Yellon S.M, Foster D.L. Alternate photoperiods time puberty in the female lamb. *Endocrinology,* 1985 May;116(5):2090-7.

[48] Kivela A, Kauppila A, Ylostalo P, Vakkuri O, Leppaluoto J. Seasonal, menstrual and circadian secretions of melatonin, gonadotropins and prolactin in women. *Acta. Physiol. Scand.,* 1988 Mar;132(3):321-7.

[49] Danilenko K.V, Samoilova E.A. Stimulatory effect of morning bright light on reproductive hormones and ovulation: results of a controlled crossover trial. *PLoS Clin. Trials,* 2007;2(2):e7.

[50] Leppamaki S.J, Partonen T.T, Hurme J, Haukka J.K, Lonnqvist JK. Randomized trial of the efficacy of bright-light exposure and aerobic exercise on depressive symptoms and serum lipids. *J. Clin. Psychiatry,* 2002 Apr;63(4):316-21.

[51] Epperson C.N, Terman M, Terman J.S, Hanusa B.H, Oren D.A, Peindl KS, et al. Randomized clinical trial of bright light therapy for antepartum depression: preliminary findings. *J. Clin. Psychiatry,* 2004 Mar;65(3):421-5.

[52] Vanecek J, Klein D.C. Melatonin inhibition of GnRH-induced LH release from neonatal rat gonadotroph: involvement of Ca2+ not cAMP. *Am. J. Physiol.,* 1995 Jul;269(1 Pt 1):E85-E90.

[53] Woo M.M, Tai C.J, Kang S.K, Nathwani P.S, Pang S.F, Leung P.C. Direct action of melatonin in human granulosa-luteal cells. *J. Clin. Endocrinol. Metab.,* 2001 Oct;86(10):4789-97.

[54] Hsueh A.J, Adashi E.Y, Jones P.B, Welsh T.H, Jr. Hormonal regulation of the differentiation of cultured ovarian granulosa cells. *Endocr. Rev.,* 1984;5(1):76-127.

[55] Richards J.S, Fitzpatrick S.L, Clemens J.W, Morris J.K, Alliston T, Sirois J. Ovarian cell differentiation: a cascade of multiple hormones, cellular signals, and regulated genes. *Recent. Prog. Horm. Res.,* 1995;50:223-54.

[56] Voordouw B.C, Euser R, Verdonk R.E, Alberda B.T, de Jong F.H, Drogendijk AC, et al. Melatonin and melatonin-progestin combinations alter pituitary-ovarian function in women and can inhibit ovulation. *J. Clin. Endocrinol. Metab.,* 1992 Jan;74(1):108-17.

[57] Brzezinski A. Melatonin in humans. *N. Engl. J. Med.,* 1997 Jan 16;336(3):186-95.

[58] Sirotkin A.V, Schaeffer H.J. Direct regulation of mammalian reproductive organs by serotonin and melatonin. *J. Endocrinol.,* 1997 Jul;154(1):1-5.

[59] Cohen M, Lippman M, Chabner B. Role of pineal gland in aetiology and treatment of breast cancer. *Lancet,* 1978 Oct 14;2(8094):814-6.

[60] Yie S.M, Niles L.P, Younglai E.V. Melatonin receptors on human granulosa cell membranes. *J. Clin. Endocrinol. Metab.,* 1995 May;80(5):1747-9.

[61] El-Raey M, Geshi M, Somfai T, Kaneda M, Hirako M, Abdel-Ghaffar AE, et al. Evidence of melatonin synthesis in the cumulus oocyte complexes and its role in enhancing oocyte maturation in vitro in cattle. *Mol. Reprod. Dev.,* 2011 Apr;78(4):250-62.

[62] Brzezinski A, Seibel M.M, Lynch H.J, Deng M.H, Wurtman R.J. Melatonin in human preovulatory follicular fluid. *J. Clin. Endocrinol. Metab.,* 1987 Apr;64(4):865-7.

[63] Ronnberg L, Kauppila A, Leppaluoto J, Martikainen H, Vakkuri O. Circadian and seasonal variation in human preovulatory follicular fluid melatonin concentration. *J. Clin. Endocrinol. Metab.,* 1990 Aug;71(2):492-6.

[64] Wurtman R.J, Axelrod J, Potter L.T. The Uptake of H3-Melatonin in Endocrine and Nervous Tissues and the Effects of Constant Light Exposure. *J. Pharmacol. Exp. Ther.,* 1964 Mar;143:314-8.

[65] Itoh M.T, Ishizuka B, Kuribayashi Y, Amemiya A, Sumi Y. Melatonin, its precursors, and synthesizing enzyme activities in the human ovary. *Mol. Hum. Reprod.,* 1999 May;5(5):402-8.

[66] Peng C, Fan N.C, Ligier M, Vaananen J, Leung PC. Expression and regulation of gonadotropin-releasing hormone (GnRH) and GnRH receptor messenger ribonucleic acids in human granulosa-luteal cells. *Endocrinology,* 1994 Nov;135(5):1740-6.

[67] Brzezinski A, Fibich T, Cohen M, Schenker J.G, Laufer N. Effects of melatonin on progesterone production by human granulosa lutein cells in culture. *Fertil. Steril.,* 1992 Sep;58(3):526-9.

[68] Webley G.E, Leidenberger F. The circadian pattern of melatonin and its positive relationship with progesterone in women. *J. Clin. Endocrinol. Metab.,* 1986 Aug;63(2):323-8.

[69] Battista P.J, Condon W.A. Serotonin-induced stimulation of progesterone production by cow luteal cells in vitro. *J. Reprod. Fertil.,* 1986 Jan;76(1):231-8.

[70] Nakamura Y, Tamura H, Takayama H, Kato H. Increased endogenous level of melatonin in preovulatory human follicles does not directly influence progesterone production. *Fertil. Steril.,* 2003 Oct; 80 (4): 1012-6.

[71] Schaeffer H.J, Sirotkin A.V. Melatonin and serotonin regulate the release of insulin-like growth factor-I, oxytocin and progesterone by cultured human granulosa cells. *Exp. Clin. Endocrinol. Diabetes,* 1997;105(2):109-12.

[72] Sirotkin A.V. Direct influence of melatonin on steroid, nonapeptide hormones, and cyclic nucleotide secretion by granulosa cells isolated from porcine ovaries. *J. Pineal. Res.,* 1994 Oct;17(3):112-7.

[73] Tamura H, Nakamura Y, Takiguchi S, Kashida S, Yamagata Y, Sugino N, et al. Melatonin directly suppresses steroid production by preovulatory follicles in the cyclic hamster. *J. Pineal. Res.,* 1998 Oct;25(3):135-41.

[74] Crisp T.M, Channing C.P. Fine structural events correlated with progestin secretion during luteinization of rhesus monkey granulosa cells in culture. *Biol. Reprod.,* 1972 Aug;7(1):55-72.

[75] Sugino N, Takiguchi S, Kashida S, Karube A, Nakamura Y, Kato H. Superoxide dismutase expression in the human corpus luteum during the menstrual cycle and in early pregnancy. *Mol. Hum. Reprod.,* 2000 Jan;6(1):19-25.

[76] Turek F.W, Joshu C, Kohsaka A, Lin E, Ivanova G, McDearmon E, et al. Obesity and metabolic syndrome in circadian Clock mutant mice. *Science,* 2005 May 13;308(5724):1043-5.

[77] Tanavde V.S, Maitra A. In vitro modulation of steroidogenesis and gene expression by melatonin: a study with porcine antral follicles. *Endocr. Res.,* 2003 Nov;29(4):399-410.

[78] Baratta M, Tamanini C. Effect of melatonin on the in vitro secretion of progesterone and estradiol 17 beta by ovine granulosa cells. *Acta. Endocrinol. (Copenh), 1992* Oct;127(4):366-70.

[79] Adriaens I, Jacquet P, Cortvrindt R, Janssen K, Smitz J. Melatonin has dose-dependent effects on folliculogenesis, oocyte maturation capacity and steroidogenesis. *Toxicology,* 2006 Dec 7;228(2-3):333-43.

[80] Tamura H, Nakamura Y, Korkmaz A, Manchester LC, Tan DX, Sugino N, et al. Melatonin and the ovary: physiological and pathophysiological implications. *Fertil. Steril.,* 2009 Jul;92(1):328-43.

[81] Webley G.E, Luck M.R. Melatonin directly stimulates the secretion of progesterone by human and bovine granulosa cells in vitro. *J. Reprod. Fertil.,* 1986 Nov;78(2):711-7.

[82] Akbulut K.G, Gonul B, Akbulut H. The role of melatonin on gastric mucosal cell proliferation and telomerase activity in ageing. *J. Pineal. Res.,* 2009 Nov;47(4):308-12.

[83] Carretero M, Escames G, Lopez LC, Venegas C, Dayoub JC, Garcia L, et al. Long-term melatonin administration protects brain mitochondria from aging. *J. Pineal. Res.,* 2009 Sep;47(2):192-200.

[84] Yamamoto H.A, Mohanan P.V. Melatonin attenuates brain mitochondria DNA damage induced by potassium cyanide *in vivo* and *in vitro. Toxicology,* 2002 Sep 30;179(1-2):29-36.

[85] Martin M, Macias M, Escames G, Leon J, Acuna-Castroviejo D. Melatonin but not vitamins C and E maintains glutathione homeostasis in t-butyl hydroperoxide-induced mitochondrial oxidative stress. *FASEB J.,* 2000 Sep;14(12):1677-9.

[86] Jou M.J, Peng T.I, Yu P.Z, Jou S.B, Reiter R.J, Chen J.Y, et al. Melatonin protects against common deletion of mitochondrial DNA-augmented mitochondrial oxidative stress and apoptosis. *J. Pineal. Res.,* 2007 Nov;43(4):389-403.

[87] Milczarek R, Hallmann A, Sokolowska E, Kaletha K, Klimek J. Melatonin enhances antioxidant action of alpha-tocopherol and ascorbate against N. *J. Pineal. Res.,* 2010 Sep;49(2):149-55.

[88] Paradies G, Petrosillo G, Paradies V, Reiter R.J, Ruggiero FM. Melatonin, cardiolipin and mitochondrial bioenergetics in health and disease. *J. Pineal. Res.,* 2010 May;48(4):297-310.

[89] Taketani T, Tamura H, Takasaki A, Lee L, Kizuka F, Tamura I, et al. Protective role of melatonin in progesterone production by human luteal cells. *J. Pineal. Res.,* 2011 Sep;51(2):207-13.

[90] Scarpellini F, Mastrone M, Sbracia M, Scarpellini L. Serum lipoperoxide level variations in normal and luteal phase defect cycles. *Gynecol. Obstet. Invest.,* 1996;42(1):28-30.

[91] Kang J.T, Koo O.J, Kwon D.K, Park H.J, Jang G, Kang S.K, et al. Effects of melatonin on in vitro maturation of porcine oocyte and expression of melatonin receptor RNA in cumulus and granulosa cells. *J. Pineal. Res.,* 2009 Jan;46(1):22-8.

[92] Takasaki A, Tamura H, Taniguchi K, Asada H, Taketani T, Matsuoka A, et al. Luteal blood flow and luteal function. *J. Ovarian. Res.,* 2009;2:1.

[93] Kang K, Lee K, Park S, Kim Y.S, Back K. Enhanced production of melatonin by ectopic overexpression of human serotonin N-acetyltransferase plays a role in cold resistance in transgenic rice seedlings. *J. Pineal. Res.,* 2010 Sep;49(2):176-82.

[94] Manjunatha B.M, Devaraj M, Gupta P.S, Ravindra J.P, Nandi S. Effect of taurine and melatonin in the culture medium on buffalo in vitro embryo development. *Reprod. Domest. Anim.,* 2009 Feb;44(1):12-6.

[95] Tamura H, Takasaki A, Miwa I, Taniguchi K, Maekawa R, Asada H, et al. Oxidative stress impairs oocyte quality and melatonin protects oocytes from free radical damage and improves fertilization rate. *J. Pineal. Res., 2008* Apr;44(3):280-7.

[96] Mahmood T.A, Templeton A. Prevalence and genesis of endometriosis. *Hum. Reprod.,* 1991 Apr;6(4):544-9.

[97] Sangi-Haghpeykar H, Poindexter A.N, III. Epidemiology of endometriosis among parous women. *Obstet. Gynecol.,* 1995 Jun;85(6):983-92.

[98] Van L.A, Casanas-Roux F, Donnez J. Oxidative stress and peritoneal endometriosis. *Fertil. Steril.*, 2002 May;77(5):861-70.
[99] Zeller J.M, Henig I, Radwanska E, Dmowski W.P. Enhancement of human monocyte and peritoneal macrophage chemiluminescence activities in women with endometriosis. *Am. J. Reprod. Immunol. Microbiol.*, 1987 Mar;13(3):78-82.
[100] Paul S, Sharma A.V, Mahapatra P.D, Bhattacharya P, Reiter R.J, Swarnakar S. Role of melatonin in regulating matrix metalloproteinase-9 via tissue inhibitors of metalloproteinase-1 during protection against endometriosis. *J. Pineal. Res.*, 2008 May;44(4):439-49.
[101] Ozcelik B, Serin IS, Basbug M, Uludag S, Narin F, Tayyar M. Effect of melatonin in the prevention of post-operative adhesion formation in a rat uterine horn adhesion model. *Hum. Reprod.*, 2003 Aug;18(8):1703-6.
[102] Guney M, Oral B, Karahan N, Mungan T. Regression of endometrial explants in a rat model of endometriosis treated with melatonin. *Fertil. Steril.*, 2008 Apr;89(4):934-42.
[103] Plachot M, Belaisch-Allart J, Mayenga J.M, Chouraqui A, Tesquier A, Serkine AM, et al. [Oocyte and embryo quality in polycystic ovary syndrome]. *Gynecol. Obstet. Fertil.*, 2003 Apr;31(4):350-4.
[104] Gonzalez F, Rote NS, Minium J, Kirwan J.P. Increased activation of nuclear factor kappaB triggers inflammation and insulin resistance in polycystic ovary syndrome. *J. Clin. Endocrinol. Metab.*, 2006 Apr;91(4):1508-12.
[105] Sabuncu T, Vural H, Harma M, Harma M. Oxidative stress in polycystic ovary syndrome and its contribution to the risk of cardiovascular disease. *Clin. Biochem.*, 2001 Jul;34(5):407-13.
[106] Yildirim B, Demir S, Temur I, Erdemir R, Kaleli B. Lipid peroxidation in follicular fluid of women with polycystic ovary syndrome during assisted reproduction cycles. *J. Reprod. Med.*, 2007 Aug;52(8):722-6.
[107] Sun C.L, Qiao J, Hu Z.X, Zhang T, Chen Y.Y. [Expression of novel apoptosis-related protein PDCD5 in granulosa cells of polysystic ovary syndrome]. *Beijing Da Xue Xue Bao,* 2005 Oct 18;37(5):476-9.
[108] Luboshitzky R, Qupti G, Ishay A, Shen-Orr Z, Futerman B, Linn S. Increased 6-sulfatoxymelatonin excretion in women with polycystic ovary syndrome. *Fertil. Steril.*, 2001 Sep;76(3):506-10.
[109] Auwerx J, Staels B. Leptin. Lancet 1998 Mar 7;351(9104):737-42.
[110] Li M.G, Ding G.L, Chen X.J, Lu X.P, Dong L.J, Dong M.Y, et al. Association of serum and follicular fluid leptin concentrations with granulosa cell phosphorylated signal transducer and activator of transcription 3 expression in fertile patients with polycystic ovarian syndrome. *J. Clin. Endocrinol. Metab.*, 2007 Dec;92(12):4771-6.
[111] Wolden-Hanson T, Mitton D.R, McCants R.L, Yellon S.M, Wilkinson CW, Matsumoto AM, et al. Daily melatonin administration to middle-aged male rats suppresses body weight, intraabdominal adiposity, and plasma leptin and insulin independent of food intake and total body fat. *Endocrinology,* 2000 Feb;141(2):487-97.
[112] Canpolat S, Sandal S, Yilmaz B, Yasar A, Kutlu S, Baydas G, et al. Effects of pinealectomy and exogenous melatonin on serum leptin levels in male rat. *Eur. J. Pharmacol.*, 2001 Sep 28;428(1):145-8.
[113] Franks S, Gharani N, McCarthy M. Candidate genes in polycystic ovary syndrome. *Hum. Reprod. Update,* 2001 Jul;7(4):405-10.

[114] Pelusi B, Gambineri A, Pasquali R. Type 2 diabetes and the polycystic ovary syndrome. *Minerva Ginecol.,* 2004 Feb;56(1):41-51.

[115] Li C, Shi Y, You L, Wang L, Chen Z.J. Association of rs10830963 and rs10830962 SNPs in the melatonin receptor (MTNR1B) gene among Han Chinese women with polycystic ovary syndrome. *Mol. Hum. Reprod.,* 2011 Mar;17(3):193-8.

[116] Ronn T, Wen J, Yang Z, Lu B, Du Y, Groop L, et al. A common variant in MTNR1B, encoding melatonin receptor 1B, is associated with type 2 diabetes and fasting plasma glucose in Han Chinese individuals. *Diabetologia,* 2009 May;52(5):830-3.

[117] Coulam C.B, Adamson S.C, Annegers J.F. Incidence of premature ovarian failure. *Obstet. Gynecol.,* 1986 Apr;67(4):604-6.

[118] Groff A.A, Covington S.N, Halverson L.R, Fitzgerald O.R, Vanderhoof V, Calis K, et al. Assessing the emotional needs of women with spontaneous premature ovarian failure. *Fertil. Steril.,* 2005 Jun;83(6):1734-41.

[119] Abir R, Ben-Haroush A, Felz C, Okon E, Raanani H, Orvieto R, et al. Selection of patients before and after anticancer treatment for ovarian cryopreservation. *Hum. Reprod.,* 2008 Apr;23(4):869-77.

[120] Larsen E.C, Muller J, Schmiegelow K, Rechnitzer C, Andersen A.N. Reduced ovarian function in long-term survivors of radiation- and chemotherapy-treated childhood cancer. *J. Clin. Endocrinol. Metab.,* 2003 Nov;88(11):5307-14.

[121] Luborsky J, Llanes B, Davies S, Binor Z, Radwanska E, Pong R. Ovarian autoimmunity: greater frequency of autoantibodies in premature menopause and unexplained infertility than in the general population. *Clin. Immunol.,* 1999 Mar;90(3):368-74.

[122] Nandedkar T.D, Wadia P. Autoimmune disorders of the ovary. *Indian. J. Exp. Biol.,* 1998 May;36(5):433-6.

[123] Narayanan M, Murthy PS, Munaf SA, Shah LC, Kini MD. Antiovarian antibodies and their effect on the outcome of assisted reproduction. *J. Assist. Reprod. Genet.,* 1995 Oct;12(9):599-605.

[124] Vijayalaxmi, Reiter R.J, Tan D.X, Herman T.S, Thomas C.R, Jr. Melatonin as a radioprotective agent: a review. *Int. J. Radiat. Oncol. Biol. Phys.,* 2004 Jul 1;59(3):639-53.

[125] Gosden R.G, Wade J.C, Fraser H.M, Sandow J, Faddy M.J. Impact of congenital or experimental hypogonadotrophism on the radiation sensitivity of the mouse ovary. *Hum. Reprod.,* 1997 Nov;12(11):2483-8.

[126] Kim J.K, Lee C.J. Effect of exogenous melatonin on the ovarian follicles in gamma-irradiated mouse. *Mutat. Res.,* 2000 Apr 3;449(1-2):33-9.

[127] Shirazi A, Ghobadi G, Ghazi-Khansari M. A radiobiological review on melatonin: a novel radioprotector. *J. Radiat. Res.,* 2007 Jul;48(4):263-72.

[128] Badr F.M, E.l Habit O.H, Harraz M.M. Radioprotective effect of melatonin assessed by measuring chromosomal damage in mitotic and meiotic cells. *Mutat. Res.,* 1999 Aug 18;444(2):367-72.

[129] Reiter R.J, Tan D.X, Osuna C, Gitto E. Actions of melatonin in the reduction of oxidative stress. A review. *J. Biomed. Sci.,* 2000 Nov;7(6):444-58.

[130] Koc M, Taysi S, Emin B.M, Bakan N. The effect of melatonin against oxidative damage during total-body irradiation in rats. *Radiat. Res.,* 2003 Aug;160(2):251-5.

[131] Lissoni P, Barni S, Meregalli S, Fossati V, Cazzaniga M, Esposti D, et al. Modulation of cancer endocrine therapy by melatonin: a phase II study of tamoxifen plus melatonin in metastatic breast cancer patients progressing under tamoxifen alone. *Br. J. Cancer,* 1995 Apr;71(4):854-6.

[132] Oz E, Erbas D, Surucu H.S, Duzgun E. Prevention of doxorubicin-induced cardiotoxicity by melatonin. *Mol. Cell Biochem.,* 2006 Jan;282(1-2):31-7.

[133] Voznesenskaya T, Makogon N, Bryzgina T, Sukhina V, Grushka N, Alexeyeva I. Melatonin protects against experimental immune ovarian failure in mice. *Reprod. Biol.,* 2007 Nov;7(3):207-20.

[134] Friedman O, Orvieto R, Fisch B, Felz C, Freud E, Ben-Haroush A, et al. Possible improvements in human ovarian grafting by various host and graft treatments. *Hum. Reprod.,* 2012 Feb;27(2):474-82.

[135] Dittrich R, Lotz L, Keck G, Hoffmann I, Mueller A, Beckmann MW, et al. Live birth after ovarian tissue autotransplantation following overnight transportation before cryopreservation. *Fertil. Steril.,* 2012 Feb;97(2):387-90.

[136] Revel A, Laufer N, Ben M.A, Lebovich M, Mitrani E. Micro-organ ovarian transplantation enables pregnancy: a case report. *Hum. Reprod.,* 2011 May;26(5):1097-103.

[137] Silber S.J. Ovary cryopreservation and transplantation for fertility preservation. *Mol. Hum. Reprod.,* 2012 Feb;18(2):59-67.

[138] Abir R, Fisch B, Jessel S, Felz C, Ben-Haroush A, Orvieto R. Improving posttransplantation survival of human ovarian tissue by treating the host and graft. *Fertil. Steril.,* 2011 Mar 15;95(4):1205-10.

[139] Molpeceres V, Mauriz JL, Garcia-Mediavilla MV, Gonzalez P, Barrio JP, Gonzalez-Gallego J. Melatonin is able to reduce the apoptotic liver changes induced by aging via inhibition of the intrinsic pathway of apoptosis. *J. Gerontol. A Biol. Sci. Med. Sci.,* 2007 Jul;62(7):687-95.

[140] Hemadi M, Shokri S, Pourmatroud E, Moramezi F, Khodadai A. Follicular dynamic and immunoreactions of the vitrified ovarian graft after host treatment with variable regimens of melatonin. *Am. J. Reprod. Immunol.,* 2012 May;67(5):401-12.

[141] Sapmaz E, Ayar A, Celik H, Sapmaz T, Kilic N, Yasar MA. Effects of melatonin and oxytetracycline in autologous intraperitoneal ovary transplantation in rats. *Neuro. Endocrinol. Lett.,* 2003 Oct;24(5):350-4.

[142] Abir R, Biron-Shental T, Orvieto R, Garor R, Krissi H, Fisch B. Transplantation of frozen-thawed late-gestational-age human fetal ovaries into immunodeficient mice. *Fertil. Steril.,* 2009 Aug; 92 (2): 770-7.

[143] Abir R, Nitke S, Ben-Haroush A, Fisch B. In vitro maturation of human primordial ovarian follicles: clinical significance, progress in mammals, and methods for growth evaluation. *Histol. Histopathol.,* 2006 Aug;21(8):887-98.

[144] Rocha R.M, Lima L.F, Alves A.M, Celestino J.J, Matos M.H, Lima-Verde IB, et al. Interaction between melatonin and follicle-stimulating hormone promotes in vitro development of caprine preantral follicles. *Domest. Anim. Endocrinol.,* 2013 Jan;44(1):1-9.

In: New Developments in Melatonin Research ISBN: 978-1-62618-843-3
Editors: D.Acuña-Castroviejo, I.Rusanova, G.Escames © 2013 Nova Science Publishers, Inc.

Chapter 9

Melatonin and Pregnancy

Camila Souza de Oliveira Guimarães, Laura Penna Rocha, Juliana Reis Machado, Marlene Antônia dos Reis and Rosana Rosa Miranda Corrêa
Triângulo Mineiro Federal University, Uberaba, Minas Gerais, Brazil

Abstract

Melatonin is an endogenously produced indoleamine involved in a variety of important physiological functions, including regulation of the circadian rhythms, reproductive physiology, and body temperature, and it has been determined to possess important antioxidant properties as well.

Several studies have suggested that in complicated pregnancies, maternal treatment with antioxidants may improve placental function and thereby fetal development; moreover, melatonin treatment in these cases has been proposed to possess numerous attractive attributes, resulting in a wide range of health benefits and helping to reduce complications in the neonatal period.

This review will focus on studies reporting the use of melatonin during pregnancy and its potential benefits of improving quality of life and reducing healthcare costs.

Introduction

Pregnancy is a physiological state accompanied by a high metabolic demand and elevated requirements for tissue oxygen, as it is associated with the increased production of reactive oxygen species (ROS) [1]. It represents a state of metabolic challenge, and even women with normal pregnancies experience increased oxidative stress and lipid peroxidation relative to nonpregnant women [1; 2]. Newborns, especially preterm infants, are especially prone to oxidative stress [3], and it likely contributes to the severity of several newborn conditions. The idea of "oxygen radical disease of neonatology" [4] suggests that oxidative stress affects a variety of organs, often simultaneously, and gives rise to different signs according to the organ that is most severely damaged. Bronchopulmonary dysplasia/chronic lung disease, retinopathy of prematurity, and necrotizing enterocolitis are included in this category. Subsequently, it became clear that free radicals are involved in periventricular leukomalacia [5] as well as in influencing the ductus arteriosus and pulmonary circulation [5; 6]. It appears that these conditions are not different diseases, but belong to the same category, yielding different symptoms according to which organs are most involved [1]. Based on this concept, studies on the influence of oxidative stress during pregnancy and possible treatments to minimize it have been shown to be very important in preventing such complications.

Oxidative Stress

Oxygen comprises 21% of the Earth's atmosphere and is essential for aerobic organisms, being used to generate energy in the form of adenosine triphosphate [7]. During life in utero, the partial pressure of oxygen is low. Thus, from early pregnancy, fetal and placental adaptations, including high fetal cardiac output, relative vasodilatation of the fetoplacental vasculature, and the high oxygen-carrying capacity of fetal blood ensure the delivery of oxygen to fetal tissues [8]. Despite being essential to aerobic organisms, certain states of oxygen can be highly toxic and deleterious to cells and tissues. A relatively large amount—approximately 5%—of inspired oxygen is converted to free radicals, many of which are extremely toxic [9]. A free radical is described as a molecular species with an unpaired electron in the outer shell that then renders it highly reactive and unstable [10]. Free radicals containing oxygen and oxygen-derived metabolites, collectively termed ROS, are normally produced in aerobic organisms. Under normal physiological conditions, oxidative reduction occurs continuously, where the mitochondria consume oxygen and reduce it to water in a process involving cytochrome oxidase in the mitochondrial respiratory chain. The rate of ROS formation is dependent on the amount of oxygen passing through the mitochondria at any given time [11]. When produced in excess, ROS mutilate molecules and are important mediators of cell and tissue damage. This resulting damage, which is unavoidable, is referred to as oxidative stress [12]. The 3 most commonly described ROS are the superoxide (O_2^-) and hydroxyl radicals (OH^-), and the non-radical hydrogen peroxide (H_2O_2). Of these, the most abundant ROS formed in the course of cellular metabolism is O_2^- [13], which is considered the primary ROS because it is produced directly when oxygen acquires an additional electron, giving rise to the secondary reactive oxygen species H_2O_2 and OH^- [14]. Along with oxygen free radicals, nitric oxide (NO) complexes are also implicated in free radical injury. NO is a weak free radical overproduced by NO synthase under hypoxic conditions. It is capable of rapidly combining with O_2^- to form peroxynitrite ($ONOO^-$), a potent free radical strongly implicated in the compromise of cellular function due to lipid peroxidation [15], which is described as a chain of reactions between free radicals and the polyunsaturated lipids contained within biological membranes, producing membrane destruction [16].

At normal rates of cellular respiration and subtoxic levels, free radicals have been shown to act as signal transduction mediators [17] and are involved in mediating certain physiological processes, including the intracellular regulation of calcium, activation of transcription factors, and protein phosphorylation [14]. In some situations, however, they can be life threatening. The accumulation of reactive free radicals beyond the capacity of the endogenous antioxidant defense system to scavenge them results in DNA damage (fragmentation, apoptosis, base modifications, and strand breaks) and oxidation of lipids, proteins, and polysaccharides [18-20] that initially compromise cell function and can ultimately lead to cell death via apoptosis or necrosis [18]. Clinically, oxidative stress is proposed as the cause of tissue damage in many pathophysiological disorders such as hypoxia, inflammation, and tissue ischemia and reperfusion [18; 21; 22]. It also has been linked to neurodegenerative diseases such as idiopathic Parkinson's disease, amyotrophic lateral sclerosis, and Alzheimer's disease [21], and has been implicated in the normal aging process [23].

Oxidative stress is also related to proinflammatory processes. It is currently well accepted that oxidative stress, infection, and inflammation are closely linked. Upon activation, many cells in the immune system generate oxygen free radicals, and equally, the overproduction of free radicals induces an inflammatory response. This is particularly true in pregnancy [24]. ROS can initiate an inflammatory response, and conversely, many proinflammatory mediators stimulate the generation of free radicals and subsequent oxidative stress. Of these mediators, the transcription factor nuclear factor-κB (NF-κB) is believed to be the key to this interaction, being upregulated by mediators of both inflammation and by hypoxia itself [25]. A role of ROS, particularly H_2O_2, has also been suggested in the activation of NF-κB [25]. Elevated IκB kinase phosphorylation and NF-κB activation have been described in the placenta, and in turn, activated NF-κB mediates the production and release of placental proinflammatory cytokines such as interleukin-1β (IL-1β) and tumor necrosis factor-α (TNFα) [26; 27]. The predisposition of the placenta to generate free radicals and proinflammatory metabolites relates in part to the high placental content of the tryptophan-dependent enzyme indoleamine 2,3-dioxygenase (IDO). The IDO-dependent metabolism of tryptophan yields a number of kynurenine metabolites that are either proinflammatory in themselves or excitotoxic by virtue of their interactions with the *N*-methyl-D-aspartic acid receptor in the brain [28]. Increased levels of these cytotoxic tryptophan metabolites in human umbilical cord blood have been reported in association with signs of clinical infection [29]. It is likely that this is due to NF-κB inducing the increase of tryptophan catabolism [28]. In addition, NF-κB activation can lead to the release of ROS [30]. These observations show that the placenta itself is an important source of reactive free radicals [31], and imply that treatments that target or include the placenta may be necessary in devising successful neuroprotective strategies for the fetal and newborn brain [8].

Antioxidant Defense

Within all organisms, there is a critical balance between free radical generation and antioxidant defenses. Therefore, oxidative stress is a result of an imbalance between pro-oxidants, free radical species, the body's scavenging ability and antioxidants [32]. To protect cells from the damage caused by free radicals and the related reactants, organisms have evolved several defense mechanisms to remove ROS rapidly and efficiently from the intracellular environment [33]. Under physiological conditions, the overproduction of free radical species and their neutralization is prevented by the activity of the antioxidative defense system, which consists of enzymatic and non-enzymatic components [32]. The oxidants that are not directly scavenged or otherwise not metabolized attack cellular components, producing useless molecular debris and occasionally cause cell death [33].

The antioxidant defense system comprises several enzymes and small–molecular weight molecules with antioxidant capabilities [34], which directly scavenge free radicals and related reactants. Antioxidants may be broadly classified as enzymatic (superoxide dismutase [SOD], catalase, and glutathione peroxidase [GPx]) or nonenzymatic (vitamins C and E, b-carotene, allopurinol, melatonin, etc.). These compounds, which prevent cellular damage caused by ROS, may act in numerous ways, ranging from preventing ROS formation (such as metal ion chelators and anti-inflammatory agents) to intercepting ROS once they are formed. Most antioxidants used clinically fall into the latter category [9]. The antioxidant enzymes represent the first line of defense against toxic reactants by metabolizing them to innocuous byproducts [33]. As a compensatory mechanism to better protect cells from the damage induced by free radicals, the activity and expression of these enzymes is increased. However, in certain cases, a large amount of free radicals is generated, and even the increased activity of the antioxidative enzymes may be insufficient to counteract the potential damage. It has been proposed that moderate levels of toxic reactants induce increases in antioxidant enzymes, whereas very high levels of reactants reduce enzyme activities as a result of damage of the molecular machinery that is required to induce these enzymes [35].

One such enzymatic defense is SOD that specifically processes O_2^- to produce H_2O_2, which is then dissociated by catalase or GPx into water and molecular oxygen. Additional small molecule antioxidants such as glutathione (GSH), ascorbic acid, and tocopherol scavengers further mediate the detoxification of these free radicals [11]. Antioxidant enzymes are regulated by multiple factors. The oxidative status of the cell is the primary factor regulating gene expression and the activity of these enzymes [36]. Both endogenous [37] and exogenous agents [38; 39] are involved in this process, acting as oxidants that alter cellular oxidative equilibrium, and thus, the expression of antioxidant enzyme genes. In addition to developmental changes, differentiation and aging influences [35; 40; 41], inflammation [42; 43], and hormonal regulation of antioxidative enzymes [44; 45] have been reported to influence antioxidant enzymes. It has been shown that the antioxidative defense system is altered during pregnancy [1]. In pregnant women, it has been reported that there is a deficiency of antioxidative enzymes such as SOD [46] and GPx [47], which may lead to elevated oxidative stress. Even in normal pregnancies, the increase in antioxidants is insufficient to offset the rise in free radical generation, which leads to increased oxidative stress and lipid peroxidation relative to nonpregnant women [1].

The placenta is very likely the site of lipid peroxide generation [48]. During pregnancy, the generation of free radicals increases with the placental mitochondria being the major source of ROS production. The peroxidation of lipids by ROS results in the formation of primary lipid peroxidation products such as lipid hydroperoxides and secondary products such as malondialdehyde and lipid peroxides. The lipid hydroperoxides formed bind to lipoproteins. These are then transported to distant sites where the hydroperoxides promote ongoing lipid peroxidation, resulting in systemic oxidative stress [49]. The capacity of placental antioxidant defenses is critical for healthy placental function, and thus, for optimal fetal growth and development. However, variations in uteroplacental blood flow, reduced placental function, or altered fetal demand can alter oxygen delivery to the placenta. Although a variety of fetal adaptations exist that enable the fetus to withstand acute or chronic reductions in oxygen availability, the developing fetus may at times be exposed to high levels of oxidative stress due to the overproduction of oxygen free radicals and a decrease in antioxidant defense capability [8].

Melatonin

Melatonin (*N*-acetyl-5-methoxytryptamine), so named because of its ability in certain fish, reptiles, and amphibians to temporarily turn the skin a dark color (produced by the chemical pigment melanin) [50], is an endogenously produced indoleamine that plays a key role in a variety of important physiological functions. It was first recognized for its multiple neurohormonal functions, including regulation of the circadian rhythms, reproductive physiology, and body temperature [51-53]. In addition, it is considered a stringent biological modulator of mood, sleep, retinal physiology, sexual behavior, seasonal reproductive physiology and behavior, and immunologic function [54-56], and there is experimental evidence of the influence of melatonin on aging and age-related processes and disease states [57]. In humans and other animals, studies have shown that melatonin also has proinflammatory actions, including the activation of proinflammatory cytokines in the early-phase response and mediation of leukocyte recruitment [58], as well as anti-inflammatory effects [58-61]. The anti-inflammatory property of melatonin arises from the fact that it prevents the translocation of NF-κB to the nucleus, thus reducing the upregulation of proinflammatory cytokines [62]. It decreases IL-6, IL-8, TNF-α, and nitrite/nitrate levels and modifies serum inflammatory parameters in surgical neonates, thus improving their clinical course [60]. Preliminary findings indicate that melatonin has in vitro antimicrobial activity against antibiotic-resistant Gram-positive and Gram-negative pathogenic microorganisms, probably by reducing intracellular substrates [63]; similarly, it has antiviral functions [64].

Melatonin is primarily produced in the pineal gland and secreted in a circadian manner, with high levels occurring in all species at night. The initial precursor of melatonin biosynthesis is the amino acid tryptophan. Pinealocytes take up tryptophan from the blood and convert it to serotonin through hydroxylation and decarboxylation; serotonin is then converted to *N*-acetyl-serotonin by the enzyme arylalkylamine *N*-acetyltransferase (NAT), and *N*-acetyl-serotonin is methylated to form melatonin by the enzyme hydroxyindole-*O*-methyltransferase [65; 66]. The period of melatonin secretion is proportional to the duration of darkness, and it thus acts as a neuroendocrine transducer of photoperiodic information [67]. The photoperiodic environment regulates its biosynthetic pathway such that in the presence of light, neuronal impulses originating in the retina are transmitted to the suprachiasmatic nuclei (SCN) of the hypothalamus and other hypothalamic structures. From the SCN, a projection descends to the intermediolateral cell column in the upper thoracic region of the spinal cord. From the spinal cord, fibers project to the superior (third) cervical ganglion, with postganglionic sympathetic fibers terminating at the pineal gland [68]. In humans, the onset of darkness leads to these sympathetic fibers releasing norepinephrine, which binds predominantly to b1-adrenergic receptors (and to a lesser extent, to a1-adrenergic receptors) to initiate the intracellular release of stored serotonin and NAT. This cascade of neuronal and intrapineal biochemical signals facilitates melatonin anabolism in humans and is responsible for the circadian synthesis and release of melatonin [54].

Melatonin exhibits a high degree of conservation across the evolutionary ladder, pointing to a critical function in all life forms [69], even in organisms devoid of a pineal gland. Clearly, the production of melatonin is not restricted to the pineal gland, as its synthesis occurs in other organs in invertebrates [70] and in unicells [71]. Additionally, melatonin has been identified in plants [72], in which it may also be synthesized [73].

During the typical light:dark cycle, circulating melatonin concentrations are low during the day and elevated at night, usually exhibiting a characteristic rapid rise in concentration after the onset of darkness [74]. With the onset of darkness, the concentrations of melatonin in the pineal gland increase, and the hormone passively diffuses into the cerebrospinal fluid and in circulation. In humans, the secretion of melatonin peaks in the middle of the night between 2:00 a.m. and 4:00 a.m., and gradually declines thereafter throughout the following 24-h period [75]. Serum melatonin concentration varies remarkably according to age, and newborns are known to secrete very little melatonin. However, concentrations begin to rise very shortly after birth and continue to increase with age. Melatonin levels peak between the ages of 1 and 3 years, after which serum concentrations have been reported to gradually fall, as its secretory pattern becomes circadian during puberty and adolescence [75]. These circadian pulses of melatonin appear to remain consistent until the individual reaches an approximate age of 25 years, and then slowly begin to decline with age until the late sixth decade of life. It was shown that human subjects over the age of 60 years secrete significantly lower day and evening levels of melatonin, indicating an association between physiological melatonin concentrations and aging [76].

Once synthesized and released, melatonin has been shown to regulate a variety of organ systems in different species. These organ-specific effects are mediated via interactions with specific melatonin receptors. Two pharmacologically distinct families of membrane-bound melatonin receptors known as ML1 and ML2 have been identified. Although on different chromosomes, the genes encoding the human melatonin receptors appear to be quite similar, and other forms of the receptors may exist as a result of alternative splicing [77].

Three kinetically distinct subtypes of ML1 receptors are known: Mel1a (*Kd*, 20–40 pM), Mel1b (*Kd*, 160 pM), and more recently, Mel1c (*Kd*, 20–60 pM), which has been found only in chickens, *Xenopus*, zebra fish, and in a human embryonic kidney (HEK293) cell line [77]. It is believed that the ML1 receptor subtypes are involved in renal function [78], sleep induction, circadian rhythms, reproduction [77], and the contractility of cerebral arteries [79], and all ML1 subtypes have been implicated in the Ca21-dependent release of dopamine in the mammalian retina as well as various light-dependent processes such as the phagocytosis of retinal photopigment discs [77; 80]. Currently, it is believed that the inhibitory influence of melatonin on the SCN and its circadian and reproductive effects are mediated via the Mel1a receptor [77]. Low-affinity ML2 receptors are believed to be coupled to G-proteins that mediate signal transduction in a fashion similar to that of the ML1 receptors [81], but the physiological importance of the ML2 receptors remains undetermined. Both MT1 and MT2 receptors are members of the 7-transmembrane G-protein–coupled receptor family [82; 83]. ML1 receptors reside predominantly in neuronal regions, including the cerebellum and hippocampus [84], as well as in the SCN, hypothalamus, thalamus, preoptic area, the plexiform layer of the retina, pars tuberalis of the pituitary, and many areas of the cerebral cortex [77]. Non-neuronal ML1 receptors are found in the cerebral and caudal arteries, the hypophyseal pars tuberalis, ovary, kidney, and the small intestine [77; 78; 80]. In contrast, ML2 receptors have no well-characterized specific distribution in mammalian tissues [80; 81]. They are most strongly expressed in the retina, and at considerably lower levels in the SCN, hippocampus, and cerebellum [85]. Melatonin receptor expression in peripheral human tissues is also well-documented [83]. The RNA and/or protein expression of melatonin receptors has been identified in human reproductive tissues, including breast epithelium [86], uterine myometrium [87], and ovarian granulosa and luteal cells [88].

Melatonin as an Antioxidant

Numerous beneficial actions have been attributed to melatonin. In addition to its role as a protector against glucocorticoid damage [89] and some degenerative neurological conditions [90], an anti-cancer agent [91; 92], and as an enhancer of immune function [93; 94], its protective effects against oxidative processes have now been identified under a very wide range of conditions both in experimental animals and in humans [59; 95; 96]. The speculation that melatonin is an effective scavenger of H_2O_2, lipid peroxides, and peroxynitrites has been substantiated by several groups [97; 98], suggesting that melatonin has a potential physiological role in facilitating the prevention of age-related neurodegeneration, DNA damage, and cell death. Furthermore, research indicating that aging is a result of oxidative stress also implies that the administration of exogenous melatonin may help to combat the damage incurred due to oxidative stress, thus aiding in the prevention of various negative aspects of the aging process [99]. The positive effects of melatonin have been reported in the nervous system [100], the prevention of cataract formation [101], free radical damage induced by toxins [102], and in cases of intestinal and gastric damage following ischemia/reperfusion or drug administration [103; 104]. It was also reported in the reduction in the severity of colitis,the prevention of multiple-organ damage resulting from therapeutic and nontherapeutic chemotherapeutic agents [105-110], and ultraviolet damage to tissues [111], as well as free radical damage in experimental diabetes [112] and in chemotherapy and radiotherapy lesions [113], suggesting that melatonin possesses antioxidant properties [114; 115]. Studies have revealed that melatonin, both endogenous and exogenous, may help to neutralize free radicals before they can exert their destructive activity [97; 98; 116; 117]. In addition, the metabolites of melatonin (i.e., cyclic 3-hydroxmelatonin, *N*1-acetyl-*N*2-formyl-5-methoxykynuramine [AFMK], and *N*1-acetyl-5-methoxykynuramine), which are products of its reaction with free radicals, are themselves also powerful antioxidants [118-121].

The antioxidant properties of melatonin and its metabolites are related to their direct and indirect antioxidant actions [118-121]. They directly scavenge reactive oxygen/nitrogen species, including the O_2^-, singlet oxygen ($^1O_2$), H_2O_2, hypochlorous acid, nitric oxide (NO^-), and $ONOO^-$ [115; 118; 122; 123], and particularly, the highly destructive OH^- [62]. It reduces oxidative stress, reduces the leakage of electrons from the mitochondrial electron transport chain, which improves mitochondria function, and restores homeostasis of GSH, an important intracellular antioxidant [53; 124; 125]. Moreover, it has indirect antioxidant effects, as it stimulates the activities of antioxidant enzymes such as SOD, GPx, and GSH reductase, which are involved in metabolizing potentially reactive species to harmless molecules or inducing the synthesis of other endogenously produced antioxidants [33; 53; 126]. In the same manner, studies have shown that melatonin downregulates pro-oxidant enzymes (NO synthases, lipoxygenases) [33; 53; 126]. Melatonin also reduces NF-κB binding to DNA, probably by preventing its translocation to the nucleus [127]. This, in turn, reduces the production of proinflammatory cytokines and chemokines that induce free radical damage and limits the recruitment of polymorphonuclear leukocytes to inflammatory sites [128].

Melatonin is highly lipophilic [116], and its ability to diffuse into intracellular compartments aids in its role as an antioxidant [99; 129]. The mechanisms of action of melatonin involve the interaction of melatonin with H_2O_2 [130] followed by the scavenging of H_2O_2 and the formation of AFMK [131]; however, the details of these interaction mechanisms are not known. Melatonin may readily diffuse into cells to activate intracellular sites through binding to cytosolic calmodulin (CaM) [80]. Once bound to CaM, melatonin can influence calcium signaling through interactions with downstream effector enzymes such as adenylyl cyclase and phosphodiesterases, as well as through associations with tubulin and microtubules [80]. Melatonin is also known to interact with a nuclear family of orphan receptors known as retinoid-Z receptors (RZR), indicating that once in the nucleus, melatonin may conceivably regulate gene expression, functioning as a free radical scavenger [9; 80]. It has been suggested that melatonin exerts its effects via the inhibition of the multifunctional oxidase cytochrome P450 [132]; however, this does not appear to be entirely the case [99]. Melatonin has also been shown to influence antioxidant enzyme gene expression [133-135]. Reports documenting the influence of melatonin on antioxidant enzyme activity were first published in the mid-1990s [133; 134; 136]. Antioxidant enzyme activities exhibit endogenous rhythms under normal light:dark conditions. This is true in terms of their activity and gene expression. These changes with time suggest that these cycles might be dependent on the circadian melatonin rhythm [137; 138].

Antioxidant enzymes are known to be regulated by several factors that induce oxidative stress [38; 39; 42]; these factors presumably activate oxidative stress–sensitive transcription factors. In addition, the transcriptional activation of antioxidant enzyme genes has been reported after the treatment of cells with protective agents [139], wherein non-oxidative stress–dependent transcription factors are found to be involved. Melatonin has been shown to regulate the activation or repression of several transcription factors [127; 140-142], all of which are present in the promoter region of the 3 antioxidant enzymes GPx, SOD, and catalase. Thus, subsequent experiments should be performed in order to shed light on the intracellular pathways and transcription factors involved in the regulation of antioxidant enzyme gene expression and activity by melatonin [119]. Despite the intracellular molecular pathways involved in the regulation of antioxidant enzyme gene expression and/or activity by melatonin being presently unknown, it is suggested that melatonin regulation of antioxidant enzymes is receptor-mediated, thereby most likely implicating the MT1/MT2 receptors via second messengers such as cAMP, phospholipase C, or intracellular calcium concentration [143]. In addition, the binding of melatonin to membrane receptors could stimulate mitogen-activated protein kinase cascades, thereby activating several transcription factors [144]. The possibility exists that retinoid Z/retinoid-related receptors (RZR/ROR) could also mediate the effects of melatonin on antioxidative enzymes [145]; if so, the pathways involved in their regulation remain unknown. One possibility may relate to MT1/MT2 melatonin binding that, through second messengers and phosphorylation cascades, activates RZR/ROR [146]. Another possibility by which melatonin may regulate RZR/ROR would be via modulation of the calcium/CaM signaling pathway, either by changing intracellular calcium concentrations by binding to MT1/MT2 receptors [147], or by direct binding to calmodulin [148]. The calcium/CaM signaling pathway has been reported to regulate transcriptional activity of RZR/ROR via CaM-dependent protein kinases [149]. It has been suggested that melatonin also potentiates free radical scavenging by a non-enzymatic process of electron donation [9]. Regardless of how melatonin inhibits the effects of free radicals, the potential clinical applications of this characteristic of the hormone are noteworthy [99].

Melatonin and Normal Pregnancy

During pregnancy, maternal plasma melatonin levels are elevated, reaching a maximum at term and then returning to basal levels soon after delivery [150; 151]. A clear diurnal rhythm in serum melatonin concentrations is found in both early and late pregnancy, and serum melatonin levels during the third trimester of pregnancy are significantly higher than that during the first and the second trimester and in non-pregnant control women [152]. Melatonin may contribute to the maintenance of pregnancy by stimulating progesterone production while inhibiting prostaglandin synthesis and uterine contractility [49]. It also plays a functional role in fetoplacental development, as suggested by studies reporting the expression of melatonin receptors in the human and rat placenta and the ability of melatonin to stimulate human chorionic gonadotropin and to downregulate rat placental lactogen II mRNA levels [153-155]. Elevated levels of melatonin may also have an essential role as an antioxidant to reduce oxidative stress, which is a consequence of placenta metabolism and polymorphonuclear leukocytes during gestation. Elevated O_2^- generation in pregnant women has been observed [31; 156], accompanied by progressively increased melatonin levels [150; 152]. Due to its potent antioxidant properties, this increase in melatonin is likely to reduce oxidative damage from ROS in the placenta and systemic endothelial cells [49].

In cases where the basal plasma melatonin concentration is higher in the maternal rather than fetal compartment [157], it is suggested that melatonin crosses the placenta, and that fetal circulating melatonin is of maternal origin [158-160]. Due to its ability to diffuse through the placenta, maternal melatonin readily passes to all fetal tissues [161]. Studies have demonstrated that the fetal rat brain synthesizes melatonin [162], and although the SCN and the pineal gland appear to be mature in early fetal life in humans [163], the neurological circuitry linking these structures is incomplete [164]. Thus, the major source of this increased melatonin in both the maternal and fetal circulation during pregnancy appears to be of maternal pineal origin [160], via the action of a yet-unidentified placental hormone [49]. Prenatally, information about day length and circadian phase, presumably mediated by the maternal melatonin rhythm, is transferred to the fetus. Thus, photoperiodic information, as perceived by the mother, plays a role in synchronizing fetal physiology [165]. It is suggested that the diurnal activity of the fetal SCN is maintained by a signal related to the external lighting regime [166] and evidence suggests that photoperiodic information via maternal melatonin provides the fetus with information regarding the time of day [167; 168]. After birth, the full-term neonate does not produce melatonin for 2–4 months, leading to a transient absence of melatonin [162; 169]. Studies in sheep [160; 170] and rats [171] have reported that the serum melatonin levels in maternal circulation exhibit a diurnal rhythm that provides an important signal for the fetus to entrain the light–dark rhythm of newborns after delivery, but the changes in serum melatonin concentrations and their roles in pregnancy in humans are not clearly understood [49].

Melatonin and Complicated Pregnancies

In complicated pregnancy, the fetoplacental unit may become compromised, with alterations in placental efficiency, fetal growth, and birth weight [172], considered a major cause of both prenatal and postnatal mortality and morbidity [173]. In these situations, oxidative stress may be increased [8; 49]. Therefore, the prevention and/or treatment of these conditions remain a major concern in perinatal practice at present, and melatonin treatment has been reported as a useful option to prevent or minimize prenatal and postnatal negative outcomes related to these complications during pregnancy. Preeclampsia is a specific syndrome of human pregnancy and is associated with high rates of maternal and fetal morbidity and mortality. It is diagnosed by new development of hypertension (≥140/90 mmHg) and proteinuria (≥0.3 g/24 h) in the second half of gestation. Other manifestations of preeclampsia include generalized vasoconstriction, increased vasoactivity, reduced perfusion to organs, and platelet activation. After delivery, these signs are not observed. The etiopathogenesis of preeclampsia is not well understood, but it is suggested that the diverse manifestations of preeclampsia are derived from pathologic changes within the maternal vascular endothelium [174]. Evidence points to the placenta as a key source of factors that lead to the maternal endothelial cell dysfunction in preeclampsia [174]. Inadequate placental trophoblast invasion of the maternal uterine spiral arteries results in poor placental perfusion, which leads to placental ischemia. This could result in the release of cytotoxic factors into the maternal circulation that can cause widespread activation/dysfunction of the endothelium. Those circulating factors might induce oxidative stress and/or elicit an inflammatory response in the maternal endothelium, which results in the altered expression of several genes involved in the regulation of vascular tone [175].

Oxidative stress and especially lipid peroxidation are abnormally increased in the placentas of preeclamptic women [48; 176; 177] and are associated with the augmented production of lipid peroxides and thromboxane [178] and higher levels of lipid peroxide metabolites [178]. The placental mitochondria is likely an important source of this oxidative stress, contributing to the abnormal increase in lipid peroxidation in preeclamptic placenta via both increased O_2^- generation and an increase in susceptibility of the mitochondrial membrane to oxidation, leading to an overall increase in placental lipid peroxidation [177]. The blood concentrations of lipid peroxides in preeclamptic women are significantly elevated, and the placenta contains an excess of lipid peroxide [178], representing a likely source of the excess in blood. Conversely, the plasma concentration of vitamin E, an important chain reaction–breaking antioxidant, as well as the placental activities of GPx and SOD, the most important antioxidative enzymes, are significantly lower [47; 48; 176; 177; 179-181]. In addition, there appears to be increased nitrotyrosine residue formation in the placentas of women with preeclampsia, suggestive of $ONOO^-$ formation—perhaps arising from local NO production coupled with increased generation of O_2^- and either regionally decreased or inadequate SOD [1; 181; 182]. Patients with severe preeclampsia exhibit significantly lower nighttime serum melatonin levels than individuals with mild preeclampsia or normal pregnant women after 32 weeks of gestation [150]. The primary insult here is likely an imbalance favoring oxidative over antioxidative processes [183]. This effect is mediated in part by O_2^-, produced in elevated amounts during preeclampsia by the placental mitochondria, which leads to an overall increase in placental lipid peroxidation [184].

Perinatal hypoxia is related to alterations in the expression of NO, whose deficiency is associated with the development of hypertension. A study demonstrated that the restoration of the NO pathway is likely to have an important role in the antihypertensive effect of melatonin [185]. Another study revealed a greater agreement between the findings from the anatomic and pathological examination of placentas and the clinical status presented by patients with hypertensive syndromes of pregnancy [186]. As fetal growth depends on placental blood supply, experimental ischemia causes oxidative damage and decreased placental blood circulation, which may be associated with fetal growth restriction. Pretreatment with melatonin reverses these immunohistochemical changes, indicating that melatonin can prevent oxidative DNA damage of the placenta [187].

Both the direct antioxidant activity and the stimulatory effect on antioxidant enzyme activity demonstrated by melatonin may have clinical implications for the treatment of preeclampsia and the prevention of intrauterine growth restriction (IUGR), in which excess free radical production may be involved [188]. The concept of treating preeclampsia, IUGR, and fetal hypoxia with antioxidant agents remains controversial. Of the various synthetic and natural antioxidants that effectively reduce lipid peroxidation, the best known is vitamin E, which readily scavenges lipoperoxide radicals (LOO). A recent report concluded that supplementation with vitamins E and C may be beneficial in preventing preeclampsia in women who are at increased risk [189]. Interestingly, it was demonstrated that melatonin might be a more efficient scavenger than vitamin E [116; 190]. In addition to direct antioxidant activity, melatonin provides indirect protection against free radical injury by stimulating GPx activity. Due to this unique action, melatonin may have potential application in the prevention of preeclampsia and possibly other clinical states involving excessive free radical production, such as IUGR and fetal hypoxia [188].

The pathogenesis of IUGR is complex and incompletely understood. One factor implicated is decreased uterine blood supply [187; 188]. A reduction in fetal oxygenation is not an uncommon event in pregnancy, arising acutely from decreases in uterine or umbilical blood flow, for example, during uterine contractions, or chronically when remodeling of the uteroplacental circulation does not keep pace with the increased oxygen demand of the fetus as it grows. It was demonstrated that placental ischemia causes fetal hypoxia and acidosis [191], and that chronic fetal hypoxemia, most commonly caused by placental insufficiency, produces an adaptive reduction of fetal growth, both resulting in IUGR [8; 191]. In addition to chronic hypoxia and poor nutrient supply from a dysfunctional placenta, the IUGR fetus must cope with prolonged elevation of inflammatory products and oxygen free radicals arising from the dysfunctional placenta. Severe hypoxia, whether acute or chronic, is also likely to lead to oxidative stress, particularly when transient changes of perfusion or oxygenation leads to free radical production due to uncoupled electron flow in the mitochondrial electron transport chain [10; 18]. In most cases, the balance between free radical production and the bioavailability of NO can regulate blood flow [192]. The increased ROS, in particular O_2^-, will react with NO to form $ONOO^-$. In addition to causing oxidative cellular damage directly, enhanced O_2^- production also promotes reductions in blood flow because it increases the sequestration of NO, reducing its bioavailability [193]. Reductions in blood flow in any circulation may therefore occur because of an increase in O_2^- production and/or a fall in antioxidant capacity. Conversely, an increase in antioxidant capacity and/or a fall in free radical production will favor vasodilatation. This tenet is particularly relevant during pregnancy, as NO is indispensable for the maintenance of blood flow in placental and umbilical circulation, and thereby for appropriate nutrient and oxygen delivery to the fetus [194].

Transient occlusion of the circulation to a single uterine horn in rat results in asymmetric restriction of fetal growth as a consequence of ischemia/reperfusion injury, which may impair placental function oxidatively by producing oxygen and nitrogen-based oxidants and subsequently lead to fetal growth restriction [195]. In these cases, the primary insult may be an imbalance favoring oxidative over antioxidative processes [183], in part mediated by elevated O_2^- production by the placental mitochondria, which leads to an overall increase in placental lipid peroxidation [184]. The overproduction of ROS and oxidative stress as a result of tissue hypoxia caused by hypoxemia, hypoperfusion, and/or ischemia/reperfusion leads to cell damage, accumulation of ROS in tissues associated with considerable lipid and protein peroxidation, and cell death via the apoptotic or necrotic pathways [14]. It has been reported that melatonin inhibits ischemia/reperfusion-induced lipid peroxidation and oxidative damage in the placental mitochondria [188], diminishes free radical–mediated lipid peroxidation in vitro, suppresses the vasospastic effects of H_2O_2 in the human umbilical artery, and can inhibit oxidative low-density lipoprotein (LDL) modification [7; 196], protecting against oxidative damage induced by ischemia/reperfusion injury in rat placenta [187; 188] and brain [197]. In very premature infants, abnormal brain development and IUGR have been related to melatonin deficiency [198; 199]. Brain mitochondria in premature fetal rats have been reported to be highly susceptible to oxidative damage [200], and in these cases, melatonin and its metabolites may be an effective neuroprotective treatment by scavenging radicals and reducing their generation [198; 199; 201] and by increasing the efficiency of mitochondrial electron transport [124; 202].

The modulatory and neuroprotective actions of melatonin may not be solely due to the scavenging of OH^- [203] and increased intracerebral antioxidant enzyme activity [159]. Melatonin directly inhibits noradrenalin-stimulated fetal cerebral artery contraction and decreases cerebral vascular permeability following hypoxia [204]. Systemically, melatonin induces umbilical vasodilatation via the stimulation of NO synthase [205], which may prove a particularly useful property in pregnancies complicated by placental insufficiency. These results indicate that maternally administered melatonin and its metabolites function as antioxidants [206; 207] and prevent ischemia/reperfusion-induced restriction in fetal growth and mitochondrial damage of the placenta. Due to these actions, melatonin may have potential application in clinical states involving excessive free radical production, such as preeclampsia, IUGR, and fetal hypoxia [188]. The choice of using melatonin alone or in combination with other antioxidants and conventional treatments may lead to the development of a new therapeutic approach for hypoxic fetal neural injury. Therefore, melatonin could become an important medication for preventing fetal brain damage.

Diabetes mellitus (DM) is characterized by a series of complications that affect the blood and tissues [208]. The combined stress of insulin-dependent DM and pregnancy creates a metabolic environment that is often life threatening to both the mother and fetus [209]. This is primarily due to the difficulty in controlling diabetes in the mother because of the natural diabetogenic state of pregnancy. Congenital anomalies occur in 6–8% of the fetuses of diabetic women (type 1) compared with 2% in non-diabetics [210]. Clinical and experimental studies have clearly demonstrated that hyperglycemia is the major teratogenic factor for embryonic malformations, although other associated factors, such as ketone bodies, branched amino acids, and triglycerides have also been shown to exert adverse effects on developing embryos [211], but the mechanisms by which maternal hyperglycemia causes embryonic malformations remain to be fully delineated.

Hyperglycemia occurring in diabetic pregnancy is one of the important factors responsible for the development of oxidative stress and ROS [211]. In diabetes, protein glycosylation and glucose auto-oxidation can lead to the formation of free radicals, and this can induce lipid peroxidation (LPO) [211]. The principal free radicals are O_2^-, OH^-, and peroxyl (ROO^-) radicals. Free radicals may play a role in DNA damage, protein modification and glycosylation, and lipid oxidative modification reactions in diabetes [212]. Oxidized LDL may be more toxic to cells. The ability of melatonin to reduce LPO may stem from its function as a preventive antioxidant (scavenging the initiating radicals) or from yet-unidentified actions. Furthermore, melatonin stimulates the activity or gene expression of several important endogenous antioxidant enzymes, including GPx, SOD, and xanthine oxidase, and $ONOO^-$ has been shown to be directly scavenged by melatonin [213]. Therefore, melatonin supplementation may be potentially beneficial in pregnancies complicated by diabetes; however, further studies are necessary to confirm this hypothesis.

Spontaneous abortion, defined by the World Health Organization as the termination of pregnancy before 20 complete gestational weeks from the last menstrual period or a fetal weight of less than 500 g, is estimated to occur in 15–20% of identified pregnancies. The causes of spontaneous abortion can be related to chromosomal anomalies or abnormalities in the intrauterine environment [214]. Studies have demonstrated that there is increased generation of O_2^- by the placental mitochondria [31] and polymorphonuclear leukocytes [156] in the first trimester of pregnancy, and it has been proposed that an oxidant/antioxidant imbalance is associated with pregnancy loss [215], suggesting that systemic and placental oxidative stress [216] associated with a deficiency in antioxidant defenses [217] may be implicated in the pathophysiology of abortion and recurrent pregnancy loss. In normal pregnant women, melatonin levels increase with gestation [150; 152], which would aid in reducing oxidative stress. Pinealectomy, which decreases circulating melatonin levels, leads to abortion in pregnant rats [218]. Based on the findings that: (a) melatonin is known as a powerful free radical scavenger and antioxidant; (b) plasma melatonin levels normally increase during pregnancy; (c) pinealectomy increases the frequency of spontaneous abortions in pregnant rats; (d) melatonin has immunomodulatory effects; (e) melatonin stimulates the secretion of progesterone, which reduces uterine contractility and prevents immunological rejection of the trophoblast; and (f) melatonin inhibits the synthesis of prostaglandins, which are potent inducers of uterine contractility and labor, it is proposed that deficient pineal melatonin production in early pregnancy may be causally related to the development of spontaneous abortions in cases where chromosomal anomalies or structural abnormalities of the uterus have been excluded [49].

Converging evidence from different lines of research suggests the possibility that in complicated pregnancy, maternal treatment with antioxidants may improve placental function and thereby diminish intrauterine growth retardation and its burden [219-222]. Maternal undernutrition during pregnancy promotes asymmetric growth retardation [223] and is associated with increased oxidative stress [219-221; 224; 225]. Oxidative stress in the placental and fetal tissues may be further aggravated by the reduced intake of thiols, transferrin, and vitamins C and E, all of which play an important role in the defense against oxidant damage. In rats, maternal undernutrition can overwhelm the endogenous placental antioxidant capacity and promote oxidative stress in the offspring [219-221; 224; 225]. In late pregnancy, it leads to decreased placental efficiency, disproportionate intrauterine growth retardation, and a reduction in birth weight. In these cases, maternal treatment with melatonin improved placental efficiency, restored birth weight, and increased the expression of placental antioxidant enzymes [157]. The mechanism of protection of melatonin in undernourished pregnancy may therefore be related to an increase in the endogenous placental antioxidant capacity, shifting the vascular oxidant ratio toward dilatation, thereby improving placental efficiency, maintaining perfusion, and nutrient and oxygen delivery to the fetus [157]. Human and rat placentas express receptors for melatonin [153-155], but whether melatonin exerts any receptor-mediated or indirect effects on placental transporters or in the concentration gradient of glucose in normal or complicated pregnancy remains unknown. Alternative explanations for the protective effect of melatonin on birth weight in undernourished pregnancy, independent of an effect on bloodflow, include its effects on the relative proportions of the transport surface within each gram of placenta, or in the density of nutrient transporters within that surface area or changes in the concentration gradients [157].

Clinical Applications of Melatonin

Melatonin is currently under investigation in a wide range of biomedical research areas including, but not limited to, heart disease [226], Alzheimer's disease [227], AIDS [228], diabetes [229], depression [230], cancer [231; 232], and environmental hazards [115]. Research showing that melatonin protects human white blood cells against radiation damage [233] and prevents cataracts in animals already indicates its potential clinically applicable benefits. As a treatment in pregnancy or the neonatal period, melatonin possesses a number of attractive attributes. It is highly lipophilic, enabling it to cross a variety of membranes readily, to enter both cytoplasmic and nuclear compartments [7]. It readily crosses the placenta and the blood–brain barrier [234], and is rapidly transferred from the maternal to fetal circulation [197]. It is reported that melatonin is transferred more effectively across the placenta than vitamin E and has a good safety profile with no known adverse effects [1; 198]. The pre-insult administration of melatonin is reported to prevent the increase in lipid peroxidation products and cerebral injury [200; 203; 234], and several lines of evidence suggest that in reducing free radical generation, melatonin may be as effective a neuroprotective treatment for the fetus [235] as it is in adults [206; 236].

Despite some researchers reporting the coincidental finding of adverse effects in the offspring of Wistar–Kyoto rats given melatonin supplementation during gestation, which caused offspring mortality and smaller size [237], there is consensus that short-term melatonin therapy has a remarkably benign safety profile even when neonates are treated with pharmacological doses [59; 95; 124; 202; 238]. Overall, significant complications with long-term melatonin therapy in children and adults have not been reported, and various animal studies on maternal melatonin treatment and postnatal life have not reported treatment-related side effects [239-242]. Taking into account all of this information, melatonin treatment might result in a wide range of health benefits, improve quality of life, reduce healthcare costs, and may help reduce complications in the neonatal period [243; 244]. As a result of its wide spectrum of actions, melatonin appears to be a highly beneficial molecule with unexploited clinical potential. Although the circadian and endocrine effects of melatonin are moderately well understood, the potential role it plays as a free radical scavenger is only beginning to be revealed [99]. It is not known whether the immunorestorative properties of the hormone are directly related to its free radical scavenging activity, but it is clear that the global antioxidant actions of melatonin are, in themselves, of great importance and interest and likely therapeutic utility [99]. Exogenously administered melatonin has a serum half-life of 0.5–5.6 min, with few or no reported side effects [80]. In view of its extensive regulatory repertoire, melatonin administration may be beneficial in treating a wide spectrum of human diseases; however, the short half-life of the parent molecule suggests that more stable (and selective) analogs may be required for the management of such medical conditions [99].

It is important to note that the safety profiles of substances proposed for human treatment should be sufficiently characterized to be considered as candidate therapies; therefore, further rigorous testing in appropriate animal models may be required before clinical trials can be recommended. It is a given that any proposal to protect the fetus by pretreatment of the mother must in itself be benign and impose no additional burden of risk on the mother or her baby. This is particularly important with respect to the fetus and the immature brain, where developmental programming resulting from antenatal changes in endocrine or cardiovascular function may have profound long-term effects [8].

To some extent, this has already been performed for melatonin, allopurinol, and vitamins C and E, for which clinical randomized clinical trial data are now available or being collected. Most commonly, experimental and clinical studies have examined antioxidant treatments in situations of acute perinatal hypoxia, but there is a clear lack of clinical studies assessing treatments aimed at reducing the burden of chronic fetal hypoxia and IUGR, whether by antioxidant therapies or other therapies [8]. It is possible that antioxidant therapy might be useful in the management of neonates with oxidative stress–related problems, but further biochemical investigations are required to define the most effective antioxidant therapy [1]. Both direct antioxidant activity and the stimulatory effect on antioxidant enzyme activity exhibited by melatonin may make this hormone a particularly suitable agent for antioxidant treatment. With its unique combination of actions, melatonin may be able to prevent preeclampsia and IUGR, in which excessive free radical production has been demonstrated [49; 188]. Insults known to increase the production of oxygen free radicals and to produce perinatal brain injury (i.e., chronic hypoxia arising from placental insufficiency, or acute severe hypoxia-ischemia as occurs with birth asphyxia) could potentially benefit from antioxidant therapies [8]. Decreasing free radicals and restoring oxidative imbalance certainly appear to benefit the brain in response to episodes of hypoxia and reperfusion, but studies to date have not adequately addressed the consequences of altering the oxidative or immune balance when no challenge is present; that is, what happens when antioxidants are administered because oxidative stress is suspected, but in fact has not occurred [8]? This again supports the idea that melatonin may have potential usefulness as a fetal protector under conditions of elevated oxidative stress. However, clinical studies are needed to determine the indications, dosage, safety, and effectiveness.

Conclusion

As demonstrated herein, the placenta is an important source of reactive free radicals [31], and even normal pregnancies are characterized by increased oxidative stress and lipid peroxidation [1; 2; 48]. In some situations, however, the fetus may be exposed to exacerbated oxidative stress, as has been demonstrated in pregnancies complicated by preeclampsia, IUGR, hypoxia, and diabetes, among others, consequently leading to prenatal and postnatal negative outcomes. Therefore, the prevention and/or treatment of these conditions remain a major concern in perinatal practice at present. Studies on the influences of oxidative stress during pregnancy and possible treatments to minimize it have been demonstrated as being very important. In this context, melatonin treatment has been reported as a useful option to prevent or minimize the negative outcomes related to these complications during pregnancy. However, the roles of melatonin in human pregnancy are not clearly understood. It has been demonstrated to be a highly beneficial molecule, but its mechanisms of action as a free radical scavenger have not been completely elucidated to date, and further studies are necessary to explain this. Nonetheless, the antioxidant actions of melatonin are of great importance and interest, with clear potential therapeutic utility, which undoubtedly may be beneficial in treating a wide spectrum of human diseases, particularly complicated pregnancies involving excessive free radical production.

Acknowledgments

Funding sources: Conselho Nacional de Desenvolvimento Científico e Tecnológico (CNPq), Coordenação de Aperfeiçoamento de Pessoal de Nível Superior (CAPES), Fundação de Amparo à Pesquisa do Estado de Minas Gerais (FAPEMIG), and Fundação de Ensino e Pesquisa de Uberaba (FUNEPU).

References

[1] Gitto E, Pellegrino S, Gitto P, Barberi I, Reiter RJ. Oxidative stress of the newborn in the pre- and postnatal period and the clinical utility of melatonin. *J. Pineal. Res.* 2009 Mar;46(2):128-39.

[2] Morris JM, Gopaul NK, Endresen MJ, Knight M, Linton EA, Dhir S, et al. Circulating markers of oxidative stress are raised in normal pregnancy and pre-eclampsia. *Br. J. Obstet. Gynaecol.* 1998 Nov;105(11):1195-9.

[3] Saugstad OD. Bronchopulmonary dysplasia-oxidative stress and antioxidants. *Semin. Neonatol.* 2003 Feb;8(1):39-49.

[4] Saugstad OD. Hypoxanthine as an indicator of hypoxia: its role in health and disease through free radical production. *Pediatr. Res.* 1988 Feb;23(2):143-50.

[5] Haynes RL, Folkerth RD, Keefe RJ, Sung I, Swzeda LI, Rosenberg PA, et al. Nitrosative and oxidative injury to premyelinating oligodendrocytes in periventricular leukomalacia. *J. Neuropathol. Exp. Neurol.* 2003 May;62(5):441-50.

[6] Clyman RI, Saugstad OD, Mauray F. Reactive oxygen metabolites relax the lamb ductus arteriosus by stimulating prostaglandin production. *Circ. Res.* 1989 Jan;64(1):1-8.

[7] Reiter RJ. Oxidative damage in the central nervous system: protection by melatonin. *Prog. Neurobiol.* 1998 Oct;56(3):359-84.

[8] Miller SL, Wallace EM, Walker DW. Antioxidant therapies: a potential role in perinatal medicine. *Neuroendocrinology* 2012;96(1):13-23.

[9] Reiter RJ. Functional diversity of the pineal hormone melatonin: its role as an antioxidant. *Exp. Clin. Endocrinol. Diabetes* 1996;104(1):10-6.

[10] Floyd RA. Role of oxygen free radicals in carcinogenesis and brain ischemia. *FASEB J.* 1990 Jun;4(9):2587-97.

[11] Delivoria-Papadopoulos M, Mishra OP. Mechanisms of cerebral injury in perinatal asphyxia and strategies for prevention. *J. Pediatr.* 1998 Mar;132(3 Pt 2):S30-S34.

[12] Fridovich I. Oxygen toxicity: a radical explanation. *J. Exp. Biol.* 1998 Apr;201(Pt 8):1203-9.

[13] Halliwell B. Reactive oxygen species in living systems: source, biochemistry, and role in human disease. *Am. J. Med.* 1991 Sep 30;91(3C):14S-22S.

[14] Buonocore G, Perrone S, Tataranno ML. Oxygen toxicity: chemistry and biology of reactive oxygen species. *Semin. Fetal. Neonatal. Med.* 2010 Aug;15(4):186-90.

[15] Rodrigo J, Fernandez AP, Serrano J, Peinado MA, Martinez A. The role of free radicals in cerebral hypoxia and ischemia. *Free Radic. Biol. Med.* 2005 Jul 1;39(1):26-50.

[16] Lewen A, Matz P, Chan PH. Free radical pathways in CNS injury. *J. Neurotrauma* 2000 Oct;17(10):871-90.

[17] Suzuki YJ, Forman HJ, Sevanian A. Oxidants as stimulators of signal transduction. *Free Radic. Biol. Med.* 1997;22(1-2):269-85.

[18] Abramov AY, Scorziello A, Duchen MR. Three distinct mechanisms generate oxygen free radicals in neurons and contribute to cell death during anoxia and reoxygenation. *J. Neurosci.* 2007 Jan 31;27(5):1129-38.

[19] Sarker AH, Watanabe S, Seki S, Akiyama T, Okada S. Oxygen radical-induced single-strand DNA breaks and repair of the damage in a cell-free system. *Mutat. Res.* 1995 Sep;337(2):85-95.

[20] Saugstad OD. Mechanisms of tissue injury by oxygen radicals: implications for neonatal disease. *Acta. Paediatr.* 1996 Jan;85(1):1-4.

[21] Coyle JT, Puttfarcken P. Oxidative stress, glutamate, and neurodegenerative disorders. *Science* 1993 Oct 29;262(5134):689-95.

[22] Reiter RJ, Tan DX, Poeggeler B, Menendez-Pelaez A, Chen LD, Saarela S. Melatonin as a free radical scavenger: implications for aging and age-related diseases. *Ann. N. Y. Acad. Sci.* 1994 May 31;719:1-12.

[23] Muscari C, Giaccari A, Giordano E, Clo C, Guarnieri C, Caldarera CM. Role of reactive oxygen species in cardiovascular aging. *Mol. Cell Biochem.* 1996 Jul;160-161:159-66.

[24] Redman CW, Sargent IL. Pre-eclampsia, the placenta and the maternal systemic inflammatory response--a review. Placenta 2003 Apr;24 *Suppl.* A:S21-S27.

[25] Li N, Karin M. Is NF-kappaB the sensor of oxidative stress? *FASEB J.* 1999 Jul;13(10):1137-43.

[26] Cindrova-Davies T, Spasic-Boskovic O, Jauniaux E, Charnock-Jones DS, Burton GJ. Nuclear factor-kappa B, p38, and stress-activated protein kinase mitogen-activated protein kinase signaling pathways regulate proinflammatory cytokines and apoptosis in human placental explants in response to oxidative stress: effects of antioxidant vitamins. *Am. J. Pathol.* 2007 May;170(5):1511-20.

[27] Cindrova-Davies T, Yung HW, Johns J, Spasic-Boskovic O, Korolchuk S, Jauniaux E, et al. Oxidative stress, gene expression, and protein changes induced in the human placenta during labor. *Am. J. Pathol.* 2007 Oct;171(4):1168-79.

[28] Dharane Nee LP, Manuelpillai U, Wallace E, Walker DW. NFkappaB-dependent increase of kynurenine pathway activity in human placenta: inhibition by sulfasalazine. *Placenta* 2010 Nov;31(11):997-1002.

[29] Manuelpillai U, Ligam P, Smythe G, Wallace EM, Hirst J, Walker DW. Identification of kynurenine pathway enzyme mRNAs and metabolites in human placenta: up-regulation by inflammatory stimuli and with clinical infection. *Am. J. Obstet. Gynecol.* 2005 Jan;192(1):280-8.

[30] Lappas M, Permezel M, Georgiou HM, Rice GE. Nuclear factor kappa B regulation of proinflammatory cytokines in human gestational tissues in vitro. *Biol. Reprod.* 2002 Aug;67(2):668-73.

[31] Myatt L, Cui X. Oxidative stress in the placenta. *Histochem. Cell Biol.* 2004 Oct;122(4):369-82.

[32] Dordevic NZ, Babic GM, Markovic SD, Ognjanovic BI, Stajn AS, Zikic RV, et al. Oxidative stress and changes in antioxidative defense system in erythrocytes of preeclampsia in women. *Reprod. Toxicol.* 2008 Feb;25(2):213-8.

[33] Rodriguez C, Mayo JC, Sainz RM, Antolin I, Herrera F, Martin V, et al. Regulation of antioxidant enzymes: a significant role for melatonin. *J. Pineal. Res.* 2004 Jan;36(1):1-9.

[34] Halliwell B. Oxygen radicals as key mediators in neurological disease: fact or fiction?. *Ann. Neurol.* 1992;32 Suppl:S10-S15.

[35] Wei YH, Lee HC. Oxidative stress, mitochondrial DNA mutation, and impairment of antioxidant enzymes in aging. *Exp. Biol. Med.* (Maywood) 2002 Oct;227(9):671-82.

[36] Warner BB, Stuart L, Gebb S, Wispe JR. Redox regulation of manganese superoxide dismutase. *Am. J. Physiol.* 1996 Jul;271(1 Pt 1):L150-L158.

[37] Nicotera TM, Notaro J, Notaro S, Schumer J, Sandberg AA. Elevated superoxide dismutase in Bloom's syndrome: a genetic condition of oxidative stress. *Cancer Res.* 1989 Oct 1;49(19):5239-43.

[38] Kim HP, Roe JH, Chock PB, Yim MB. Transcriptional activation of the human manganese superoxide dismutase gene mediated by tetradecanoylphorbol acetate. *J. Biol. Chem.* 1999 Dec 24;274(52):37455-60.

[39] Yoo HY, Chang MS, Rho HM. The activation of the rat copper/zinc superoxide dismutase gene by hydrogen peroxide through the hydrogen peroxide-responsive element and by paraquat and heat shock through the same heat shock element. *J. Biol. Chem.* 1999 Aug 20;274(34):23887-92.

[40] Hayashibe H, Asayama K, Dobashi K, Kato K. Prenatal development of antioxidant enzymes in rat lung, kidney, and heart: marked increase in immunoreactive superoxide dismutases, glutathione peroxidase, and catalase in the kidney. *Pediatr. Res.* 1990 May;27(5):472-5.

[41] Vanella A, Villa RF, Gorini A, Campisi A, Giuffrida-Stella AM. Superoxide dismutase and cytochrome oxidase activities in light and heavy synaptic mitochondria from rat cerebral cortex during aging. *J. Neurosci. Res.* 1989 Mar;22(3):351-5.

[42] Jones PL, Ping D, Boss JM. Tumor necrosis factor alpha and interleukin-1beta regulate the murine manganese superoxide dismutase gene through a complex intronic enhancer involving C/EBP-beta and NF-kappaB. *Mol. Cell Biol.* 1997 Dec;17(12):6970-81.

[43] Rogers RJ, Chesrown SE, Kuo S, Monnier JM, Nick HS. Cytokine-inducible enhancer with promoter activity in both the rat and human manganese-superoxide dismutase genes. *Biochem. J.* 2000 Apr 1;347 Pt 1:233-42.

[44] Dougall WC, Nick HS. Manganese superoxide dismutase: a hepatic acute phase protein regulated by interleukin-6 and glucocorticoids. *Endocrinology* 1991 Nov;129(5):2376-84.

[45] Sugino N, Hirosawa-Takamori M, Zhong L, Telleria CM, Shiota K, Gibori G. Hormonal regulation of copper-zinc superoxide dismutase and manganese superoxide dismutase messenger ribonucleic acid in the rat corpus luteum: induction by prolactin and placental lactogens 3. *Biol. Reprod.* 1998 Sep;59(3):599-605.

[46] Wisdom SJ, Wilson R, McKillop JH, Walker JJ. Antioxidant systems in normal pregnancy and in pregnancy-induced hypertension. *Am. J. Obstet. Gynecol.* 1991 Dec;165(6 Pt 1):1701-4.

[47] Walsh SW, Wang Y. Deficient glutathione peroxidase activity in preeclampsia is associated with increased placental production of thromboxane and lipid peroxides. *Am. J. Obstet. Gynecol.* 1993 Dec;169(6):1456-61.

[48] Vanderlelie J, Venardos K, Clifton VL, Gude NM, Clarke FM, Perkins AV. Increased biological oxidation and reduced anti-oxidant enzyme activity in pre-eclamptic placentae. *Placenta* 2005 Jan;26(1):53-8.

[49] Tamura H, Nakamura Y, Terron MP, Flores LJ, Manchester LC, Tan DX, et al. Melatonin and pregnancy in the human. *Reprod. Toxicol.* 2008 Apr;25(3):291-303.

[50] Carlson JC, Sawada M, Boone DL, Stauffer JM. Stimulation of progesterone secretion in dispersed cells of rat corpora lutea by antioxidants. *Steroids* 1995 Mar;60(3):272-6.

[51] Inui Y, Hazeki O. Acute effects of melatonin and its time of administration on core body temperature and heart rate in cynomolgus monkeys. *J. Toxicol. Sci.* 2010 Jun;35(3):383-91.

[52] Jarzynka MJ, Passey DK, Johnson DA, Konduru NV, Fitz NF, Radio NM, et al. Microtubules modulate melatonin receptors involved in phase-shifting circadian activity rhythms: in vitro and in vivo evidence. *J. Pineal. Res.* 2009 Mar;46(2):161-71.

[53] Reiter RJ, Paredes SD, Manchester LC, Tan DX. Reducing oxidative/nitrosative stress: a newly-discovered genre for melatonin. *Crit. Rev. Biochem. Mol. Biol.* 2009 Jul;44(4):175-200.

[54] Brzezinski A. Melatonin in humans. N Engl J Med 1997 Jan 16;336(3):186-95.

[55] Cahill GM, Besharse JC. Circadian clock functions localized in xenopus retinal photoreceptors. *Neuron* 1993 Apr;10(4):573-7.

[56] Reppert SM, Weaver DR, Ebisawa T. Cloning and characterization of a mammalian melatonin receptor that mediates reproductive and circadian responses. *Neuron* 1994 Nov;13(5):1177-85.

[57] Pierpaoli W, Regelson W. Pineal control of aging: effect of melatonin and pineal grafting on aging mice. *Proc. Natl. Acad. Sci. USA* 1994 Jan 18;91(2):787-91.

[58] Radogna F, Diederich M, Ghibelli L. Melatonin: a pleiotropic molecule regulating inflammation. *Biochem. Pharmacol.* 2010 Dec 15;80(12):1844-52.

[59] Gitto E, Reiter RJ, Cordaro SP, La RM, Chiurazzi P, Trimarchi G, et al. Oxidative and inflammatory parameters in respiratory distress syndrome of preterm newborns: beneficial effects of melatonin. *Am. J. Perinatol.* 2004 May;21(4):209-16.

[60] Gitto E, Romeo C, Reiter RJ, Impellizzeri P, Pesce S, Basile M, et al. Melatonin reduces oxidative stress in surgical neonates. *J. Pediatr. Surg.* 2004 Feb;39(2):184-9.

[61] Rodriguez MI, Escames G, Lopez LC, Lopez A, Garcia JA, Ortiz F, et al. Chronic melatonin treatment reduces the age-dependent inflammatory process in senescence-accelerated mice. *J. Pineal. Res.* 2007 Apr;42(3):272-9.

[62] Reiter RJ, Tan DX, Osuna C, Gitto E. Actions of melatonin in the reduction of oxidative stress. A review. *J. Biomed. Sci.* 2000 Nov;7(6):444-58.

[63] Tekbas OF, Ogur R, Korkmaz A, Kilic A, Reiter RJ. Melatonin as an antibiotic: new insights into the actions of this ubiquitous molecule. *J. Pineal. Res.* 2008 Mar;44(2):222-6.

[64] Bonilla E, Valero N, Chacin-Bonilla L, Medina-Leendertz S. Melatonin and viral infections. *J. Pineal. Res.* 2004 Mar;36(2):73-9.

[65] Hardeland R, Reiter RJ, Poeggeler B, Tan DX. The significance of the metabolism of the neurohormone melatonin: antioxidative protection and formation of bioactive substances. *Neurosci. Biobehav. Rev.* 1993;17(3):347-57.

[66] Tamura H, Takasaki A, Miwa I, Taniguchi K, Maekawa R, Asada H, et al. Oxidative stress impairs oocyte quality and melatonin protects oocytes from free radical damage and improves fertilization rate. J. *Pineal. Res.* 2008 Apr;44(3):280-7.

[67] Reiter RJ, Manchester LC, Tan DX. Melatonin in walnuts: influence on levels of melatonin and total antioxidant capacity of blood. *Nutrition* 2005 Sep;21(9):920-4.

[68] Haines DE, Dietrichs E, Mihailoff GA, McDonald EF. The cerebellar-hypothalamic axis: basic circuits and clinical observations. *Int. Rev. Neurobiol.* 1997;41:83-107.

[69] Tan DX, Hardeland R, Manchester LC, Paredes SD, Korkmaz A, Sainz RM, et al. The changing biological roles of melatonin during evolution: from an antioxidant to signals of darkness, sexual selection and fitness. *Biol. Rev. Camb. Philos. Soc.* 2010 Aug;85(3):607-23.

[70] Hardeland R, Poeggeler B. Non-vertebrate melatonin. J Pineal Res 2003 May;34(4):233-41.

[71] Poeggeler B, Hardeland R. Detection and quantification of melatonin in a dinoflagellate, Gonyaulax polyedra: solutions to the problem of methoxyindole destruction in non-vertebrate material. *J. Pineal. Res.* 1994 Aug;17(1):1-10.

[72] Hattori A, Migitaka H, Iigo M, Itoh M, Yamamoto K, Ohtani-Kaneko R, et al. Identification of melatonin in plants and its effects on plasma melatonin levels and binding to melatonin receptors in vertebrates. *Biochem. Mol. Biol. Int.* 1995 Mar;35(3):627-34.
[73] Murch SJ, Alan AR, Cao J, Saxena PK. Melatonin and serotonin in flowers and fruits of Datura metel L. *J. Pineal. Res.* 2009 Oct;47(3):277-83.
[74] Mirick DK, Davis S. Melatonin as a biomarker of circadian dysregulation. *Cancer Epidemiol. Biomarkers Prev.* 2008 Dec;17(12):3306-13.
[75] Waldhauser F, Weiszenbacher G, Frisch H, Zeitlhuber U, Waldhauser M, Wurtman RJ. Fall in nocturnal serum melatonin during prepuberty and pubescence. *Lancet* 1984 Feb 18;1(8373):362-5.
[76] Humbert W, Pevet P. The decrease of pineal melatonin production with age. Causes and consequences. *Ann. N. Y. Acad. Sci.* 1994 May 31;719:43-63.
[77] Reppert SM, Weaver DR, Godson C. Melatonin receptors step into the light: cloning and classification of subtypes. *Trends. Pharmacol. Sci.* 1996 Mar;17(3):100-2.
[78] Song Y, Chan CW, Brown GM, Pang SF, Silverman M. Studies of the renal action of melatonin: evidence that the effects are mediated by 37 kDa receptors of the Mel1a subtype localized primarily to the basolateral membrane of the proximal tubule. *FASEB J.* 1997 Jan;11(1):93-100.
[79] Geary GG, Krause DN, Duckles SP. Melatonin directly constricts rat cerebral arteries through modulation of potassium channels. *Am. J. Physiol.* 1997 Sep;273(3 Pt 2):H1530-H1536.
[80] Brzezinski A. Melatonin in humans. *N. Engl. J. Med.* 1997 Jan 16;336(3):186-95.
[81] Dubocovich ML. Melatonin receptors: are there multiple subtypes?. *Trends. Pharmacol. Sci.* 1995 Feb;16(2):50-6.
[82] Reppert SM. Melatonin receptors: molecular biology of a new family of G protein-coupled receptors. *J. Biol. Rhythms* 1997 Dec;12(6):528-31.
[83] von GC, Stehle JH, Weaver DR. Mammalian melatonin receptors: molecular biology and signal transduction. *Cell Tissue Res.* 2002 Jul;309(1):151-62.
[84] Mazzucchelli C, Pannacci M, Nonno R, Lucini V, Fraschini F, Stankov BM. The melatonin receptor in the human brain: cloning experiments and distribution studies. *Brain Res. Mol. Brain Res.* 1996 Jul;39(1-2):117-26.
[85] Dubocovich ML, Rivera-Bermudez MA, Gerdin MJ, Masana MI. Molecular pharmacology, regulation and function of mammalian melatonin receptors. *Front Biosci.* 2003 Sep 1;8:d1093-d1108.
[86] Sanchez-Barcelo EJ, Cos S, Mediavilla D, Martinez-Campa C, Gonzalez A, Alonso-Gonzalez C. Melatonin-estrogen interactions in breast cancer. *J. Pineal. Res.* 2005 May;38(4):217-22.
[87] Schlabritz-Loutsevitch N, Hellner N, Middendorf R, Muller D, Olcese J. The human myometrium as a target for melatonin. *J. Clin. Endocrinol. Metab.* 2003 Feb;88(2):908-13.
[88] Woo MM, Tai CJ, Kang SK, Nathwani PS, Pang SF, Leung PC. Direct action of melatonin in human granulosa-luteal cells. *J. Clin. Endocrinol. Metab.* 2001 Oct;86(10):4789-97.

[89] Aoyama H, Mori W, Mori N. Anti-glucocorticoid effects of melatonin in young rats. *Acta. Pathol. Jpn.* 1986 Mar;36(3):423-8.

[90] Sandyk R, Kay SR. The relationship of pineal calcification and melatonin secretion to the pathophysiology of tardive dyskinesia and Tourette's syndrome. *Int. J. Neurosci.* 1991 Jun;58(3-4):215-47.

[91] Burns JK. Administration of melatonin to non-human primates and to women with breast carcinoma. *J. Physiol.* 1973 Feb;229(1):38P-9P.

[92] el-Domeiri AA, Das Gupta TK. Reversal by melatonin of the effect of pinealectomy on tumor growth. *Cancer Res.* 1973 Nov;33(11):2830-3.

[93] Maestroni GJ, Conti A, Pierpaoli W. Role of the pineal gland in immunity: II. Melatonin enhances the antibody response via an opiatergic mechanism. *Clin. Exp. Immunol.* 1987 May;68(2):384-91.

[94] Pierpaoli W. The pineal gland as ontogenetic scanner of reproduction, immunity, and aging. The aging clock. *Ann. N. Y. Acad. Sci.* 1994 Nov 25;741:46-9.

[95] Gitto E, Karbownik M, Reiter RJ, Tan DX, Cuzzocrea S, Chiurazzi P, et al. Effects of melatonin treatment in septic newborns. *Pediatr. Res.* 2001 Dec;50(6):756-60.

[96] Jahovic N, Cevik H, Sehirli AO, Yegen BC, Sener G. Melatonin prevents methotrexate-induced hepatorenal oxidative injury in rats. *J. Pineal. Res.* 2003 May;34(4):282-7.

[97] Gilad E, Cuzzocrea S, Zingarelli B, Salzman AL, Szabo C. Melatonin is a scavenger of peroxynitrite. *Life Sci.* 1997;60(10):L169-L174.

[98] Matuszak Z, Reszka K, Chignell CF. Reaction of melatonin and related indoles with hydroxyl radicals: EPR and spin trapping investigations. *Free Radic. Biol. Med.* 1997;23(3):367-72.

[99] Beyer CE, Steketee JD, Saphier D. Antioxidant properties of melatonin--an emerging mystery. *Biochem. Pharmacol.* 1998 Nov 15;56(10):1265-72.

[100] Cagnoli CM, Atabay C, Kharlamova E, Manev H. Melatonin protects neurons from singlet oxygen-induced apoptosis. *J. Pineal. Res.* 1995 May;18(4):222-6.

[101] Abe M, Reiter RJ, Orhii PB, Hara M, Poeggeler B. Inhibitory effect of melatonin on cataract formation in newborn rats: evidence for an antioxidative role for melatonin. *J. Pineal. Res.* 1994 Sep;17(2):94-100.

[102] Meki AR, Hussein AA. Melatonin reduces oxidative stress induced by ochratoxin A in rat liver and kidney. *Comp. Biochem. Physiol. C Toxicol. Pharmacol.* 2001 Nov;130(3):305-13.

[103] Bandyopadhyay D, Bandyopadhyay A, Das PK, Reiter RJ. Melatonin protects against gastric ulceration and increases the efficacy of ranitidine and omeprazole in reducing gastric damage. *J. Pineal. Res.* 2002 Aug;33(1):1-7.

[104] Ustundag B, Kazez A, Demirbag M, Canatan H, Halifeoglu I, Ozercan IH. Protective effect of melatonin on antioxidative system in experimental ischemia-reperfusion of rat small intestine. *Cell Physiol. Biochem.* 2000;10(4):229-36.

[105] Arslan SO, Zerin M, Vural H, Coskun A. The effect of melatonin on bleomycin-induced pulmonary fibrosis in rats. *J. Pineal. Res.* 2002 Jan;32(1):21-5.

[106] El-Missiry MA. Prophylactic effect of melatonin on lead-induced inhibition of heme biosynthesis and deterioration of antioxidant systems in male rats. *J. Biochem. Mol. Toxicol.* 2000;14(1):57-62.

[107] Gultekin F, Delibas N, Yasar S, Kilinc I. In vivo changes in antioxidant systems and protective role of melatonin and a combination of vitamin C and vitamin E on oxidative damage in erythrocytes induced by chlorpyrifos-ethyl in rats. *Arch. Toxicol.* 2001 Apr;75(2):88-96.

[108] Lankoff A, Banasik A, Nowak M. Protective effect of melatonin against nodularin-induced oxidative stress. *Arch. Toxicol.* 2002 Apr;76(3):158-65.

[109] Oner-Iyidogan Y, Gurdol F, Oner P. The effects of acute melatonin and ethanol treatment on antioxidant enzyme activities in rat testes. *Pharmacol. Res.* 2001 Aug;44(2):89-93.

[110] Ozbek E, Turkoz Y, Sahna E, Ozugurlu F, Mizrak B, Ozbek M. Melatonin administration prevents the nephrotoxicity induced by gentamicin. *BJU Int.* 2000 Apr;85(6):742-6.

[111] Anwar MM, Moustafa MA. The effect of melatonin on eye lens of rats exposed to ultraviolet radiation. *Comp. Biochem. Physiol. C Toxicol. Pharmacol.* 2001 May;129(1):57-63.

[112] Vural H, Sabuncu T, Arslan SO, Aksoy N. Melatonin inhibits lipid peroxidation and stimulates the antioxidant status of diabetic rats. *J. Pineal. Res.* 2001 Oct;31(3):193-8.

[113] Kaya H, Delibas N, Serteser M, Ulukaya E, Ozkaya O. The effect of melatonin on lipid peroxidation during radiotherapy in female rats. *Strahlenther Onkol.* 1999 Jun;175(6):285-8.

[114] Hardeland R. Antioxidative protection by melatonin: multiplicity of mechanisms from radical detoxification to radical avoidance. *Endocrine* 2005 Jul;27(2):119-30.

[115] Reiter RJ, Tan DX, Gitto E, Sainz RM, Mayo JC, Leon J, et al. Pharmacological utility of melatonin in reducing oxidative cellular and molecular damage. *Pol. J. Pharmacol.* 2004 Mar;56(2):159-70.

[116] Pieri C, Marra M, Gaspar R, Damjanovich S. Melatonin protects LDL from oxidation but does not prevent the apolipoprotein derivatization. Biochem. Biophys. Res. Commun. 1996 May 15;222(2):256-60.

[117] Tan DX, Poeggeler B, Reiter RJ, Chen LD, Chen S, Manchester LC, et al. The pineal hormone melatonin inhibits DNA-adduct formation induced by the chemical carcinogen safrole in vivo. *Cancer Lett.* 1993 Jun 15;70(1-2):65-71.

[118] Hardeland R. Antioxidative protection by melatonin: multiplicity of mechanisms from radical detoxification to radical avoidance. *Endocrine* 2005 Jul;27(2):119-30.

[119] Rodriguez C, Mayo JC, Sainz RM, Antolin I, Herrera F, Martin V, et al. Regulation of antioxidant enzymes: a significant role for melatonin. *J. Pineal. Res.* 2004 Jan;36(1):1-9.

[120] Tan DX, Manchester LC, Terron MP, Flores LJ, Tamura H, Reiter RJ. Melatonin as a naturally occurring co-substrate of quinone reductase-2, the putative MT3 melatonin membrane receptor: hypothesis and significance. *J. Pineal. Res.* 2007 Nov;43(4):317-20.

[121] Velkov ZA, Velkov YZ, Galunska BT, Paskalev DN, Tadjer AV. Melatonin: Quantum-chemical and biochemical investigation of antioxidant activity. *Eur. J. Med. Chem.* 2009 Jul;44(7):2834-9.

[122] Allegra M, Reiter RJ, Tan DX, Gentile C, Tesoriere L, Livrea MA. The chemistry of melatonin's interaction with reactive species. *J. Pineal. Res.* 2003 Jan;34(1):1-10.
[123] Tan DX, Manchester LC, Sainz RM, Mayo JC, Leon J, Reiter RJ. Physiological ischemia/reperfusion phenomena and their relation to endogenous melatonin production: a hypothesis. *Endocrine* 2005 Jul;27(2):149-58.
[124] Leon J, Acuna-Castroviejo D, Escames G, Tan DX, Reiter RJ. Melatonin mitigates mitochondrial malfunction. *J. Pineal. Res.* 2005 Jan;38(1):1-9.
[125] Lopez A, Garcia JA, Escames G, Venegas C, Ortiz F, Lopez LC, et al. Melatonin protects the mitochondria from oxidative damage reducing oxygen consumption, membrane potential, and superoxide anion production. *J. Pineal. Res.* 2009 Mar;46(2):188-98.
[126] Reiter RJ. Melatonin: Lowering the High Price of Free Radicals. *News Physiol. Sci.* 2000 Oct;15:246-50.
[127] Mohan N, Sadeghi K, Reiter RJ, Meltz ML. The neurohormone melatonin inhibits cytokine, mitogen and ionizing radiation induced NF-kappa B. *Biochem. Mol. Biol. Int.* 1995 Dec;37(6):1063-70.
[128] Sewerynek E, Reiter RJ, Melchiorri D, Ortiz GG, Lewinski A. Oxidative damage in the liver induced by ischemia-reperfusion: protection by melatonin. *Hepatogastroenterology* 1996 Jul;43(10):898-905.
[129] Reiter RJ. Interactions of the pineal hormone melatonin with oxygen-centered free radicals: a brief review. *Braz. J. Med. Biol. Res.* 1993 Nov;26(11):1141-55.
[130] Zang LY, Cosma G, Gardner H, Vallyathan V. Scavenging of reactive oxygen species by melatonin. *Biochim. Biophys. Acta.* 1998 Nov 27;1425(3):469-77.
[131] Tan DX, Manchester LC, Reiter RJ, Qi WB, Karbownik M, Calvo JR. Significance of melatonin in antioxidative defense system: reactions and products. *Biol. Signals Recept.* 2000 May;9(3-4):137-59.
[132] Tan D, Reiter RJ, Chen LD, Poeggeler B, Manchester LC, Barlow-Walden LR. Both physiological and pharmacological levels of melatonin reduce DNA adduct formation induced by the carcinogen safrole. *Carcinogenesis* 1994 Feb;15(2):215-8.
[133] Barlow-Walden LR, Reiter RJ, Abe M, Pablos M, Menendez-Pelaez A, Chen LD, et al. Melatonin stimulates brain glutathione peroxidase activity. *Neurochem. Int.* 1995 May;26(5):497-502.
[134] Kotler M, Rodriguez C, Sainz RM, Antolin I, Menendez-Pelaez A. Melatonin increases gene expression for antioxidant enzymes in rat brain cortex. *J. Pineal. Res.* 1998 Mar;24(2):83-9.
[135] Mayo JC, Sainz RM, Antoli I, Herrera F, Martin V, Rodriguez C. Melatonin regulation of antioxidant enzyme gene expression. *Cell Mol. Life Sci.* 2002 Oct;59(10):1706-13.
[136] Pablos MI, Agapito MT, Gutierrez R, Recio JM, Reiter RJ, Barlow-Walden L, et al. Melatonin stimulates the activity of the detoxifying enzyme glutathione peroxidase in several tissues of chicks. *J. Pineal.* Res. 1995 Oct;19(3):111-5.
[137] Diaz-Munoz M, Hernandez-Munoz R, Suarez J, Chagoya dS, V. Day-night cycle of lipid peroxidation in rat cerebral cortex and their relationship to the glutathione cycle and superoxide dismutase activity. *Neuroscience* 1985 Dec;16(4):859-63.

[138] Martin V, Sainz RM, Mayo JC, Antolin I, Herrera F, Rodriguez C. Daily rhythm of gene expression in rat superoxide dismutases. *Endocr. Res.* 2003 Feb;29(1):83-95.

[139] Kim YH, Park KH, Rho HM. Transcriptional activation of the Cu,Zn-superoxide dismutase gene through the AP2 site by ginsenoside Rb2 extracted from a medicinal plant, Panax ginseng. *J. Biol. Chem.* 1996 Oct 4;271(40):24539-43.

[140] Gilad E, Wong HR, Zingarelli B, Virag L, O'Connor M, Salzman AL, et al. Melatonin inhibits expression of the inducible isoform of nitric oxide synthase in murine macrophages: role of inhibition of NFkappaB activation. *FASEB J.* 1998 Jun;12(9):685-93.

[141] Ross AW, Barrett P, Mercer JG, Morgan PJ. Melatonin suppresses the induction of AP-1 transcription factor components in the pars tuberalis of the pituitary. *Mol. Cell Endocrinol.* 1996 Oct 14;123(1):71-80.

[142] Won JS, Song DK, Huh SO, Kim YH, Suh HW. Effect of melatonin on the regulation of proenkephalin and prodynorphin mRNA levels induced by kainic acid in the rat hippocampus. *Hippocampus* 2000;10(3):236-43.

[143] Mayo JC, Sainz RM, Antoli I, Herrera F, Martin V, Rodriguez C. Melatonin regulation of antioxidant enzyme gene expression. *Cell Mol. Life Sci.* 2002 Oct;59(10):1706-13.

[144] Chan AS, Lai FP, Lo RK, Voyno-Yasenetskaya TA, Stanbridge EJ, Wong YH. Melatonin mt1 and MT2 receptors stimulate c-Jun N-terminal kinase via pertussis toxin-sensitive and -insensitive G proteins. *Cell Signal* 2002 Mar;14(3):249-57.

[145] Pablos MI, Reiter RJ, Ortiz GG, Guerrero JM, Agapito MT, Chuang JI, et al. Rhythms of glutathione peroxidase and glutathione reductase in brain of chick and their inhibition by light. *Neurochem. Int.* 1998 Jan;32(1):69-75.

[146] Ram PT, Dai J, Yuan L, Dong C, Kiefer TL, Lai L, et al. Involvement of the mt1 melatonin receptor in human breast cancer. *Cancer Lett.* 2002 May 28;179(2):141-50.

[147] Vanecek J. Cellular mechanisms of melatonin action. *Physiol. Rev.* 1998 Jul;78(3):687-721.

[148] Benitez-King G, Huerto-Delgadillo L, Anton-Tay F. Binding of 3H-melatonin to calmodulin. *Life Sci.* 1993;53(3):201-7.

[149] Kane CD, Means AR. Activation of orphan receptor-mediated transcription by Ca(2+)/calmodulin-dependent protein kinase IV. *EMBO J.* 2000 Feb 15;19(4):691-701.

[150] Nakamura Y, Tamura H, Kashida S, Takayama H, Yamagata Y, Karube A, et al. Changes of serum melatonin level and its relationship to feto-placental unit during pregnancy. *J. Pineal. Res.* 2001 Jan;30(1):29-33.

[151] Wierrani F, Grin W, Hlawka B, Kroiss A, Grunberger W. Elevated serum melatonin levels during human late pregnancy and labour. *J. Obstet. Gynaecol.* 1997 Sep;17(5):449-51.

[152] Kivela A. Serum melatonin during human pregnancy. *Acta. Endocrinol.* (Copenh) 1991 Mar;124(3):233-7.

[153] Iwasaki S, Nakazawa K, Sakai J, Kometani K, Iwashita M, Yoshimura Y, et al. Melatonin as a local regulator of human placental function. *J. Pineal. Res.* 2005 Oct;39(3):261-5.

[154] Lanoix D, Beghdadi H, Lafond J, Vaillancourt C. Human placental trophoblasts synthesize melatonin and express its receptors. *J. Pineal. Res.* 2008 Aug;45(1):50-60.
[155] Lee CK, Moon DH, Shin CS, Kim H, Yoon YD, Kang HS, et al. Circadian expression of Mel1a and PL-II genes in placenta: effects of melatonin on the PL-II gene expression in the rat placenta. *Mol. Cell Endocrinol.* 2003 Feb 28;200(1-2):57-66.
[156] Fait V, Sela S, Ophir E, Khoury S, Nissimov J, Tkach M, et al. Hyperemesis gravidarum is associated with oxidative stress. *Am. J. Perinatol.* 2002 Feb;19(2):93-8.
[157] Richter HG, Hansell JA, Raut S, Giussani DA. Melatonin improves placental efficiency and birth weight and increases the placental expression of antioxidant enzymes in undernourished pregnancy. *J. Pineal. Res.* 2009 May;46(4):357-64.
[158] McMillen IC, Nowak R. Maternal pinealectomy abolishes the diurnal rhythm in plasma melatonin concentrations in the fetal sheep and pregnant ewe during late gestation. *J. Endocrinol.* 1989 Mar;120(3):459-64.
[159] Okatani Y, Wakatsuki A, Kaneda C. Melatonin increases activities of glutathione peroxidase and superoxide dismutase in fetal rat brain. *J. Pineal. Res.* 2000 Mar;28(2):89-96.
[160] Yellon SM, Longo LD. Effect of maternal pinealectomy and reverse photoperiod on the circadian melatonin rhythm in the sheep and fetus during the last trimester of pregnancy. *Biol. Reprod.* 1988 Dec;39(5):1093-9.
[161] Okatani Y, Okamoto K, Hayashi K, Wakatsuki A, Tamura S, Sagara Y. Maternal-fetal transfer of melatonin in pregnant women near term. *J. Pineal. Res.* 1998 Oct;25(3):129-34.
[162] Jimenez-Jorge S, Guerrero JM, Jimenez-Caliani AJ, Naranjo MC, Lardone PJ, Carrillo-Vico A, et al. Evidence for melatonin synthesis in the rat brain during development. *J. Pineal. Res.* 2007 Apr;42(3):240-6.
[163] Seron-Ferre M, Torres-Farfan C, Forcelledo ML, Valenzuela GJ. The development of circadian rhythms in the fetus and neonate. *Semin. Perinatol.* 2001 Dec;25(6):363-70.
[164] Macchi MM, Bruce JN. Human pineal physiology and functional significance of melatonin. *Front Neuroendocrinol.* 2004 Sep;25(3-4):177-95.
[165] Reppert SM. Maternal entrainment of the developing circadian system. *Ann. N. Y. Acad. Sci.* 1985;453:162-9.
[166] Breen S, Rees S, Walker D. The development of diurnal rhythmicity in fetal suprachiasmatic neurons as demonstrated by fos immunohistochemistry. *Neuroscience* 1996 Oct;74(3):917-26.
[167] McMillen IC, Nowak R, Walker DW, Young IR. Maternal pinealectomy alters the daily pattern of fetal breathing in sheep 8. *Am. J. Physiol.* 1990 Jan;258(1 Pt 2):R284-R287.
[168] McMillen IC, Walker DW. Effects of different lighting regimes on daily hormonal and behavioural rhythms in the pregnant ewe and sheep fetus. *J. Physiol.* 1991 Oct;442:465-76.
[169] Tauman R, Zisapel N, Laudon M, Nehama H, Sivan Y. Melatonin production in infants. *Pediatr. Neurol.* 2002 May;26(5):379-82.
[170] McMillen IC, Houghton DC, Young IR. Melatonin and the development of circadian and seasonal rhythmicity. *J. Reprod. Fertil. Suppl.* 1995;49:137-46.
[171] Deguchi T. Ontogenesis of a biological clock for serotonin:acetyl coenzyme A N-acetyltransferase in pineal gland of rat. *Proc. Natl. Acad. Sci. USA* 1975 Jul;72(7):2814-8.

[172] Regnault TR, Galan HL, Parker TA, Anthony RV. Placental development in normal and compromised pregnancies-- a review. *Placenta* 2002 Apr;23 Suppl A:S119-S129.
[173] Alberry M, Soothill P. Management of fetal growth restriction. *Arch. Dis. Child Fetal. Neonatal. Ed.* 2007 Jan;92(1):F62-F67.
[174] Roberts JM, Lain KY. Recent Insights into the pathogenesis of pre-eclampsia. *Placenta* 2002 May;23(5):359-72.
[175] Zhou Y, McMaster M, Woo K, Janatpour M, Perry J, Karpanen T, et al. Vascular endothelial growth factor ligands and receptors that regulate human cytotrophoblast survival are dysregulated in severe preeclampsia and hemolysis, elevated liver enzymes, and low platelets syndrome. *Am. J. Pathol.* 2002 Apr;160(4):1405-23.
[176] Atamer Y, Kocyigit Y, Yokus B, Atamer A, Erden AC. Lipid peroxidation, antioxidant defense, status of trace metals and leptin levels in preeclampsia. *Eur. J. Obstet. Gynecol. Reprod. Biol.* 2005 Mar 1;119(1):60-6.
[177] Walsh SW, Vaughan JE, Wang Y, Roberts LJ. Placental isoprostane is significantly increased in preeclampsia. *FASEB J.* 2000 Jul;14(10):1289-96.
[178] Walsh SW, Wang Y. Trophoblast and placental villous core production of lipid peroxides, thromboxane, and prostacyclin in preeclampsia. *J. Clin. Endocrinol. Metab.* 1995 Jun;80(6):1888-93.
[179] Aydin S, Benian A, Madazli R, Uludag S, Uzun H, Kaya S. Plasma malondialdehyde, superoxide dismutase, sE-selectin, fibronectin, endothelin-1 and nitric oxide levels in women with preeclampsia. *Eur. J. Obstet. Gynecol. Reprod. Biol.* 2004 Mar 15;113(1):21-5.
[180] Palan PR, Shaban DW, Martino T, Mikhail MS. Lipid-soluble antioxidants and pregnancy: maternal serum levels of coenzyme Q10, alpha-tocopherol and gamma-tocopherol in preeclampsia and normal pregnancy. *Gynecol. Obstet. Invest.* 2004;58(1):8-13.
[181] Poranen AK, Ekblad U, Uotila P, Ahotupa M. Lipid peroxidation and antioxidants in normal and pre-eclamptic pregnancies. *Placenta* 1996 Sep;17(7):401-5.
[182] Beckman JS, Koppenol WH. Nitric oxide, superoxide, and peroxynitrite: the good, the bad, and ugly. *Am. J. Physiol.* 1996 Nov;271(5 Pt 1):C1424-C1437.
[183] Hubel CA, Roberts JM, Taylor RN, Musci TJ, Rogers GM, McLaughlin MK. Lipid peroxidation in pregnancy: new perspectives on preeclampsia. *Am. J. Obstet. Gynecol.* 1989 Oct;161(4):1025-34.
[184] Wang Y, Walsh SW. Placental mitochondria as a source of oxidative stress in pre-eclampsia. *Placenta* 1998 Nov;19(8):581-6.
[185] Paulis L, Pechanova O, Zicha J, Barta A, Gardlik R, Celec P, et al. Melatonin interactions with blood pressure and vascular function during L-NAME-induced hypertension. *J. Pineal. Res.* 2010 Mar;48(2):102-8.
[186] Correa RR, Gilio DB, Cavellani CL, Paschoini MC, Oliveira FA, Peres LC, et al. Placental morphometrical and histopathology changes in the different clinical presentations of hypertensive syndromes in pregnancy. *Arch. Gynecol. Obstet.* 2008 Mar;277(3):201-6.
[187] Nagai R, Watanabe K, Wakatsuki A, Hamada F, Shinohara K, Hayashi Y, et al. Melatonin preserves fetal growth in rats by protecting against ischemia/reperfusion-induced oxidative/nitrosative mitochondrial damage in the placenta. *J. Pineal. Res.* 2008 Oct;45(3):271-6.

[188] Okatani Y, Wakatsuki A, Shinohara K, Taniguchi K, Fukaya T. Melatonin protects against oxidative mitochondrial damage induced in rat placenta by ischemia and reperfusion. *J. Pineal. Res.* 2001 Sep;31(2):173-8.

[189] Chappell LC, Seed PT, Briley AL, Kelly FJ, Lee R, Hunt BJ, et al. Effect of antioxidants on the occurrence of pre-eclampsia in women at increased risk: a randomised trial. *Lancet* 1999 Sep 4;354(9181):810-6.

[190] Pieri C, Marra M, Moroni F, Recchioni R, Marcheselli F. Melatonin: a peroxyl radical scavenger more effective than vitamin E. *Life Sci.* 1994;55(15):L271-L276.

[191] Soothill PW, Nicolaides KH, Campbell S. Prenatal asphyxia, hyperlacticaemia, hypoglycaemia, and erythroblastosis in growth retarded fetuses. *Br. Med. J. (Clin. Res. Ed.)* 1987 Apr 25;294(6579):1051-3.

[192] Chen K, Keaney J. Reactive oxygen species-mediated signal transduction in the endothelium. *Endothelium* 2004 Mar;11(2):109-21.

[193] Schulz E, Anter E, Keaney JF, Jr. Oxidative stress, antioxidants, and endothelial function. *Curr. Med. Chem.* 2004 May;11(9):1093-104.

[194] Vatish M, Randeva HS, Grammatopoulos DK. Hormonal regulation of placental nitric oxide and pathogenesis of pre-eclampsia. *Trends. Mol. Med.* 2006 May;12(5):223-33.

[195] Tanaka M, Natori M, Ishimoto H, Miyazaki T, Kobayashi T, Nozawa S. Experimental growth retardation produced by transient period of uteroplacental ischemia in pregnant Sprague-Dawley rats. *Am. J. Obstet. Gynecol.* 1994 Nov;171(5):1231-4.

[196] Okatani Y, Watanabe K, Hayashi K, Wakatsuki A, Sagara Y. Melatonin suppresses vasospastic effect of hydrogen peroxide in human umbilical artery: relation to calcium influx. *J. Pineal. Res.* 1997 May;22(4):232-7.

[197] Wakatsuki A, Okatani Y, Izumiya C, Ikenoue N. Melatonin protects against ischemia and reperfusion-induced oxidative lipid and DNA damage in fetal rat brain. *J. Pineal. Res.* 1999 Apr;26(3):147-52.

[198] Fulia F, Gitto E, Cuzzocrea S, Reiter RJ, Dugo L, Gitto P, et al. Increased levels of malondialdehyde and nitrite/nitrate in the blood of asphyxiated newborns: reduction by melatonin. *J. Pineal. Res.* 2001 Nov;31(4):343-9.

[199] Hamrick SE, Ferriero DM. The injury response in the term newborn brain: can we neuroprotect?. *Curr. Opin. Neurol.* 2003 Apr;16(2):147-54.

[200] Watanabe K, Wakatsuki A, Shinohara K, Ikenoue N, Yokota K, Fukaya T. Maternally administered melatonin protects against ischemia and reperfusion-induced oxidative mitochondrial damage in premature fetal rat brain. *J. Pineal. Res.* 2004 Nov;37(4):276-80.

[201] Wakatsuki A, Okatani Y, Shinohara K, Ikenoue N, Kaneda C, Fukaya T. Melatonin protects fetal rat brain against oxidative mitochondrial damage. *J. Pineal. Res.* 2001 Jan;30(1):22-8.

[202] Leon J, Acuna-Castroviejo D, Sainz RM, Mayo JC, Tan DX, Reiter RJ. Melatonin and mitochondrial function. *Life Sci.* 2004 Jul 2;75(7):765-90.

[203] Miller SL, Yan EB, Castillo-Melendez M, Jenkin G, Walker DW. Melatonin provides neuroprotection in the late-gestation fetal sheep brain in response to umbilical cord occlusion. *Dev. Neurosci.* 2005 Mar;27(2-4):200-10.

[204] Kaur C, Sivakumar V, Ling EA. Melatonin protects periventricular white matter from damage due to hypoxia. *J. Pineal. Res.* 2010 Apr;48(3):185-93.

[205] Thakor AS, Herrera EA, Seron-Ferre M, Giussani DA. Melatonin and vitamin C increase umbilical blood flow via nitric oxide-dependent mechanisms. *J. Pineal. Res.* 2010 Nov;49(4):399-406.

[206] Maldonado MD, Murillo-Cabezas F, Terron MP, Flores LJ, Tan DX, Manchester LC, et al. The potential of melatonin in reducing morbidity-mortality after craniocerebral trauma. *J. Pineal. Res.* 2007 Jan;42(1):1-11.

[207] Reiter RJ, Tan DX, Terron MP, Flores LJ, Czarnocki Z. Melatonin and its metabolites: new findings regarding their production and their radical scavenging actions. *Acta. Biochim. Pol.* 2007;54(1):1-9.

[208] Guney M, Erdemoglu E, Mungan T. Selenium-vitamin E combination and melatonin modulates diabetes-induced blood oxidative damage and fetal outcomes in pregnant rats. *Biol. Trace. Elem. Res.* 2011 Nov;143(2):1091-102.

[209] Vanheest JL, Rodgers CD. Effects of exercise in diabetic rats before and during gestation on maternal and neonatal outcomes. *Am. J. Physiol.* 1997 Oct;273(4 Pt 1):E727-E733.

[210] Damasceno DC, Volpato GT, de Mattos PC, I, Cunha Rudge MV. Oxidative stress and diabetes in pregnant rats. *Anim. Reprod. Sci.* 2002 Aug 15;72(3-4):235-44.

[211] Zhao Z, Reece EA. Experimental mechanisms of diabetic embryopathy and strategies for developing therapeutic interventions. *J. Soc. Gynecol. Investig.* 2005 Dec;12(8):549-57.

[212] Simsek M, Naziroglu M, Erdinc A. Moderate exercise with a dietary vitamin C and e combination protects against streptozotocin-induced oxidative damage to the kidney and lens in pregnant rats. *Exp. Clin. Endocrinol. Diabetes.* 2005 Jan;113(1):53-9.

[213] Oktem F, Ozguner F, Yilmaz HR, Uz E, Dundar B. Melatonin reduces urinary excretion of N-acetyl-beta-D-glucosaminidase, albumin and renal oxidative markers in diabetic rats. *Clin. Exp. Pharmacol. Physiol.* 2006 Jan;33(1-2):95-101.

[214] Sandyk R. The influence of the pineal gland on migraine and cluster headaches and effects of treatment with picoTesla magnetic fields. *Int. J. Neurosci.* 1992 Nov;67(1-4):145-71.

[215] Lagod L, Paszkowski T, Sikorski R, Rola R. [The antioxidant-prooxidant balance in pregnancy complicated by spontaneous abortion]. *Ginekol. Pol.* 2001 Dec;72(12):1073-8.

[216] Gupta S, Agarwal A, Banerjee J, Alvarez JG. The role of oxidative stress in spontaneous abortion and recurrent pregnancy loss: a systematic review. *Obstet. Gynecol. Surv.* 2007 May;62(5):335-47.

[217] Simsek M, Naziroglu M, Simsek H, Cay M, Aksakal M, Kumru S. Blood plasma levels of lipoperoxides, glutathione peroxidase, beta carotene, vitamin A and E in women with habitual abortion. *Cell Biochem. Funct.* 1998 Dec;16(4):227-31.

[218] Guerra MO, Silva NO, Guimaraes CS, Souza JP, Andrade AT. Pinealectomy and blindness during pregnancy in the rat. *Am. J. Obstet. Gynecol.* 1973 Feb 15;115(4):582-3.

[219] Franco MC, Akamine EH, Reboucas N, Carvalho MH, Tostes RC, Nigro D, et al. Long-term effects of intrauterine malnutrition on vascular function in female offspring: implications of oxidative stress. *Life Sci.* 2007 Jan 30;80(8):709-15.

[220] Franco MC, Akamine EH, Di Marco GS, Casarini DE, Fortes ZB, Tostes RC, et al. NADPH oxidase and enhanced superoxide generation in intrauterine undernourished rats: involvement of the renin-angiotensin system. *Cardiovasc. Res.* 2003 Sep 1;59(3):767-75.

[221] Nuyt AM. Mechanisms underlying developmental programming of elevated blood pressure and vascular dysfunction: evidence from human studies and experimental animal models. *Clin. Sci. (Lond)* 2008 Jan;114(1):1-17.

[222] Wang Y, Walsh SW. Antioxidant activities and mRNA expression of superoxide dismutase, catalase, and glutathione peroxidase in normal and preeclamptic placentas. *J. Soc. Gynecol. Investig.* 1996 Jul;3(4):179-84.

[223] Fowden AL, Giussani DA, Forhead AJ. Intrauterine programming of physiological systems: causes and consequences. *Physiology (Bethesda)* 2006 Feb;21:29-37.

[224] Halliwell B, Gutteridge JMC. *Free radicals in biology and medicine.* 2007;4th ed.

[225] Luo ZC, Fraser WD, Julien P, Deal CL, Audibert F, Smith GN, et al. Tracing the origins of "fetal origins" of adult diseases: programming by oxidative stress?. *Med. Hypotheses* 2006;66(1):38-44.

[226] Brugger P, Marktl W, Herold M. Impaired nocturnal secretion of melatonin in coronary heart disease. *Lancet* 1995 Jun 3;345(8962):1408.

[227] Beal MF. Energy, oxidative damage, and Alzheimer's disease: clues to the underlying puzzle. *Neurobiol. Aging* 1994;15 Suppl 2:S171-S174.

[228] Balter M. Filtering a river of cancer data. *Science* 1995 Feb 24;267(5201):1084-6.

[229] O'Brien IA, Lewin IG, O'Hare JP, Arendt J, Corrall RJ. Abnormal circadian rhythm of melatonin in diabetic autonomic neuropathy. *Clin. Endocrinol. (Oxf.)* 1986 Apr;24(4):359-64.

[230] Rosenthal NE, Sack DA, Gillin JC, Lewy AJ, Goodwin FK, Davenport Y, et al. Seasonal affective disorder. A description of the syndrome and preliminary findings with light therapy. *Arch. Gen. Psychiatry* 1984 Jan;41(1):72-80.

[231] Lissoni P, Barni S, Crispino S, Tancini G, Fraschini F. Endocrine and immune effects of melatonin therapy in metastatic cancer patients. *Eur. J. Cancer Clin. Oncol.* 1989 May;25(5):789-95.

[232] Reiter RJ, Melchiorri D, Sewerynek E, Poeggeler B, Barlow-Walden L, Chuang J, et al. A review of the evidence supporting melatonin's role as an antioxidant. *J. Pineal. Res.* 1995 Jan;18(1):1-11.

[233] Vijayalaxmi, Reiter RJ, Meltz ML. Melatonin protects human blood lymphocytes from radiation-induced chromosome damage. *Mutat. Res.* 1995 Jan;346(1):23-31.

[234] Welin AK, Svedin P, Lapatto R, Sultan B, Hagberg H, Gressens P, et al. Melatonin reduces inflammation and cell death in white matter in the mid-gestation fetal sheep following umbilical cord occlusion. *Pediatr. Res.* 2007 Feb;61(2):153-8.

[235] Munoz-Hoyos A, Rodriguez-Cabezas T, Molina-Carballo A, Martinez-Sempere JJ, Ruiz-Cosano C, Acuna-Castroviejo D. Melatonin concentration in the umbilical artery and vein in human preterm and term neonates and neonates with acute fetal distress. *J. Pineal. Res.* 1992 Nov;13(4):184-91.

[236] Jou MJ, Peng TI, Yu PZ, Jou SB, Reiter RJ, Chen JY, et al. Melatonin protects against common deletion of mitochondrial DNA-augmented mitochondrial oxidative stress and apoptosis. *J. Pineal. Res.* 2007 Nov;43(4):389-403.

[237] Singh HJ, Keah LS, Kumar A, Sirajudeen KN. Adverse effects of melatonin on rat pups of Wistar-Kyoto dams receiving melatonin supplementation during pregnancy. *Exp. Toxicol. Pathol.* 2012 Nov;64(7-8):751-2.

[238] Gitto E, Reiter RJ, Sabatino G, Buonocore G, Romeo C, Gitto P, et al. Correlation among cytokines, bronchopulmonary dysplasia and modality of ventilation in preterm newborns: improvement with melatonin treatment. *J. Pineal. Res.* 2005 Oct;39(3):287-93.

[239] Cervantes M, Morali G, Letechipia-Vallejo G. Melatonin and ischemia-reperfusion injury of the brain. *J. Pineal. Res.* 2008 Aug;45(1):1-7.

[240] Jahnke G, Marr M, Myers C, Wilson R, Travlos G, Price C. Maternal and developmental toxicity evaluation of melatonin administered orally to pregnant Sprague-Dawley rats. *Toxicol. Sci.* 1999 Aug;50(2):271-9.

[241] Peschke E. Melatonin, endocrine pancreas and diabetes. *J. Pineal. Res.* 2008 Jan;44(1):26-40.

[242] Tengattini S, Reiter RJ, Tan DX, Terron MP, Rodella LF, Rezzani R. Cardiovascular diseases: protective effects of melatonin. *J. Pineal. Res.* 2008 Jan;44(1):16-25.

[243] Nahleh Z, Pruemer J, Lafollette J, Sweany S. Melatonin, a promising role in taxane-related neuropathy. *Clin. Med. Insights. Oncol.* 2010;4:35-41.

[244] Reiter RJ, Tan DX, Sainz RM, Mayo JC, Lopez-Burillo S. Melatonin: reducing the toxicity and increasing the efficacy of drugs. *J. Pharm. Pharmacol.* 2002 Oct;54(10):1299-321.

In: New Developments in Melatonin Research ISBN: 978-1-62618-843-3
Editors: D.Acuña-Castroviejo, I.Rusanova, G.Escames © 2013 Nova Science Publishers, Inc.

Chapter 10

By Receptors, Binding Sites or Free Radical Scavenger Action: Is There a Pivotal Action Mechanism for Melatonin in Retinal Pathologies?

Lucia de Fatima Sobral Sampaio*
Lab Biochemistry of the CNS Development,
Biological Sciences Institute,
Federal do Pará University do Pará, Belém, PA, Brazil

Abstract

Melatonin is the hormone nightly secreted by pineal gland and photoreceptors; conversely it is also secreted in non-rhythmic faction by leukocytes. Further to its forming images functions, in the retina occurs entrainment of circadian cycle by light, due to light-inhibition of the melatonin synthesis in photoreceptors, and to light sensitizing circadian photoreceptors, located in a subset of ganglion cells. As known, melatonin acts through Gi protein coupled receptors, a nuclear receptor, and two cytoplasmic binding sites, the first is located in the protein calmodulin, and the second is the active site of the QR2 enzyme (NRH: Quinone oxidoreductase 2 enzyme, EC 1.10.99.2).

A direct free radical scavenger action, and an indirect antioxidant action, by increase in synthesis of the antioxidant cascades enzymes, are also observed. Concerning membrane receptors, melatonin chronobiological effects appear to be mainly triggered by MT1 (Mel1a for avian), while those non-rhythmic are by MT2 (Mel1b for avian). Our biochemical and autoradiographic studies indicated not only developmentally regulated melatonin membrane receptors, but also the QR2 enzyme presence in the retina. These

* Lucia de Fatima Sobral Sampaio: Rua Augusto Corrêa No. 1. Belém. PA. CEP: 66075-110, lsampaio@ufpa.br.

studies were confirmed by the presence of the immunoreactivity to melatonin receptors and to QR2 enzyme in whole mounted embryonic and post-hatched retinas. We assumed that the melatonin machinery present in the retina is a scenery, in which a myriad of mechanisms underlying the therapeutic effects of this neurohormone in mitochondrial optic neuropathies and acute retinal damages can be discussed. As a consequence, we propose a model for melatonin pharmacological action in retinal pathologies.

Introduction

The environmental light excites two different types of translators in mammalian and in avian retinas. The first type comprises rods and cones photoreceptors, the first step of the clearly established image-forming pathway; and the second type comprises photopigments, located in a subtype of ganglion cells named intrinsically photosensitive retinal ganglion cells (pRGCs), where the non-image-forming pathway starts The circadian photo entrainment, the pupillary light reflex and the pineal melatonin suppression are non-image photic responses. In pRGCs, the light is received by the photopigment melanopsin that signalizes by a mechanistic not completely understood, up to the present time [1-6]. It has been described pRGCs expressing five different melanopsin subtypes in the mammalian retina, each one presumably triggered by a different luminance input.

Each one melanopsin subtype displays signal, with different output properties, that is propagated by a different pathway [7]. The suprachiasmatic nucleus (SCN) translates light signals switching off melatonin secretion by pineal gland. In function of the intrinsic resistance of the pRGC to neurodegeneration [8], the loss of non-forming image pathway occurs only with the advancement of the retinal disease; and their clinical symptoms are used for screening of the retinopathy severity [9].

In a retinopathy, the progress to total blindness have been showed to occur in the same fashion in infant preterm, in children, in youth, in adults and in ancient. At total blindness is observed free-runner. It is a endogenous sleep-walk rhythm, characterized by have a duration larger than 24 h. Blind free-runners humans often effort to maintain a 24 h sleep-wake schedule, and, consequently, are suffering from recurrent sleep disruption and daytime somnolence.

In absence of the photic entrainment on light-dark cycle, non-photic zeitgeibers synchronize their rest-activity cycle, however with effectiveness lower than photic ones [10]. In addition to the hereditary retinopathy, local or systemic free radicals surges can be causal factors of retinal degenerative diseases. Highlighting retinitis, glaucoma, systemic hypertension, neural degeneration, diabetes; and the progressive reduction in antioxidant defenses in the aging process occurring with melatonin-deficient pineal secretion. Finally, hard addition of alcohol and tobacco can be pointed out as retinopathies' risk factors, and in case of the pregnant women, the risk will be surrounding the fetus.

In this chapter, in view of the new founds about how the signal of the environmental luminance is addressed to the SCN [11;12], our aim was transform the retinal melatoninergic system in scenery, in which the melatonin action on retinal pathologies will be discussed.

Melatonin in Vertebrate Retina

Metabolism

The second major surge of melatonin in human beings occurs in the retina. However, the amount of melatonin produced in the eye is far less than that produced in the pineal body. Consequently, the retinal melatonin contribution for total amount of melatonin in blood stream is not taken in account for systemic melatonin effects, having only paracrine functions [13-17]. It is also showed to occur non-rhythmic melatonin syntheses in activated leukocytes that effluxes melatonin up to μM concentration range in inflammatory response, without relationship with melatonin circadian surges [18].

Melatonin is biosynthesized from tryptophan by a four steps pathway. In general, the serotonin (arylalkylamine) N-acetyltransferase (EC 2.3.1.87) is the rate-limiting enzyme; therefore the first step enzyme tryptophan hydroxylase (EC 1.14.16.4) has been suggested as a second point of the modulation of the melatonin synthesis in the retina [19]. Melatonin paracrine action in the retina is finished by deacetylation, resulting in 5-methoxytryptamine. Forward, 5-methoxytryptamine metabolism is influenced by the amount of the free radical and nitrogen species surrounded it. As some others melatonin metabolits, it may be found in the middle of compounds with radical scavenger properties, having also pharmacological actions (14;20). The inhibition of melatonin synthesis by light and by clock genes located in photoreceptors is very well studied [21].

Physiology

Melatonin paracrine action in the eye implies in a net comprising hormone and receptors functioning in opposite form in relation to dopamine, specifically adapting the retina to darkness. This implies in the inhibition of the dopamine release, modulation of the nocturnal vision, and improvement of the circadian photoreceptors outer segment disc shedding. Melatonin binds to membrane receptors named MT1 and MT2, or named Mel1a, Mel1b and Mel1c, if we are considering non-mammalian retinas [22-24]. The Mel1c melatonin receptor evolution in mammals is the orphan GPR50, in which melatonin does not bind. But, MT1 and MT2 can be under GPR50 modulation by protein-protein binding [25]. These melatonin membrane receptors function mainly by Gi inhibition of the adenylate cyclase activity [26], and their distribution in retinal layers appears to be well conserved in evolution [27;28]. Beyond melatonin dark adapting function, it has the capability to cross the internal mitochondrial membrane, functioning in a direct antioxidant manner against the production of the free radicals in the mitochondrial matrix of the pigmented and neural retinal cells, protecting them against neurodegeneration [29-34].

Melatonin Receptors and Binding Sites

In mammalian, the MT1 and MT2 melatonin receptors expression is in antiphase in relation to melatonin circadian pineal surge [35], the same occur for Mel1a and Mel1b, but does not was observed for Mel 1c in chicken [36]. In function of the melatonin importance in retinal physiology, effort has been done to characterize melatonin membrane receptors in the retina, at different neurodevelopmental stages, aiming to insert melatoninergic pathways in retinal physiology square. Till now, melatonin receptors were mapped by many authors in the retina of several species by immunohistochemistry, and it was observed their distribution in almost all retinal layers [22]. As part of the effort to understand melatoninergic system in retinal physiology and pathology, we have showed inhibition by melatonin of the cAMP accumulation in the neurodevelopment, using chick retina as model. The results show differential expression of GPCRs [37;38]. In addition, the presence of the previously named MT3 melatonin binding site, actual QR2 (NRH: Quinone oxidoreductase 2 enzyme, EC 1.10.99.2), was suggested for the first time by results showing increase in cAMP accumulation as a bypass QR2 effect in the retina development [39].

A qualitative study using whole mounted chick retinas was done to show the developmental profile of the immunoreactivity appearing for melatonin GPCRs and for QR2 in this tissue.

Materials and Methods

Materials

The antibodies used herein were purchased from Santa Cruz Biotechnology (Mel1a, Mel1b, MT3 and Texas Red), and Sigma Chemical Co., St. Louis, MO, USA. All others products were from analytic grade.

Animals

The eggs were from a local producer. They were housed in natural light/dark cycle, and experiments were done always in the afternoon. The Brazilian law regarding treatment of animals in research was observed.

Immunohistochemistry

Retinas from 8 and 14 days embryonic stages (E8 and E14), and 2-5 days post-hatched (PH) were dissected at 4 ^{o}C in a calcium magnesium free saline solution, and then they were submitted to following protocol: paraformaldehyde solution (PFA) 4%, 15 min; Tween 20 0.5%, 30 min; primary antibody (1:200) for 72 h; secondary antibody (1:400) 2 h. The retinas were rinsed with PBS by 3 times of the 10 min, before each step. No immune reactivity was observed after elimination of the primary antibodies. The image was captured by fluorescence microscopy (Olympus BX41). The ImajeJ software was used only for adjust of the brightness and contrast.

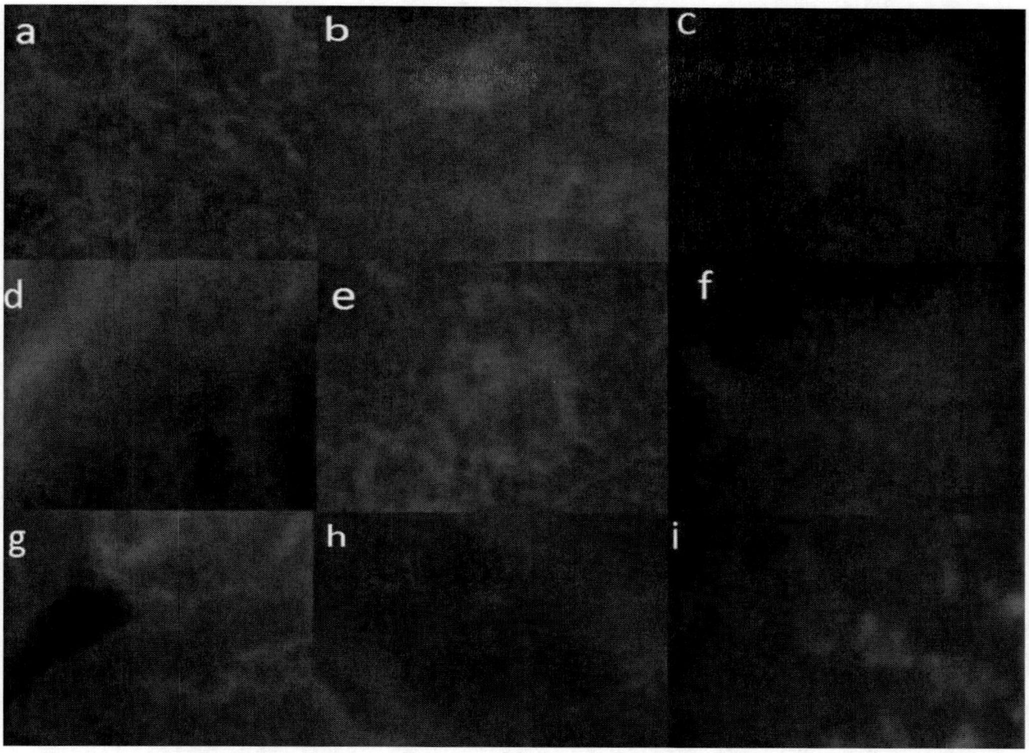

Figure 1. Different Immune fluorescent signals for Mel1a (a, b, c), Mel1b (d, e, f) and QR2 (g, h, i) in embryonic (E8, left; E14, middle) and post-hatched (PH, right) in whole-mounted chick retinas. Texas Red immunolabeling, X 400.

Results

It was done a qualitative immunohistochemistry study of Mel1a, Mel1b melatonin receptors and QR2 in whole-mounted chick retinas from E8, E14 days and 2-5 days PH. Regarding Mel1a, it was observed high immunoreactivity in retinas from E8, E14 and PH (Figure 1 a, b, and c). The Mel1b signal also was impressively observed in E14 whole retinas and in PH (Figure 1 e and f), though, when we compared it with Mel1a and QR2 immunoreactivities in E8, it was considered poorly labeled (Figure 1 d). Mel1b immunoreactivity, such Mel1a, was observed in the same fashion as in cellular body as is fibers.

We observed astonishing immunoreactivity for QR2 in retinal cells bodies in all developmental stages tested (Figure 1 g, h and i).

Melatonininergic System and Retinal Pathologies

Melatonin has chronobiotic and non-chronobiotic effects. If such in others tissues, in the retina the non-chronobiotic action should be mainly by MT2, while the chronobiotic effects should be mainly by MT1. Therefore the melatonin effect in glaucoma has been point out as triggered by MT1 receptors, showing that a border between the mechanisms underlying melatonin effects is not a simple task to outline. Another point is the importance of the melatonin free radical scavenger function, which is the unique that will be occurring, during the time before melatonin functions by membrane receptors starting. Membrane melatonin GPCRs trigger up regulation of the antioxidant enzymes (glutathione peroxidase; glutathione reductase, y-glutamylcysteine synthase, glucose-6-phosphate dehydrogenase) and down regulation of the pro-oxidant enzyme (NO synthases, lipoxygenases). Sometimes, up regulation of the Cu-, Zn- and Mn- superoxide dismutase's and of the catalase is also observed [27;40-43].

At aging, with failure of the melatonin surges from pineal gland, is observed increase in free radicals accumulation, that induces the age related macular degeneration (AMD). It occurs without co-morbidity with diabetes and hypertension [44]. Such a neurological disorder, AMD curses with inflammatory process, which is responsive to melatonin [18;23;45-47].

The most common genetic retinal pathology is retinitis pigmentosa, which is characterized by progressive degeneration of neural retina that starts in rod photoreceptors. The time course of the disease can became slower by a supplementation of the vitamin A associated with the presence of the oil in the diet. Obviously the progressive lack of photoreceptors leads to lower levels of melatonin in the retina [48]. Thus, the progressive incapability to form image is accompanied with the reduced protection against free radicals, increasing the retinal susceptibility to neurodegenerative processes. The advancement of the degeneration until ganglion cells layer affects the non-image forming function of the eye. The patient losses the capability to perceive environmental light, with loss of the zeitgeiber setting.

Two others inherit optic neuropathies are characterized by loss of retinal ganglion cells leading to optic atrophy and blindness. These neuropathies are due to hereditary mitochondrial dysfunction. Leber hereditary optic neuropathy and Kjer type dominant optic atrophy are known for initially affecting the parvocellular RGCs (papillomacular bundle), which causes dyschromatopsia, loss of visual acuity, cecocentral scotomas and temporal optic atrophy. Interestingly, the ganglion cells responsible by non-image forming vision are more resistant to death than others, implying in delayed evolution to total blindness, characterized by loss of the entrainment in sleep-walking cycle. Appearing mainly in adulthood, the progress to total blindness can be monitored by means of morphological diagnostic techniques such as Optic Coherence Tomography, and functional techniques such as Multifocal Electroretinography [9;49].

While in those optic diseases related above the non-image forming vision is only gradually lost, in children who are born blind, the absence of this kind of vision is included in general signals. Melatonin becoming a prompt therapeutic to ameliorate the general well-being [40;50;51], which has a pivotal importance in children general development, being obligatory the therapeutic pediatric use for melatonin, not only in children with total blindness, but also in children with neurological syndromes, mental retardation and epilepsy, one time clinical signs of internal desynchronization have been observed [52-57].

The immunohistochemistry evidence showed in this chapter is in agreement with our previous biochemical research, where Mel1a (MT1) melatonin receptor and QR2 effects are observed since E8, when differentiation process starts; and Mel1b (MT2) receptor effects occur mainly by E14, when synaptogenesis arises [37]. The expression of the QR2 during all developmental stages, increasing cAMP accumulation in the retina, is suggestive of a function in retinal metabolism [39].

MT1 (Mel1a) has a pivotal role in retinal cell differentiation, qualifying this receptor as a pharmacological target to development of the neurodegenerative disorders' therapeutic. Above all, those cursing with progressive failure of the neuronal plasticity, such as genetic retinopathies.

In the context of the clinical importance, the aim of the melatonin therapeutic use in children with severe disabilities, including blindness, is restore the photic zeitgeiber, improving the general well-being and development. Regarding youth and adulthood with inherit retinopathies, and ancient with AMD, depending on retinal degeneration level, the addition of the melatonin also protects the retina by antioxidant action, and /or inhibiting NO production. The acute direct scavenger action completes the scenery of the mechanisms underlying melatonin pharmacological action. This scavenger action occurs while the improvement in synthesis of antioxidant cascade, in response to melatonin receptor activation, is being initiated. Taken together, melatonin acts triggering by receptors and binding sites a diversity of effects complying with the severity of the retinopathy.

Conclusion

In light of the new facts, the subcellular mechanisms triggered by melatonin receptors are underlying pharmacological melatonin effects, being extremely important the development of selective agonists, and the approval all the word of the melatonin administration to practicing prescription for retinal and others neurodegenerative disorders [18]. The drug-candidate selectivity to GPCR target is important to avoid off target effects through QR2, which is present since non-differentiated stages in the retina.

Acknowledgments

Data presented in this chapter were supported by funds from CNPq. The experiments were done with the participation of undergraduate students Anaelle dos Santos Souza, Deborah Terra de Oliveira, Erika Thaiane Couto Canelas and Felipe Pantoja Mesquita.

References

[1] Blasic JR, Jr., Lane BR, Robinson PR. Light-dependent phosphorylation of the carboxy tail of mouse melanopsin. *Cell Mol. Life Sci.* 2012 May;69(9):1551-62.

[2] Contin MA, Verra DM, Guido ME. An invertebrate-like phototransduction cascade mediates light detection in the chicken retinal ganglion cells. *FASEB J.* 2006 Dec;20(14):2648-50.

[3] Perez-Leighton CE, Schmidt TM, Abramowitz J, Birnbaumer L, Kofuji P. Intrinsic phototransduction persists in melanopsin-expressing ganglion cells lacking diacylglycerol-sensitive TRPC subunits. *Eur. J. Neurosci.* 2011 Mar;33(5):856-67.

[4] Van Hook MJ, Wong KY, Berson DM. Dopaminergic modulation of ganglion-cell photoreceptors in rat. *Eur. J. Neurosci.* 2012 Feb;35(4):507-18.

[5] Verra DM, Contin MA, Hicks D, Guido ME. Early onset and differential temporospatial expression of melanopsin isoforms in the developing chicken retina. *Invest. Ophthalmol. Vis. Sci.* 2011 Jul;52(8):5111-20.

[6] Zele AJ, Feigl B, Smith SS, Markwell EL. The circadian response of intrinsically photosensitive retinal ganglion cells. PLoS One 2011;6(3):e17860.

[7] Sand A, Schmidt TM, Kofuji P. Diverse types of ganglion cell photoreceptors in the mammalian retina. *Prog. Retin. Eye Res.* 2012 Jul;31(4):287-302.

[8] La MC, Ross-Cisneros FN, Sadun AA, Hannibal J, Munarini A, Mantovani V, et al. Melanopsin retinal ganglion cells are resistant to neurodegeneration in mitochondrial optic neuropathies. *Brain* 2010 Aug;133(Pt 8):2426-38.

[9] Perez-Rico C, de l, V, Blanco R, Germain F, Paz-Moreno J, Arribas-Gomez I. [Alterations in nocturnal melatonin secretion in patients with optic neuropathies]. *Arch. Soc. Esp. Oftalmol.* 2009 May;84(5):251-7.

[10] Emens J, Lewy AJ, Laurie AL, Songer JB. Rest-activity cycle and melatonin rhythm in blind free-runners have similar periods. *J. Biol. Rhythms* 2010 Oct;25(5):381-4.

[11] Dinet V, Ansari N, Torres-Farfan C, Korf HW. Clock gene expression in the retina of melatonin-proficient (C3H) and melatonin-deficient (C57BL) mice. *J. Pineal. Res.* 2007 Jan;42(1):83-91.

[12] Lucas RJ, Foster RG. Neither functional rod photoreceptors nor rod or cone outer segments are required for the photic inhibition of pineal melatonin. *Endocrinology* 1999 Apr;140(4):1520-4.

[13] Haque R, Chong NW, Ali F, Chaurasia SS, Sengupta T, Chun E, et al. Melatonin synthesis in retina: cAMP-dependent transcriptional regulation of chicken arylalkylamine N-acetyltransferase by a CRE-like sequence and a TTATT repeat motif in the proximal promoter. *J. Neurochem.* 2011 Oct;119(1):6-17.

[14] Hardeland R. Melatonin metabolism in the central nervous system. *Curr. Neuropharmacol.* 2010 Sep;8(3):168-81.

[15] Nowak R, McMillen IC, Redman J, Short RV. The correlation between serum and salivary melatonin concentrations and urinary 6-hydroxymelatonin sulphate excretion rates: two non-invasive techniques for monitoring human circadian rhythmicity. *Clin. Endocrinol.* (Oxf) 1987 Oct;27(4):445-52.

[16] Pang SF, Cheng KM, Allen AE, Tsang CW, Wong CO, Nichols CR. Inherited changes in concentrations of retinal and serum melatonin in the chicken. *Gen. Comp. Endocrinol.* 1989 Dec;76(3):427-36.

[17] Zmijewski MA, Sweatman TW, Slominski AT. The melatonin-producing system is fully functional in retinal pigment epithelium (ARPE-19). *Mol. Cell Endocrinol.* 2009 Aug 13;307(1-2):211-6.

[18] Cecon E, Markus RP. Relevance of the chronobiological and non-chronobiological actions of melatonin for enhancing therapeutic efficacy in neurodegenerative disorders. *Recent Pat. Endocr. Metab. Immune Drug Discov.* 2011 May;5(2):91-9.

[19] Valenciano AI, Alonso-Gomez AL, Iuvone PM. Regulation of tryptophan hydroxylase activity in Xenopus laevis photoreceptor cells by cyclic AMP. *J. Neurochem.* 2000 May;74(5):1961-7.

[20] Mondaca M, Hernandez A, Valladares L, Sierralta W, Noseda R, Soto-Moyano R. Involvement of melatonin metabolites in the long-term inhibitory effect of the hormone on rat spinal nociceptive transmission. *Pharmacol. Biochem. Behav.* 2004 Feb;77(2):275-9.

[21] Voisin P, Cailleau V, Naud N, Cantereau A, Bernard M. Visual photoreceptor subtypes in the chicken retina: melatonin-synthesizing activity and in vitro differentiation. *Cell Tissue Res.* 2012 Jun;348(3):417-27.

[22] Alarma-Estrany P, Pintor J. Melatonin receptors in the eye: location, second messengers and role in ocular physiology. *Pharmacol. Ther.* 2007 Mar;113(3):507-22.

[23] Bok D. Retinal researchers have reasons to be optimistic. *Retina* 2005 Dec;25(8 Suppl):S43.

[24] Dubocovich ML. Modulation of [3H]dopamine release from rabbit retina. *Fed. Proc.* 1984 Sep;43(12):2714-8.

[25] Dufourny L, Levasseur A, Migaud M, Callebaut I, Pontarotti P, Malpaux B, et al. GPR50 is the mammalian ortholog of Mel1c: evidence of rapid evolution in mammals. *BMC Evol. Biol.* 2008;8:105.

[26] Dubocovich ML, Delagrange P, Krause DN, Sugden D, Cardinali DP, Olcese J. International Union of Basic and Clinical Pharmacology. LXXV. Nomenclature, classification, and pharmacology of G protein-coupled melatonin receptors. *Pharmacol. Rev.* 2010 Sep;62(3):343-80.

[27] Sengupta A, Baba K, Mazzoni F, Pozdeyev NV, Strettoi E, Iuvone PM, et al. Localization of melatonin receptor 1 in mouse retina and its role in the circadian regulation of the electroretinogram and dopamine levels. PLoS One 2011;6(9):e24483.

[28] Wiechmann AF, Sherry DM. Melatonin receptors are anatomically organized to modulate transmission specifically to cone pathways in the retina of Xenopus laevis. *J. Comp. Neurol.* 2012 Apr 15;520(6):1115-27.

[29] Baba K, Pozdeyev N, Mazzoni F, Contreras-Alcantara S, Liu C, Kasamatsu M, et al. Melatonin modulates visual function and cell viability in the mouse retina via the MT1 melatonin receptor. *Proc. Natl. Acad. Sci. U S A* 2009 Sep 1;106(35):15043-8.

[30] Fu Y, Tang M, Fan Y, Zou H, Sun X, Xu X. Anti-apoptotic effects of melatonin in retinal pigment epithelial cells. *Front Biosci.* 2012;17:1461-8.

[31] Kaur C, Sivakumar V, Foulds WS, Luu CD, Ling EA. Cellular and vascular changes in the retina of neonatal rats after an acute exposure to hypoxia. *Invest. Ophthalmol. Vis. Sci.* 2009 Nov;50(11):5364-74.

[32] Lundmark PO, Pandi-Perumal SR, Srinivasan V, Cardinali DP. Role of melatonin in the eye and ocular dysfunctions. *Vis. Neurosci.* 2006 Nov;23(6):853-62.

[33] Wiechmann AF, Summers JA. Circadian rhythms in the eye: the physiological significance of melatonin receptors in ocular tissues. *Prog. Retin. Eye Res.* 2008 Mar;27(2):137-60.

[34] Wiechmann AF, Chignell CF, Roberts JE. Influence of dietary melatonin on photoreceptor survival in the rat retina: an ocular toxicity study. *Exp. Eye Res.* 2008 Feb;86(2):241-50.

[35] Roka F, Brydon L, Waldhoer M, Strosberg AD, Freissmuth M, Jockers R, et al. Tight association of the human Mel(1a)-melatonin receptor and G(i): precoupling and constitutive activity. *Mol. Pharmacol.* 1999 Nov;56(5):1014-24.

[36] Masana MI, Witt-Enderby PA, Dubocovich ML. Melatonin differentially modulates the expression and function of the hMT1 and hMT2 melatonin receptors upon prolonged withdrawal. *Biochem. Pharmacol.* 2003 Mar 1;65(5):731-9.

[37] Sampaio LF. Melatonin inhibitory effect on cAMP accumulation in the chick retina development. Int J Dev Neurosci 2008 May;26(3-4):277-82.

[38] Sampaio LF, Markus RP. Melatonin and the time window for the expression of the alpha8 nicotinic acetylcholine receptor in the membrane of chick retinal cells in culture. *Int. J. Dev. Neurosci.* 2010 May;28(3):245-9.

[39] Sampaio LF. An unexpected effect of 5-MCA-NAT in chick retinal development. *Int. J. Dev. Neurosci.* 2009 Oct;27(6):511-5.

[40] Alcantara-Contreras S, Baba K, Tosini G. Removal of melatonin receptor type 1 increases intraocular pressure and retinal ganglion cells death in the mouse. *Neurosci. Lett.* 2011 Apr 20;494(1):61-4.

[41] Pandi-Perumal SR, Bahammam AS, Brown GM, Spence DW, Bharti VK, Kaur C, et al. Melatonin Antioxidative Defense: Therapeutical Implications for Aging and Neurodegenerative Processes. *Neurotox. Res.* 2012 Jun 28.

[42] Rodriguez C, Mayo JC, Sainz RM, Antolin I, Herrera F, Martin V, et al. Regulation of antioxidant enzymes: a significant role for melatonin. *J. Pineal Res.* 2004 Jan;36(1):1-9.

[43] Rosenstein RE, Pandi-Perumal SR, Srinivasan V, Spence DW, Brown GM, Cardinali DP. Melatonin as a therapeutic tool in ophthalmology: implications for glaucoma and uveitis. *J. Pineal Res.* 2010 Aug;49(1):1-13.

[44] Rosen R, Hu DN, Perez V, Tai K, Yu GP, Chen M, et al. Urinary 6-sulfatoxymelatonin level in age-related macular degeneration patients. *Mol. Vis.* 2009;15:1673-9.

[45] Hardeland R. Melatonin in aging and disease -multiple consequences of reduced secretion, options and limits of treatment. *Aging Dis.* 2012 Apr;3(2):194-225.

[46] Johnson LV, Forest DL, Banna CD, Radeke CM, Maloney MA, Hu J, et al. Cell culture model that mimics drusen formation and triggers complement activation associated with age-related macular degeneration. *Proc. Natl. Acad. Sci. U S A* 2011 Nov 8;108(45):18277-82.

[47] Vojnikovic B, Vojnikovic D. Chromotherapy of macular degeneration with transitions lenses and green-yellow medical filters and special programme for psychoorganic disturbances. *Coll. Antropol.* 2010 Apr;34 Suppl 2:89-93.

[48] Banas I, Buntner B, Niebroj T, Ostrowska Z. [Levels of melatonin in serum of patients with retinitis pigmentosa]. *Klin. Oczna.* 1995 Nov;97(11-12):321-3.

[49] de ZN, Plano SA, Fernandez DC, Lanzani MF, Salido E, Belforte N, et al. Effect of experimental glaucoma on the non-image forming visual system. *J. Neurochem.* 2011 Jun;117(5):904-14.

[50] Altun A, Ugur-Altun B. Melatonin: therapeutic and clinical utilization. *Int. J. Clin. Pract.* 2007 May;61(5):835-45.

[51] Ramstad K, Loge JH. [Melatonin treatment of a blind child with serious sleep disorders]. Tidsskr Nor Laegeforen 2002 Apr 20;122(10):1005-6.

[52] Cavallo A. The pineal gland in human beings: relevance to pediatrics. *J. Pediatr.* 1993 Dec;123(6):843-51.

[53] Ito J, Saijo H, Tanaka H, Tasaki T, Chou K. [Melatonin treatment for sleep-wake disorder--an experience for a severely mental retarded patient with blindness]. No To Hattatsu 1995 Sep;27(5):401-3.

[54] Lapierre O, Dumont M. Melatonin treatment of a non-24-hour sleep-wake cycle in a blind retarded child. Biol Psychiatry 1995 Jul 15;38(2):119-22.

[55] Palm L, Blennow G, Wetterberg L. Correction of non-24-hour sleep/wake cycle by melatonin in a blind retarded boy. *Ann. Neurol.* 1991 Mar;29(3):336-9.

[56] Tzischinsky O, Skene D, Epstein R, Lavie P. Circadian rhythms in 6-sulphatoxymelatonin and nocturnal sleep in blind children. *Chronobiol. Int.* 1991;8(3):168-75.

[57] Zucconi M, Bruni O. Sleep disorders in children with neurologic diseases. *Semin. Pediatr. Neurol.* 2001 Dec;8(4):258-75.

In: New Developments in Melatonin Research ISBN: 978-1-62618-843-3
Editors: D.Acuña-Castroviejo, I.Rusanova, G.Escames © 2013 Nova Science Publishers, Inc.

Chapter 11

Therapeutic Benefit of Melatonin for Glaucoma

Ruth E. Rosenstein**, *María C. Moreno, Pablo Sande, Magdalena Miranda, Marcos Aranda, María F. González Fleitas and Nicolás Belforte

Laboratory of Retinal Neurochemistry and Experimental Ophthalmology, Department of Human Biochemistry, School of Medicine/CEFyBO/, University of Buenos Aires/CONICET, Buenos Aires, Argentina

Abstract

Glaucoma is a leading cause of blindness, characterized by specific visual field defects due to the loss of retinal ganglion cells and damage to the optic nerve head. Ocular hypertension is probably the most important risk factor in primary angle open glaucoma, the more frequent form of glaucoma. Besides ocular hypertension, several concomitant factors such as elevation of synaptic glutamate levels and decrease in GABA levels, altered NO metabolism, and oxidative damage could significantly contribute to the neurodegeneration. Although the current management of glaucoma is mainly directed at the control of intraocular pressure, a therapy that prevents the death of retinal ganglion cells and optic nerve head fiber loss should be the main goal of treatment. Several lines of evidence strongly support that melatonin behaves as a neuroprotector in experimental animal models of various neurological and neurodegenerative disorders. In this chapter, we will consider evidence supporting that melatonin which decreases glutamate synaptic levels, NO production, and oxidative damage, increases GABA synaptic levels, and prevents retinal ganglion cell and optic nerve fiber loss induced by chronic ocular hypertension, could be considered as a new therapeutic resource for the management of glaucoma.

* Corresponding Author: Dr. Ruth E. Rosenstein, Department of Human Biochemistry, School of Medicine, CEFyBO, University of Buenos Aires, CONICET, Paraguay 2155, 5th floor, (1121), Buenos Aires, ARGENTINA. Tel: 54-11-45083672 (ext 31); Fax: 54-11-45083672 (ext 317); e-mail: ruthr@fmed.uba.ar.

Introduction

Melatonin in the Retina

Numerous studies have firmly established that melatonin synthesis occurs in the retina of vertebrates, including mammals [1]. Although available data indicate that photoreceptors synthesize melatonin independently of the rest of the retina [2], recent evidence indicates that melatonin could be also synthesized in chick retinal ganglion cells [3].

In the vertebrate species studied so far, melatonin synthesis in the retina is elevated at night and reduced during the day in a fashion similar to events in the pineal gland. Melatonin synthesis in the retina is under the control of a circadian oscillator, and circadian rhythms in melatonin synthesis have been described in several species. These rhythms occur *in vivo*, persist *in vit*ro, and are entrained by the light/dark signal [4;5].

Retinal biosynthesis of melatonin has been extensively studied and revised [1]. In contrast, although a mutual inhibitory relationship between melatonin and dopamine [6;7], as well as the involvement of melatonin in the regulation of photoreceptor disc shedding and phagocytosis [8], melanosome aggregation in pigment epithelium and cone photoreceptor retinomotor movements [9] were conclusively demonstrated, the full range of physiological actions of melatonin in the retina is far from being completely known. Retinal melatonin does not contribute to circulating levels, suggesting that it acts locally as a neurohormone and/or neuromodulator. The present chapter focuses on the therapeutic effect of melatonin for ther treatment of glaucoma, a highly prevalent ocular disease.

Glaucoma

Glaucoma is a leading cause of blindness worldwide, characterized by specific visual field defects due to the loss retinal ganglion cells (RGCs) and damage to the optic nerve head (ONH).

More than 60 million people around the world are affected by glaucoma, and it has been estimated that ~8 million suffer from bilateral blindness caused by this disease [10]. Visual loss often starts in the periphery and advances to involve the central vision, with devastating consequences to the patient´s quality of life [11]. It is estimated that half of those affected may be not aware of their condition because symptoms may not occur during the early stages of the disease. When vision loss appears, considerable and permanent damage has already occurred. Medications and surgery can help to slow the progression of some forms of the disease, but at present, there is no cure. An increase in intracoular pressure [IOP] definitely plays a causal role in glaucomatous neuropathy. However, although ocular hypertension is common among open-angle glaucoma patients, only a limited subset of individuals with ocular hypertension will develop this disease [12]. Moreover, a significant number of patients presenting with glaucoma continue to lose vision despite responding well to therapies that lower eye pressure [13-16]. What then leads to RGC death in glaucoma? Glaucoma is a complex, multifactorial disease, thus it is likely that several molecular pathways converge to induce RGC loss. Signals that promote RGC death in glaucoma might be exacerbated by risks factors, tilting the neuron´s fate toward dysfunction and demise. In recent years, there has been considerable progress in our understanding of multiple pathways that lead to RGC degeneration following optic nerve injury. This body of work has notably increased our knowledge of RGC neurobiology [11]. In this vein, several factors such as a glutamate excitotoxicity [17], decrease in GABA levels [18], reduced antioxidant defense system activity [19;20], and an increase in the nitridergic pathway activity [21;22] have been suggested as possible additional causes for early or advanced stages of glaucomatous damage. The current management of glaucoma is mainly directed at the control of IOP; however, a therapy that prevents the death of ganglion cells should be the main goal of treatment.

Unraveling which are the most critical mechanisms involved in glaucoma is unlikely to be achieved in studies which are limited to the clinically observable changes to the retina and optic nerve head (ON) that are seen in human glaucoma. Far more detailed and invasive studies are required, preferably in a readily available animal model. An experimental model system of pressure-induced optic nerve damage would greatly facilitate the understanding of the cellular events leading to RGC death, and how they are influenced by IOP and other risk factors associated to glaucoma. Several groups have developed various ways to increase IOP in the rat eye, generally by impeding the outflow of aqueous humor [23-25]. All of these models have both advantages and disadvantages. We have developed a model of glaucoma in rats through the intracameral injection of 1% hyaluronic acid (HA). Weekly injections of HA in the rat anterior chamber significantly increase IOP as compared with vehicle-injected contralateral eye [26;27]. Although multiple injections of HA may be needed to obtain a sustained hypertension, we have shown that the injection procedure itself does not affect IOP and retinal function and histology. On the contrary, several advantages support our model:

1) a highly consistent hypertension is achieved,
2) it may have a reasonably long course,
3) daily variations in IOP persist in HA-injected eyes,
4) in contrast to other models, in all likelihood, HA does not impede the blood flow out of the eye, and
5) it is easy to perform. Furthermore, we have shown that this model may also be utilized for pharmacological studies since the HA-induced hypertension was significantly reduced by the topic and acute application of hypotensive drugs [26].

We have demonstrated that the chronic administration of HA significantly decreases the scotopic electroretinographic activity and provokes a significant loss of RGCs and optic nerve fibers [27]. Based on both functional and histological evidence, these results indicate that the intracameral injections of HA in the rat eye anterior chamber appear to mimic some key features of primary open-angle glaucoma (POAG), and therefore it may be a useful tool to understand this ocular disease and to develop new therapeutic strategies. In particular, using this model, recent results indicate that melatonin could be a new therapy for glaucoma treatment.

Oxidative Damage in Glaucoma and Melatonin as a Retinal Antioxidant

There is a considerable variety of free radicals in the organism that are produced as byproducts of molecular oxygen and that are able to exert extensive damage, particularly over time. Free radicals may destroy virtually any molecule they encounter. Oxidative damage may be considered as the cytopathic consequence of the generation of excess reactive oxygen species [ROS] beyond the cell's defensive capacity [28]. The retina is especially susceptible to oxidative stress because of its high oxygen consumption, its high proportion of polyunsaturated fatty acids, and its exposure to light. Among others, glutathione, and antioxidant enzymes such as superoxide dismutase [SOD], catalase, and glutathione peroxidase [GPX] provide a powerful antioxidant defense in the retina [29-31]. However, despite having high levels of antioxidants, the retina is still susceptible to oxidative stress which has been observed in several retinal conditions [32-35].

As for a link between oxidative damage and glaucoma, it has been reported that the level of lipid peroxidation products increases more than two fold and that the ocular antioxidant defense mechanism decreases in the anterior chamber humor of patients with advanced glaucoma [36].

Glaucoma is an optic neuropathy in which RGCs die individually or in small groups, typically over many years, and probably through an apoptotic process. The control of apoptosis is known to involve free radicals in several systems, including the retina [37;38]. In fact, antioxidant agents suppress retinal apoptosis induced by various insults, such as axotomy or photic injury [33;39]. Mounting evidence points to the involvement of these molecules in a broad range of neuropathologic disorders, probably by increasing the peroxidation of fatty acids or nucleic acids and protein cross-linking. SOD catalyzes the conversion of superoxide radicals (O_2) to hydrogen peroxide (H_2O_2), which is the first step in the metabolic defense against cellular oxidative stress. Although H_2O_2 is not a free radical, it is highly reactive, membrane permeable, and can be converted to highly reactive metabolites of oxygen such as hydroxyl radical. Under normal conditions, most of the H_2O_2 molecules generated by SOD are further metabolized to water by catalase and GPX. Thus, it is critical for the cellular survival that SOD activity should be coupled with similar GPX and catalase activities to safely detoxify H_2O_2. We have demonstrated that SOD and catalase [but not GPX] activities decrease in eyes with ocular hypertension induced by HA [40]. Although in normal physiological conditions, GPX seems to be more efficient compared to catalase in reducing organic peroxides [41;42], Spector et al. [43] reported that under conditions of knocked out or inhibited GPX, catalase is able to provide protection against oxidative stress. Furthermore, during acute oxidative stress, catalase induction has been shown to be many folds higher than the increase of GPX activity [44]. It was demonstrated that especially in structures like the eye, catalase has a significant contribution to H_2O_2 detoxification. The inhibition of catalase activity in the eyes of rabbits increases H_2O_2 concentration 2.5-fold, which is not compensated by GPX activity [31]. Although the mechanism[s] involved in the changes of these retinal enzymatic activities from hypertensive eyes is not yet understood, it is highly probable that a decrease of SOD and catalase activities could provoke an imbalance of the endogenous antioxidant defense system. This hypothesis is strongly supported by a significant increase in retinal lipid peroxidation observed in the retinas from hypertensive eyes [40].

The possibility that melatonin could detoxify highly reactive oxygen species was originally suggested by Ianas et al. [45]. Three years later, Reiter and coworkers [46] using spin trapping and electron resonance spectroscopy, demonstrated that melatonin has capacity to directly scavenge highly reactive hydroxyl radicals. Since then, several reports have shown that melatonin acts as a free radical scavenger and an efficient antioxidant [47-52]. Not only melatonin, but also several of its metabolites generated during its free radical scavenging action may act as antioxidants [53]. The kynurenic pathway of melatonin metabolism includes a series of radical scavengers with the possible sequence: Melatonin → cyclic 3-hydroxymelatonin → N^1-acetyl-N^2-formyl-5-methoxykynuramine (AFMK) → N^1-acetyl-5-methoxykynuramine (AMK). In the metabolic step from melatonin to AFMK, up to four free radicals can be consumed [53-56]. Because of this pathway, melatonin's efficacy as an antioxidant is greatly increased. Melatonin has been shown to scavenge free radicals generated in mitochondria, reduce electron leakage from the respiratory complexes and improve ATP synthesis [57;58]. Moreover, melatonin preserves mitochondrial glutathione levels, thereby enhancing the antioxidant potential [59]. By scavenging free radicals, increasing the antioxidant defense system activity, and improving the electron transport chain at the mitochondrial level, melatonin is able to protect ocular tissues from oxidative damage [60;61].

It was demonstrated that the low affinity MT3 melatonin receptor binding site is identical with quinone reductase 2 (QR2) [62], and that melatonin inhibits the activity of this enzyme [63;64] and there is evidence that, contrary to previous belief [65], QR2 is an activating enzyme [66;67] since its deletion from living organisms leads to increased toxicity of quinones [67]. Thus, inhibition of QR2 could have antioxidant effects. Moreover, it was recently demonstrated that melatonin significantly increases SOD activity and GSH levels whereas it decreases retinal lipid peroxidation in the rat retina [68]. In the experimental model of glaucoma induced by injections of HA, we have demonstrated a significant decrease in retinal melatonin levels [40]. Taking into account the conclusive evidence on the role of melatonin as antioxidant, together with the fall in retinal melatonin levels and with the decrease in the antioxidant defense system activity in hypertensive eyes, it is tempting to speculate about a causal relationship between these latter phenomena.

Whether retinal oxidative damage is involved in glaucomatous RGC death is far from being understood. Compared with other retinal cells, neonatal ganglion cells are remarkably resistant to cell death induced by superoxide anion, hydrogen peroxide, or hydroxyl radical, and it was postulated that this resistance may be mediated by the possession of sufficient constitutive levels of one or more peroxidases, probably catalase and/or GPX [69]. Thus, it seems possible that a decrease of some of these enzymatic activities may overcome the capacity of these cells to resist oxidative damage. In summary, these results support the involvement of oxidative stress in glaucomatous damage. Thus, manipulation of intracellular redox status using antioxidants such as melatonin may be a new therapeutic tool to prevent glaucomatous cell death.

Nitrosative stress in Glaucoma and Anti-Nitridergic Effects of Melatonin

NO is a ubiquitous signaling molecule that participates in a variety of cellular functions. However, in concert with reactive oxygen species, NO can be transformed into a highly potent and effective cytotoxic entity of pathophysiological significance. NO may also signal through the interaction with reduced cysteines of proteins changing protein function [70]. As an intracellular signaling molecule, NO modulates the activity of various proteins that contribute to apoptosis [71]. Furthermore, it was demonstrated that an extracellular proteolytic pathway in the retina contributes to RGC death *via* NO-activated metalloproteinase-9 [72]. Several lines of evidence support a link between NO and glaucoma.

In that sense, an increased presence of neuronal NOS [NOS-1 or nNOS] and inducible NOS (NOS-2 or iNOS), was reported in astrocytes of the lamina cribrosa and ONH of patients with POAG [73;74]. In rats whose extraocular veins were cauterized to produce chronic ocular hypertension and retinal damage, expression of NOS-2 but not NOS-1 increases in ONH astrocytes [75;76]. Moreover, elevation of hydrostatic pressure *in vitro* upregulates the expression of NOS-2 in human astrocytes derived from the ONH [77]. Most important, inhibition of NOS-2 by aminoguanidine or L-N[6]-[1-iminoethyl]lysine 5-tetrazole amide protects against RGC loss in the rat cautery model of glaucoma [78;79]. These data support that activation of NOS, especially NOS-2, may play a significant role in glaucomatous optic neuropathy. However, later on, Pang et al. [80] showed that chronically elevated IOP in the rat induced by episcleral injection of hypertonic saline does not increase NOS-2 immunoreactivity in the optic nerve, ONH, or ganglion cell layer. Moreover, retinal and ONH NOS-2 mRNA levels did not correlate with either IOP level or severity of optic nerve injury. In addition, there was no difference in NOS-2 immunoreactivity in the optic nerve or ONH between POAG and nonglaucomatous eyes [80], and aminoguanidine treatment did not affect the development of pressure-induced optic neuropathy in rats [80]. A significant activation of the retinal nitridergic pathway was described in the experimental model of glaucoma induced by intracameral injections of HA [21]. Despite that other studies [mostly based on Western blotting or immunohistochemical analysis] previously addressed the issue of NO involvement in human or experimental glaucoma, they did not assessed changes in the functional capacity of the retinal nitridergic pathway. Although no changes in the levels of NOS isoforms were observed in HA-treated eyes, a significant increase of the retinal arginine to citrulline conversion was demonstrated in HA-injected eyes [21]. The intracellular events triggered by ocular hypertension that could explain the increase in retinal NOS activity, remain to be established. However, since glutamate acting through NMDA receptors is one of the most conspicuous activators of NOS-1 activity, the raise in glutamate synaptic levels in HA-treated eyes [as discussed below] could account for it. In this sense, it was shown that RGCs in the nNOS-deficient mouse were relatively resistant to NMDA, while damage in the retina of the endothelial NOS-deficient mouse was not distinguishable from that observed in control animals [81]. Moreover, it was demonstrated that intravitreal injection of NMDA in rats induces accumulation of nitrite/nitrate [82].

A significant increase in the retinal uptake of L-arginine (a NOS substrate) was demonstrated in HA-treated eyes. Purified NOS from different sources has been reported to have a low half-saturating L-arginine concentration (EC_{50}) ~ 10 μM. Since high levels of intracellular L-arginine ranging from 0.1 - 1 mM have been measured in many systems [83], it is expected that endogenous L-arginine would support maximal activation of NOS. However, a number of *in vivo* and *in vitro* studies indicate that NO production under physiological conditions can be increased by extracellular L-arginine, despite saturating intracellular L-arginine concentrations. This has been termed "the arginine paradox" [84]. One possible explanation could be that intracellular L-arginine is sequestered in one or more pools that are poorly, if at all, accessible to NOS, whereas extracellular L-arginine transported into the cells is preferentially delivered to NO biosynthesis [84]. Accordingly, it was demonstrated that L-arginine availability controls NMDA-induced NO synthesis in the rat central nervous system [85]. Therefore, it seems likely that to induce the activation of NOS, an obligatory influx of L-arginine is required. The coordination between NOS activity and L-arginine uptake has been demonstrated in several systems such as rat brain [86], and diabetic rat retina [87]. A similar coordination between NO biosynthesis and intracellular L-arginine availability seems to occur in hypertensive eyes. It was demonstrated that activation of NMDA receptors in cultured retinal cells promotes an increase of the intracellular L-arginine pool available for NO synthesis [88]. This way, the increase in both NOS activity and L-arginine influx, could be triggered by higher levels of synaptic glutamate levels.

Four amino acid transport systems (denoted by y^+, $b^{o,+}$, $B^{o,+}$ or y^+L) have been defined on the basis of substrate specificity and sodium dependence [89]. Only one of them (y^+) is selective for cationic amino acids and sodium-independent. It was demonstrated that the uptake of L-arginine in retinas from rats and hamsters occurs through a transporter resembling the y^+ system [90;91]. This transport system encompasses three homologous proteins [named cationic amino acid transporter (CAT)-1, CAT-2, and CAT-3) that have been characterized in several tissues. RT-PCR analysis using primers for the aforementioned isoforms demonstrated an increase of mRNAs for both CAT-1 and CAT-2 in retinas from hypertensive eyes, suggesting that ocular hypertension could induce an upregulation of L-arginine transporters [21;90].

It was demonstrated that melatonin inhibits the nitridergic pathway activity in the golden hamster [92] and rat retina [68]. Melatonin significantly decreases retinal NOS activity and L-arginine uptake, and inhibits the accumulation of cGMP induced by both L-arginine and a NO donor. The inhibitory effect of melatonin on retinal NOS activity is consistent with the previously described effect of melatonin on this enzyme from other neural structures [93-95]. However, while the effect of melatonin in those tissues was evident up to 1 nM, a much higher sensitivity to the methoxyindole was evident in the hamster retina, since it is effective even at 1 pM, suggesting that the retinal nitridergic pathway is regulated by physiological concentrations of melatonin [92]. In addition to inhibiting NOS activity, melatonin is able to directly scavenge NO, generating at least one stable product, i.e., N-nitrosomelatonin [96]. Moreover, melatonin reduces NO-induced lipid peroxidation in rat retinal homogenates and ileum tissue sections [97;98]. Taken together, these results indicate that melatonin modulates the nitridergic pathway in an opposite way to that induced by ocular hypertension.

Excitotoxic Damage in Glaucoma and the Effect of Melatonin on Glutamate Clearance

Glutamate is the main excitatory neurotransmitter in the retina, but it is toxic when present in excessive amounts. Retinal tissue is in fact, an established paradigm for glutamate neurotoxicity for several reasons:

(i) insult leads to accumulation of relatively high levels of glutamate in the extracellular fluid [99],
(ii) administration of glutamate leads to neuronal cell death [100]; and
(iii) glutamate receptor antagonists can protect against neuronal degeneration [101].

Thus, an appropriate clearance of synaptic glutamate is required for the normal function of retinal excitatory synapses and for prevention of neurotoxicity. Glial cells, mainly astrocytes and Müller glia, surround glutamatergic synapses, and express glutamate transporters and the glutamate-metabolizing enzyme, glutamine synthetase (GS) [102;103].

Glutamate is transported into glial cells and amidated by GS to the non-toxic aminoacid glutamine. Glutamine is then released by the glial cells and taken up by neurons, where it is hydrolyzed by glutaminase to form glutamate again, completing the retinal glutamate/glutamine cycle [103;104]. In this way, the neurotransmitter pool is replenished and glutamate neurotoxicity is prevented. Glutamatergic injury has been proposed to contribute to the RGC death in glaucoma. This hypothesis is supported by the demonstration that vitreal glutamate is elevated in glaucomatous dogs [105], and quail with congenital glaucoma [105;106]. In addition, high glutamine levels were been found in retinal Müller cells of glaucomatous rat eyes [105;107]. In contrast, other authors showed no significant elevation of glutamate in the vitreous of patients with glaucoma [108], or in rats [109], and monkeys with experimental glaucoma [110;111]. In any case, it seems limited a viewpoint to assume that high levels of glutamate in the vitreous are a necessary condition for excitotoxicity to be involved in glaucomatous neuropathy. The local concentration of glutamate at the membrane receptors of RGCs is the important issue for toxicity. This could be very different from the level in samples of vitreous. Vitreous humor must be removed for experimental measurement by a process that inevitably disturbs its state before removal. These manipulations could themselves alter the measured amount of glutamate. At present, there are no available tools to directly assess retinal glutamate synaptic concentrations *in vivo*. However, glutamate synaptic concentrations could be estimated by studying the retinal mechanisms that regulate glutamate clearance and recycling.

We have demonstrated a significant alteration of the retinal glutamate/glutamine cycle activity in rats exposed to experimentally elevated IOP [17]. Since no enzymes exist extracellularly that degrade glutamate, glutamate transporters are responsible for maintaining low synaptic glutamate concentrations. Retinal glutamate uptake significantly decreases in HA-treated eyes. In agreement, a significant reduction in the amount of the main retinal glutamate transporter [excitatory amino acid transporter type 1, [EAAT-1]] assessed by Western blot analysis in a rat glaucoma model [112], and a downregulation of this transporter in retinal Müller cells from glaucoma patients [113] were demonstrated. While these studies did not assess changes in the functional capacity of glutamate transporters, our results demonstrated a removing glutamate disability in retinas from hypertensive eyes. The synaptically released glutamate is taken up into glial cells, where GS converts it into glutamine. Since Müller cells rapidly convert glutamate to glutamine, the driving force for glutamate uptake would be stronger in these cells than in neurons, which have much higher intracellular free glutamate concentrations [114]. In fact, although glutamate uptake is controlled by the expression and post-translational modifications, physiological measurements suggest that glutamate uptake may also depend on its metabolism [115-117]. Indeed, an increase in internal glutamate concentrations significantly slows down the net transport of glutamate, and it was suggested that instantaneous intracellular glutamate metabolism may be needed for efficient glutamate clearance of the extracellular milieu [118;119]. Thus, a decrease in GS activity could account for a decrease in glutamate uptake. Glutamine is released from Müller cells and could be a precursor for neuronal glutamate synthesis. The increase in the basal release and the uptake of glutamine in HA-treated eyes could provoke a raise in the availability of substratum for glutamate synthesis. Moreover, this increase in glutamate production could be further potentiated by the augment of GS. Decreasing the levels of expression of the EAAT1 increases vitreal glutamate, and is toxic to RGCs [120]. Thus, the decrease in glutamate influx could provoke an increase in synaptic glutamate levels. In addition, a decrease of GS activity, as well as in increase in glutaminase activity in retinas form hypertensive eyes could contribute synergically and/or redundantly to an excessive increase in synaptic glutamate levels [18].

Nanomolar concentrations of melatonin significantly modulate the glutamate/glutamine cycle activity in the golden hamster [121] and rat retina [68]. In that sense, it was demonstrated that low concentrations of melatonin significantly increase retinal glutamate uptake and GS activity, and decrease glutaminase activity. This way, melatonin may contribute to the conversion of glutamate to glutamine through a possibly redundant mechanism. The physiological consequences of a modulation by melatonin of the retinal glutamate/glutamine cycle are yet to be determined, although this effect could provide new insights into the neuroprotective potential of melatonin. In that respect, it was demonstrated that an increase in GS provides neuroprotection in experimental models of neurodegeneration [122;123]. Induction of GS *in vivo* or *in vitro* by glucocorticoids was clearly demonstrated in different tissues, including the retina [124;125]. Physiological levels of glucocorticoids regulate GS expression by stimulating the gene transcription. This effect of glucocorticoids has been associated to their ability to protect against neuronal degeneration [122], as shown in animal models of brain injury [126], as well as after retinal photic injury [127]. However, since induction of GS expression by glucocorticoids takes about 24 h, there are some potential weaknesses in glucocorticoid treatment. In contrast, since the effect of melatonin is much faster [in the range of minutes] a treatment with the methoxyindole may circumvent this obstacle. Furthermore, this beneficial effect of melatonin may be further improved by its effect on glutamate uptake, and glutaminase activity. In summary, these findings suggest that a treatment with melatonin could be considered as a new approach to handling glutamate-mediated neuronal degeneration, such as that induced by glaucoma.

GABAergic Dysfunction in Glaucoma and the Effect of Melatonin on the Retinal Gabaergic System

The neurochemical organization maintained throughout vertebrate retinas is that glutamate is the neurotransmitter in the photoreceptor cell→ bipolar cell→ ganglion cell chain, whereas GABA is used by numerous horizontal and amacrine cells in the lateral pathway, modulating neural transmission in both synaptic layers [128;129]. Retinal output neurons communicate by liberating glutamate, while tonically or phasically active inhibitory neurons (mostly GABAergic) modulate the passage of information, offering resistance against which the firing tendencies, which results in variable levels of neural activity. The prevailing view is that the balance between excitatory and inhibitory signaling plays a pivotal role in mechanisms underlying the modulation and maintenance of a variety of retinal functions and sensory information encoding. In fact, the loss of this balance could provoke cell death. Despite the putative involvement of glutamate in glaucomatous cell death previously discussed, and the key role of GABA in retinal function, the GABAergic activity was not extensively examined in experimental models of glaucoma. Recently, a significant dysfunction of the retinal GABAergic system was demonstrated in rats exposed to experimentally elevated IOP [18]. These results indicate that retinal GABA steady state concentrations, GABA turnover rate, glutamic acid decarboxylase (GAD) activity, GABA transporters (GATs), and GABA receptors are susceptible to ocular hypertension.

Retinal GABA release involves two distinct components; one requires extracellular calcium, while the other is calcium-independent and involves reversal of the operating direction of a high affinity GABA carrier [130]. Although differences in retinal GABA release were observed among species, glutamate induces GABA release mostly *via* a Ca^{2+}-independent Na^{+}-dependent carrier mechanism, while high K^{+}-induced GABA release is partially calcium-dependent [131-133]. Retinal GABA release induced by both stimuli significantly decreases in the retina from HA-injected eyes, supporting that ocular hypertension affects the carrier-mediated component. As significant changes in GABA influx are also observed in HA-treated eyes [18], ocular hypertension may influence the preferred direction of GABA transporters provoking a switch from release to uptake. Indeed, since GAD activity significantly decreases in HA-treated eyes, the driving force for GABA uptake would be stronger in cells with lower intracellular GABA concentrations, favoring its uptake over its release.

GATs in cells surrounding the release site are responsible for terminating GABA signals within the retina [134]. GATs were mainly localized in amacrine, displaced amacrine, RGCs, and Müller cells [135;136]. GABA uptake is significantly higher in retinas from eyes injected with HA, which could contribute synergically and/or redundantly to a significant decrease of synaptic GABA levels in retinas exposed to ocular hypertension.

To our knowledge, there is no other retinal pathological condition in which a GABAergic deficit has been previously described. However, a decrease in GABAergic neurotransmission has been implicated in the pathophysiology of several central nervous system disorders, particularly in epilepsy. In this case, excessive glutamate-mediated neurotransmission and impaired GABA-mediated inhibition, among other mechanisms, may trigger a cascade of events leading to neuronal damage and cell death. Excitotoxicity is a common pathogenetic mechanism in neurodegenerative diseases, including probably glaucoma, which may result from the failure of normal compensatory antiexcitatory mechanisms, necessary to maintain cellular homeostasis. An abnormal glutamate outflow may play a crucial role in triggering cellular events leading to excitotoxic neuronal death. Reduced synaptic inhibition as a result of a GABAergic dysfunction could be one of the major causes for this imbalance. In this way, ocular hypertension may greatly shift the balance between retinal excitation and inhibition. As mentioned before, we have demonstrated an increase in glutamate synaptic concentrations in retinas from eyes injected with HA [18]. Since an increase in synaptic glutamate or its residence time in the synaptic region is toxic to RGCs [137;138], the decrease in GABAergic activity could make worse glutamate toxicity. In this way, the deficit in GABAergic activity could contribute to glaucomatous neuropathy.

It was demonstrated that melatonin increases retinal GABA levels, as shown by its effect on GABA turnover rate and GAD activity [68]. The effect of melatonin on the GABAergic activity seems not to be exclusive for the retina, since it was previously demonstrated that melatonin increases GABA turnover rate and GAD activity in rat hypothalamus, cerebellum, and cerebral cortex [139;140]. These results indicate that glaucomatous damage may involve a decrease in GABA synaptic levels, which can be restored by a treatment with melatonin.

Effect of Melatonin on Glaucomatous Damage

As already discussed in this chapter, previous results indicate that melatonin is able to impair retinal glutamate neurotoxicity, decrease NO levels, increase GABA concentrations, and reduce oxidative stress, and that an increase in glutamate and NO levels, a decrease in the GABAergic activity, and oxidative damage could be involved in glaucomatous neuropathy. Thus, it seems likely that melatonin could have a beneficial effect against glaucoma. This hypothesis was recently analyzed in the glaucoma model induced by HA injections [68]. For this purpose, a pellet of melatonin was implanted subcutaneously 24 h before the first injection of HA. Melatonin, which did not affect IOP, prevented the effect of ocular hypertension on retinal function (assessed by electroretinography), and diminished the vulnerability of RGCs to the deleterious effects of ocular hypertension [68]. Although melatonin conferred neuroprotection in the experimental model of glaucoma induced by HA, the translational relevance of this result is limited by the fact that melatonin was administered before the induction of ocular hypertension (e.g. 24 h before the first injection of HA).

Human open angle glaucoma is a progressive optic neuropathy. In agreement, different stages were identified in the experimental model of glaucoma induced by HA, showing the following characteristics:

(i) 3 weeks of ocular hypertension: increase in glutamate and NO levels, decrease in GABA levels, and incipient oxidative stress, without changes in the ERG and retinal morphology (e.g. *asymptomatic ocular hypertension*);
(ii) 6 weeks of ocular hypertension: increase in NO levels, higher oxidative stress, and decrease in the ERG without histological changes (e.g. *moderated glaucoma*); and
(iii) 10 weeks of ocular hypertension: higher oxidative stress, further decrease in the ERG (vs. 6 weeks), and loss of RGCs and optic nerve fibers (e.g. *advanced glaucoma*) [27].

To analyze the therapeutic effect, a pellet of melatonin was implanted at 6 weeks of ocular hypertension, a time point in which functional alterations are already evident, and the results indicate that the delayed treatment with melatonin of eyes with ocular hypertension resulted in similar protection when compared with eyes treated from the onset of ocular hypertension. We do not have any clear explanation for these results. We have shown that an increase in synaptic glutamate concentrations [17] and NO production, as well as a GABAergic dysfunction [17] occur mostly prior to 6 weeks of ocular hypertension induced by HA. Based on these results, it seems possible that alterations in glutamate, NO, and GABA may trigger an initial insult responsible for initiation of damage that is followed by a slower secondary degeneration that ultimately results in cell death. In that sense, we showed that oxidative stress is a longer lasting phenomenon which can be observed even at 10 weeks of ocular hypertension [40]. In this scenario, the preventive effect of melatonin (shown by the administration of melatonin before the first injection of HA) could be explained by the decrease in glutamate and NO levels and an increase in GABA concentrations, while its therapeutic effect (shown by the administration of melatonin at 6 weeks of ocular hypertension) can be explained essentially by its antioxidant effect. In this context, the fact that melatonin was similarly effective in the chronically treated animals and the delayed treatment, could support the hypothesis that in both cases melatonin is able to reverse oxidative damage which could be a key factor in glaucomatous dysfunction and cell death.

Neuroprotection in glaucoma implies the use of drugs or chemicals to slow down whatever causes loss of vision (RGC death), without influencing IOP. In order to be effective, a neuroprotectant must reach the ONH and/or RGCs and will therefore probably have to be taken orally [141]. Because it will reach other parts of the body, any side-effect of an appropriate neuroprotectant must be reduced to a minimum. Melatonin, a very safe compound for human use, is highly lipophilic and readily diffuses into tissues. In fact, subcutaneously administered, melatonin reaches the retina [142], increasing the local levels of the methoxyindole. RGCs are induced to die by different triggers in glaucoma, suggesting that neuroprotectants with multiple modes of actions are likely be effective in the therapeutic management of glaucoma [143].

Besides the mechanisms already described, there are other beneficial mechanisms of melatonin which can support its usefulness for glaucoma treatment. Several lines of evidence support that the obstruction of retrograde transport at the ONH results in the deprivation of neurotrophic support to RGCs, leading to apoptotic cell death in glaucoma [144]. An important corollary to this concept is the implication that appropriate enhancement of neurotrophic support will prolong the survival of injured RGCs. Of particular importance is the fact that brain-derived neurotrophic factor (BDNF) not only promotes RGC survival following damage to the ON, but also helps to preserve the structural integrity of the surviving neurons, which in turn results in enhanced visual function [145]. As for the link between melatonin and neurotrophins, it has been suggested that melatonin may participate in neurodevelopment and in the regulation of neurotrophic factors [146;147]. *In vitro*, melatonin promotes the viability and neuronal differentiation of neural stem cells and increases their production of BDNF [148]. Moreover, ramelteon [a melatonin receptor agonist] is capable of increasing BDNF protein in primary cultures of cerebellar granule cells [149].

In addition to ocular hypertension, the majority of glaucoma patients show signs of reduced ocular blood flow as well as ischemic signs in the eye, supporting that hemodynamic factors are involved as well in glaucomatous neuropathy. Several animal and human studies have indicated that vascular dysregulation and ischemia play a role in glaucoma pathogenesis [150-153]. Retinal ischemia develops when retinal blood flow is insufficient to match the metabolic needs of the retina, one of the highest oxygen-consuming tissues. Ischemia impairs retinal energy metabolism, and triggers a reaction cascade which can result in cell death. Oxidative stress, excitotoxicity, calcium influx, and others mechanisms acting in tandem are of considerable importance in retinal ischemic damage [154]. Notably, most of these mechanisms are also involved in glaucomatous neuropathy [40]. In this sense, it was shown that melatonin could increase the survival rate and rescue and restore injured RGCs in an experimental model of ischemia/reperfusion in rats [144], and it counteracts ischemia induced apoptosis in human retinal pigment epithelial cells [154]. Finally, while the cellular mechanisms involved in RGC loss observed in glaucomatous neuropathy are based on apoptosis phenomenon, melatonin was shown to have antiapoptotic properties acting through several mechanisms, such as reduction of caspases, cytochrome c release, and modulation of Bcl-2 and Bax genes, among others. Taking together, these data indicate that melatonin seems to fulfill all the requirements to be considered a promissory neuroprotectant for glaucoma treatment. Alone or combined with an ocular hypotensive therapy, a treatment with melatonin, a very safe compound for human use, could be a new therapeutic tool helping the challenge faced by ophthalmologists treating glaucoma.

Glaucoma, Circadian Rhythms, and Melatonin

Circadian rhythms are controlled by a biological clock that in humans is located in the suprachiasmatic nuclei [SCN] and have a period of approximately 24 hours [155]. Because SCN neurons contain an internal pacemaker which generates an endogenous rhythmic electrical activity [156] changes supervised by the SCN occur even in the absence of external stimuli. Nevertheless, the SCN are influenced by environmental changes, especially by the light-dark cycle [157]. The inherited period of the human circadian clock is not precisely 24 hours, however, the light-dark and other cyclic environmental and behavioral clues modify the period to precisely 24 hours, thereby supporting the circadian daytime activity-nocturnal sleep routine, among many other biological rhythms [158;159].

Although the eye has been largely recognized as the organ of sight (in man and animals), over the past decade, a second role for the eye has been uncovered: even in the absence of "cognitive" vision, the eye can serve as a sensor for ambient lighting, akin to the light meter in a camera [160]. A host of light-regulated functions, including entrainment of circadian clocks, suppression of activity by light, photic suppression of pineal melatonin synthesis, and pupillary light responses are retained in animals that are blind as a result of mutations causing complete or near-complete degeneration of the classical photoreceptors, the rods and cones [161-163]. These light-regulated functions are controlled by non classical retinal photoreceptors because animals lacking RGCs lose circadian photoresponses, behavioral masking, and pupillary light responses [164]. The discovery of intrinsically photosensitive RGCs has given non-visual phototransduction an anatomical basis [165-167]. A subtype of RGCs [mRGCs] containing a novel photopigment, melanopsin, responds to light independently of the input from rods and cones, and project their axons through the retinohypothalamic tract to the SCN. A strong body of evidence supports that mRGCs are involved in modulating circadian rhythms [168-170]. In addition, mRGCs send monosynaptic projections to the olivary pretectal nucleus, responsible for the pupil light reflex [PLR] [171]. In that sense, although it was originally assumed that the light-evoked neural signals driving the PLR originated exclusively from rods and cones, it was later shown that mRGCs significantly contribute to the pupil constriction [172-174].

Most studies on glaucoma have focused on RGCs involved in conscious visual functions, and have found that a chronic increase in IOP causes a progressive loss of these cells. However, clinical studies in glaucomatous patients show a high prevalence of sleep-disordered breathing, characterized by snoring, excessive daytime sleepiness, and insomnia accompanied by large swings in blood pressure and repetitive hypoxic periods during sleep [175]. Moreover, an abnormal light-induced nocturnal melatonin suppression in glaucoma patients was described [176], and afferent pupillary defects during the early stages of the disease were reported [177;178]. In addition, it was recently shown that the post-illumination pupil response is dysfunctional in patients with early, moderate, or severe glaucoma [179].

The involvement of mRGCs in glaucoma has been postulated, and two studies in animal models of glaucoma demonstrate a loss of mRGCs [180;181]. These clues imply that mRGCs as other RGCs can be damaged in glaucomatous patients. However, other studies have shown that mRGCs may be spared in some animal models of chronic ocular hypertension [182;183]. In an experimental model of glaucoma in rats induced by chronic injections of chondroitin sulfate [CS] in the eye anterior chamber [184], we have recently demonstrated that a similar decrease in the number of RGCs projecting to the superior colliculus [which are involved in the image-forming visual system] and in the number of mRGCs [which participate in the non-image forming visual system] occurs in glaucomatous eyes. In addition, we have demonstrated that experimental glaucoma induces a significant decrease in the afferent pupil light reflex, and alterations in the light-induced nocturnal melatonin suppression [185]. These results indicate that experimental glaucoma can affect the non-image forming visual system.

Notwithstanding, further studies are warranted to clarify the involvement of mRGCs in the natural history of human glaucoma, and to investigate the occurrence of circadian rhythm abnormalities in patients with advanced glaucoma. In this regard, we have recently analyzed the circadian rhythm in locomotor activity and the sleep/wake cycle, estimated by wrist actigraphy, in patients with advanced stages of glaucoma [184]. The results of this pilot study indicate significant changes in the sleep pattern of advanced glaucoma patients, which showed more awakenings at night, and a decrease in the amount of sleep duration and sleep efficiency, as compared with control subjects. Although no significant changes were found for circadian parameters such as period, amplitude or acrophase of locomotor activity, the general pattern of actimetry, from which sleep parameters were estimated, indicated alterations in its robustness, suggesting a disrupted sleep-wake cycle. In particular, clear differences between control and glaucoma patients were observed in the sleep, but not in the wakefulness state, which supports that circadian misalignment in glaucomatous patients could be attributed to sleep disturbances.

Although several groups have examined the involvement of mRGCs or melanopsin in experimental glaucoma in rodents [180-182], to date, few studies investigated the mRGCs-system directly in human glaucoma [176;186]. In that sense, a disturbance of the autonomic nervous system circadian rhythm was shown in patients with glaucoma [187]. It was demonstrated that the light-induced suppression of melatonin secretion is substantially unaffected in other neurodegenerative optic neuropathies such as Leber hereditary optic neuropathy and dominant optic atrophy [188], in which the pupil light reflex is also preserved [189;190]. Thus, it is tempting to speculate that mRGCs are particularly susceptible to glaucomatous damage, and that glaucoma is a key model that needs to be further investigated in regards to circadian photoreception in optic neuropathies. These results suggest that the effects of glaucoma on the circadian timing system might be twofold:

1) a direct impact through degeneration of RGCs and eventually, also of mRGCs;
2) an indirect impact through social isolation due to blindness, as is the case for other ophthalmic diseases [164].

Although these findings should be replicated in large-scale studies before definitive conclusions can be reached, these results are consistent with sleep alterations in advanced glaucoma, suggesting that attention should be paid to non-image-forming visual functions, such as control of circadian rhythms and its clinical impact in patients with glaucoma, even when most of them retains some residual visual function.

Besides the already discussed beneficial effects of melatonin on retinal glaucomatous damage, a treatment with melatonin could also be usefull to treat sleep alterations in patients with glaucoma. Treatment of circadian rhythm disorders, whether precipitated by intrinsic factors (e.g., sleep disorders, blindness, mental disorders, aging) or by extrinsic factors (e.g., shift work, jet-lag) has led to the development of a new type of agents called “chronobiotics”. The term “chronobiotic” defines a substance displaying the therapeutic activity of shifting the phase or increasing the amplitude of the circadian rhythms. The prototype of this therapeutic group is melatonin, whose administration synchronizes the sleep-wake cycle in blind people and in individuals suffering from circadian rhythm sleep disorders, like delayed sleep phase syndrome, jet lag or shift-work [191]. Melatonin and melatoninergic drugs have hypnotic effects mediated through specific receptors, especially those in the SCN, which acts on the hypothalamic sleep switch. They favor sleep initiation and reset the circadian clock allowing persistent sleep, a requirement in circadian rhythm sleep alterations. The action of melatonin on sleep is mainly of a chronobiological nature; melatonin acts in a dual way, resetting the circadian clock, and suppressing neuronal firing [191-193]. In this regard, it was demonstrated that melatonin is effective in advancing sleep-wake rhythm and endogenous melatonin rhythm in delayed sleep phase disorder [194] and that melatonin administration significantly improves sleep and behavioral disorders in the elderly and facilitates discontinuation of therapy with conventional hypnotic drugs [195].

Conclusion

Glaucoma may affect the quality of life in several ways. These include the visual effects of the disease itself (decreased visual field), the psychological effects of diagnosis (specifically fear of blindness), the potential side effects of treatment (either medical or surgical), and financial effects (as the cost of visits and therapy). Recent results suggest another risk to the quality of life of patients with glaucoma, i.e. alterations of the circadian physiology. Circadian rhythm disorders may include poor concentration, sleep problems, impaired performance, and decrease in cognitive skills, poor psychomotor coordination, and headaches, among many others. Based on all the considerations discussed in this chapter, melatonin appears as a highly attractive resource for glaucoma treatment, because besides its properties as a retinal neuroprotectant, it could also contribute to restore circadian balance, and in this way, significantly help to improve the quality of life of patients with this ocular disease.

References

[1] Tosini G, Fukuhara C. Photic and circadian regulation of retinal melatonin in mammals. *J Neuroendocrinol* 2003 Apr;15(4):364-9.

[2] Cahill GM, Besharse JC. Circadian clock functions localized in xenopus retinal photoreceptors. *Neuron* 1993 Apr;10(4):573-7.

[3] Garbarino-Pico E, Carpentieri AR, Contin MA, Sarmiento MI, Brocco MA, Panzetta P, et al. Retinal ganglion cells are autonomous circadian oscillators synthesizing N-acetylserotonin during the day. *J Biol Chem* 2004 Dec 3;279(49):51172-81.

[4] Iuvone PM, Tosini G, Pozdeyev N, Haque R, Klein DC, Chaurasia SS. Circadian clocks, clock networks, arylalkylamine N-acetyltransferase, and melatonin in the retina. *Prog Retin Eye Res* 2005 Jul;24(4):433-56.

[5] Tosini G, Menaker M. Circadian rhythms in cultured mammalian retina. *Science* 1996 Apr 19;272(5260):419-21.

[6] Dubocovich ML. Melatonin is a potent modulator of dopamine release in the retina 1. *Nature* 1983 Dec 22;306(5945):782-4.

[7] Jaliffa CO, Lacoste FF, Llomovatte DW, Sarmiento MI, Rosenstein RE. Dopamine decreases melatonin content in golden hamster retina. *J Pharmacol Exp Ther* 2000 Apr;293(1):91-5.

[8] Besharse JC, Dunis DA. Methoxyindoles and photoreceptor metabolism: activation of rod shedding. *Science* 1983 Mar 18;219(4590):1341-3.

[9] Pierce ME, Besharse JC. Circadian regulation of retinomotor movements. I. Interaction of melatonin and dopamine in the control of cone length. *J Gen Physiol* 1985 Nov;86(5):671-89.

[10] Quigley HA, Broman AT. The number of people with glaucoma worldwide in 2010 and 2020. *Br J Ophthalmol* 2006 Mar;90(3):262-7.

[11] Almasieh M, Wilson AM, Morquette B, Cueva Vargas JL, Di PA. The molecular basis of retinal ganglion cell death in glaucoma. *Prog Retin Eye Res* 2012 Mar;31(2):152-81.

[12] Friedman DS, Wilson MR, Liebmann JM, Fechtner RD, Weinreb RN. An evidence-based assessment of risk factors for the progression of ocular hypertension and glaucoma. *Am J Ophthalmol* 2004 Sep;138(3 Suppl):S19-S31.

[13] Caprioli J. Neuroprotection of the optic nerve in glaucoma. *Acta Ophthalmol Scand* 1997 Aug;75(4):364-7.

[14] Georgopoulos G, Andreanos D, Liokis N, Papakonstantinou D, Vergados J, Theodossiadis G. Risk factors in ocular hypertension. *Eur J Ophthalmol* 1997 Oct;7(4):357-63.

[15] Harbin TS, Jr., Podos SM, Kolker AE, Becker B. Visual field progression in open-angle glaucoma patients presenting with monocular field loss. *Trans Sect Ophthalmol Am Acad Ophthalmol Otolaryngol* 1976 Mar;81(2):253-7.

[16] Leske MC. Glaucoma and mortality: a connection?. *Ophthalmology* 2003 Aug;110(8):1473-5.

[17] Moreno MC, Sande P, Marcos HA, de ZN, Keller Sarmiento MI, Rosenstein RE. Effect of glaucoma on the retinal glutamate/glutamine cycle activity. *FASEB J* 2005 Jul;19(9):1161-2.

[18] Moreno MC, de ZN, Sande P, Jaliffa CO, Fernandez DC, Keller Sarmiento MI, et al. Effect of ocular hypertension on retinal GABAergic activity. *Neurochem Int* 2008 Mar;52(4-5):675-82.

[19] Aslan M, Cort A, Yucel I. Oxidative and nitrative stress markers in glaucoma. *Free Radic Biol Med* 2008 Aug 15;45(4):367-76.

[20] Tezel G. Oxidative stress in glaucomatous neurodegeneration: mechanisms and consequences. *Prog Retin Eye Res* 2006 Sep;25(5):490-513.

[21] Belforte N, Moreno MC, Cymeryng C, Bordone M, Keller Sarmiento MI, Rosenstein RE. Effect of ocular hypertension on retinal nitridergic pathway activity. *Invest Ophthalmol Vis Sci* 2007 May;48(5):2127-33.

[22] Neufeld AH, Sawada A, Becker B. Inhibition of nitric-oxide synthase 2 by aminoguanidine provides neuroprotection of retinal ganglion cells in a rat model of chronic glaucoma. *Proc Natl Acad Sci U S A* 1999 Aug 17;96(17):9944-8.

[23] Morrison JC, Moore CG, Deppmeier LM, Gold BG, Meshul CK, Johnson EC. A rat model of chronic pressure-induced optic nerve damage. Exp Eye Res 1997 Jan;64(1):85-96.

[24] Shareef SR, Garcia-Valenzuela E, Salierno A, Walsh J, Sharma SC. Chronic ocular hypertension following episcleral venous occlusion in rats. *Exp Eye Res* 1995 Sep;61(3):379-82.

[25] Ueda J, Sawaguchi S, Hanyu T, Yaoeda K, Fukuchi T, Abe H, et al. Experimental glaucoma model in the rat induced by laser trabecular photocoagulation after an intracameral injection of India ink. *Jpn J Ophthalmol* 1998 Sep;42(5):337-44.

[26] Benozzi J, Nahum LP, Campanelli JL, Rosenstein RE. Effect of hyaluronic acid on intraocular pressure in rats. *Invest Ophthalmol Vis Sci* 2002 Jul;43(7):2196-200.

[27] Moreno MC, Marcos HJ, Oscar CJ, Sande PH, Campanelli J, Jaliffa CO, et al. A new experimental model of glaucoma in rats through intracameral injections of hyaluronic acid. *Exp Eye Res* 2005 Jul;81(1):71-80.

[28] Simonian NA, Coyle JT. Oxidative stress in neurodegenerative diseases. *Annu Rev Pharmacol Toxicol* 1996;36:83-106.

[29] Armstrong D, Santangelo G, Connole E. The distribution of peroxide regulating enzymes in the canine eye. *Curr Eye Res* 1981;1(4):225-42.

[30] Castorina C, Campisi A, Di GC, Sorrenti V, Russo A, Vanella A. Lipid peroxidation and antioxidant enzymatic systems in rat retina as a function of age. *Neurochem Res* 1992 Jun;17(6):599-604.

[31] Ohta Y, Yamasaki T, Niwa T, Niimi K, Majima Y, Ishiguro I. Role of catalase in retinal antioxidant defence system: its comparative study among rabbits, guinea pigs, and rats. *Ophthalmic Res* 1996;28(6):336-42.

[32] Rajesh M, Sulochana KN, Punitham R, Biswas J, Lakshmi S, Ramakrishnan S. Involvement of oxidative and nitrosative stress in promoting retinal vasculitis in patients with Eales' disease 4. *Clin Biochem* 2003 Jul;36(5):377-85.

[33] Tanito M, Nishiyama A, Tanaka T, Masutani H, Nakamura H, Yodoi J, et al. Change of redox status and modulation by thiol replenishment in retinal photooxidative damage. *Invest Ophthalmol Vis Sci* 2002 Jul;43(7):2392-400.

[34] van Reyk DM, Gillies MC, Davies MJ. The retina: oxidative stress and diabetes. *Redox Rep* 2003;8(4):187-92.

[35] Wu GS, Zhang J, Rao NA. Peroxynitrite and oxidative damage in experimental autoimmune uveitis. *Invest Ophthalmol Vis Sci* 1997 Jun;38(7):1333-9.

[36] Kurysheva NI, Vinetskaia MI, Erichev VP, Demchuk ML, Kuryshev SI. [Contribution of free-radical reactions of chamber humor to the development of primary open-angle glaucoma]. *Vestn Oftalmol* 1996 Sep;112(4):3-5.

[37] Giardino I, Fard AK, Hatchell DL, Brownlee M. Aminoguanidine inhibits reactive oxygen species formation, lipid peroxidation, and oxidant-induced apoptosis. *Diabetes* 1998 Jul;47(7):1114-20.

[38] Liversidge J, Dick A, Gordon S. Nitric oxide mediates apoptosis through formation of peroxynitrite and Fas/Fas-ligand interactions in experimental autoimmune uveitis. *Am J Pathol* 2002 Mar;160(3):905-16.

[39] Castagne V, Clarke PG. Neuroprotective effects of a new glutathione peroxidase mimetic on neurons of the chick embryo's retina. *J Neurosci Res* 2000 Feb 15;59(4):497-503.

[40] Moreno MC, Campanelli J, Sande P, Sanez DA, Keller Sarmiento MI, Rosenstein RE. Retinal oxidative stress induced by high intraocular pressure. *Free Radic Biol Med* 2004 Sep 15;37(6):803-12.

[41] Holmgren A. Thioredoxin and glutaredoxin systems. *J Biol Chem* 1989 Aug 25;264(24):13963-6.

[42] Sen CK. Redox signaling and the emerging therapeutic potential of thiol antioxidants. *Biochem Pharmacol* 1998 Jun 1;55(11):1747-58.

[43] Spector A, Yang Y, Ho YS, Magnenat JL, Wang RR, Ma W, et al. Variation in cellular glutathione peroxidase activity in lens epithelial cells, transgenics and knockouts does not significantly change the response to H2O2 stress. *Exp Eye Res* 1996 May;62(5):521-40.

[44] Verkerk A, Jongkind JF. Vascular cells under peroxide induced oxidative stress: a balance study on in vitro peroxide handling by vascular endothelial and smooth muscle cells. *Free Radic Res Commun* 1992;17(2):121-32.

[45] Ianas O, Olinescu R, Badescu I. Melatonin involvement in oxidative processes. *Endocrinologie* 1991;29(3-4):147-53.

[46] Reiter RJ, Tan DX, Poeggeler B, Menendez-Pelaez A, Chen LD, Saarela S. Melatonin as a free radical scavenger: implications for aging and age-related diseases. *Ann N Y Acad Sci* 1994 May 31;719:1-12.

[47] Hardeland R, Balzer I, Poeggeler B, Fuhrberg B, Uria H, Behrmann G, et al. On the primary functions of melatonin in evolution: mediation of photoperiodic signals in a unicell, photooxidation, and scavenging of free radicals. *J Pineal Res* 1995 Mar;18(2):104-11.

[48] Pandi-Perumal SR, Srinivasan V, Maestroni GJ, Cardinali DP, Poeggeler B, Hardeland R. Melatonin: Nature's most versatile biological signal?. *FEBS J* 2006 Jul;273(13):2813-38.

[49] Reiter RJ, Guerrero JM, Escames G, Pappolla MA, Acuna-Castroviejo D. Prophylactic actions of melatonin in oxidative neurotoxicity. *Ann N Y Acad Sci* 1997 Oct 15;825:70-8.

[50] Reiter RJ. Oxidative damage in the central nervous system: protection by melatonin. *Prog Neurobiol* 1998 Oct;56(3):359-84.

[51] Reiter RJ, Tan DX, Osuna C, Gitto E. Actions of melatonin in the reduction of oxidative stress. A review. *J Biomed Sci* 2000 Nov;7(6):444-58.

[52] Turjanski AG, Rosenstein RE, Estrin DA. Reactions of melatonin and related indoles with free radicals: a computational study. *J Med Chem* 1998 Sep 10;41(19):3684-9.

[53] Tan DX, Manchester LC, Terron MP, Flores LJ, Reiter RJ. One molecule, many derivatives: a never-ending interaction of melatonin with reactive oxygen and nitrogen species?. *J Pineal Res* 2007 Jan;42(1):28-42.

[54] Adler LJ, Gyulai FE, Diehl DJ, Mintun MA, Winter PM, Firestone LL. Regional brain activity changes associated with fentanyl analgesia elucidated by positron emission tomography. *Anesth Analg* 1997 Jan;84(1):120-6.

[55] Guenther AL, Schmidt SI, Laatsch H, Fotso S, Ness H, Ressmeyer AR, et al. Reactions of the melatonin metabolite AMK (N1-acetyl-5-methoxykynuramine) with reactive nitrogen species: formation of novel compounds, 3-acetamidomethyl-6-methoxycinnolinone and 3-nitro-AMK. *J Pineal Res* 2005 Oct;39(3):251-60.

[56] Hardeland R. Antioxidative protection by melatonin: multiplicity of mechanisms from radical detoxification to radical avoidance. *Endocrine* 2005 Jul;27(2):119-30.

[57] Acuna-Castroviejo D, Escames G, Leon J, Carazo A, Khaldy H. Mitochondrial regulation by melatonin and its metabolites. *Adv Exp Med Biol* 2003;527:549-57.

[58] Leon J, Acuna-Castroviejo D, Escames G, Tan DX, Reiter RJ. Melatonin mitigates mitochondrial malfunction. *J Pineal Res* 2005 Jan;38(1):1-9.

[59] Leon J, Acuna-Castroviejo D, Sainz RM, Mayo JC, Tan DX, Reiter RJ. Melatonin and mitochondrial function. *Life Sci* 2004 Jul 2;75(7):765-90.

[60] Lundmark PO, Pandi-Perumal SR, Srinivasan V, Cardinali DP. Role of melatonin in the eye and ocular dysfunctions. *Vis Neurosci* 2006 Nov;23(6):853-62.

[61] Siu AW, Maldonado M, Sanchez-Hidalgo M, Tan DX, Reiter RJ. Protective effects of melatonin in experimental free radical-related ocular diseases. *J Pineal Res* 2006 Mar;40(2):101-9.

[62] Nosjean O, Ferro M, Coge F, Beauverger P, Henlin JM, Lefoulon F, et al. Identification of the melatonin-binding site MT3 as the quinone reductase 2. *J Biol Chem* 2000 Oct 6;275(40):31311-7.

[63] Boutin JA, Marcheteau E, Hennig P, Moulharat N, Berger S, Delagrange P, et al. MT3/QR2 melatonin binding site does not use melatonin as a substrate or a co-substrate. *J Pineal Res* 2008 Nov;45(4):524-31.

[64] Calamini B, Santarsiero BD, Boutin JA, Mesecar AD. Kinetic, thermodynamic and X-ray structural insights into the interaction of melatonin and analogues with quinone reductase 2. *Biochem J* 2008 Jul 1;413(1):81-91.

[65] Tan DX, Manchester LC, Terron MP, Flores LJ, Tamura H, Reiter RJ. Melatonin as a naturally occurring co-substrate of quinone reductase-2, the putative MT3 melatonin membrane receptor: hypothesis and significance. *J Pineal Res* 2007 Nov;43(4):317-20.

[66] Celli CM, Tran N, Knox R, Jaiswal AK. NRH:quinone oxidoreductase 2 (NQO2) catalyzes metabolic activation of quinones and anti-tumor drugs. *Biochem Pharmacol* 2006 Jul 28;72(3):366-76.

[67] Long DJ, Iskander K, Gaikwad A, Arin M, Roop DR, Knox R, et al. Disruption of dihydronicotinamide riboside:quinone oxidoreductase 2 (NQO2) leads to myeloid hyperplasia of bone marrow and decreased sensitivity to menadione toxicity. *J Biol Chem* 2002 Nov 29;277(48):46131-9.

[68] Belforte NA, Moreno MC, de ZN, Sande PH, Chianelli MS, Keller Sarmiento MI, et al. Melatonin: a novel neuroprotectant for the treatment of glaucoma. *J Pineal Res* 2010 May;48(4):353-64.

[69] Kortuem K, Geiger LK, Levin LA. Differential susceptibility of retinal ganglion cells to reactive oxygen species. *Invest Ophthalmol Vis Sci* 2000 Sep;41(10):3176-82.

[70] Martinez-Ruiz A, Lamas S. S-nitrosylation: a potential new paradigm in signal transduction 1. *Cardiovasc Res* 2004 Apr 1;62(1):43-52.

[71] Melino G, Bernassola F, Knight RA, Corasaniti MT, Nistico G, Finazzi-Agro A. S-nitrosylation regulates apoptosis. *Nature* 1997 Jul 31;388(6641):432-3.

[72] Manabe S, Gu Z, Lipton SA. Activation of matrix metalloproteinase-9 via neuronal nitric oxide synthase contributes to NMDA-induced retinal ganglion cell death. *Invest Ophthalmol Vis Sci* 2005 Dec;46(12):4747-53.

[73] Liu B, Neufeld AH. Expression of nitric oxide synthase-2 (NOS-2) in reactive astrocytes of the human glaucomatous optic nerve head. *Glia* 2000 Apr;30(2):178-86.

[74] Neufeld AH, Hernandez MR, Gonzalez M. Nitric oxide synthase in the human glaucomatous optic nerve head. *Arch Ophthalmol* 1997 Apr;115(4):497-503.

[75] Neufeld AH, Liu B. Glaucomatous optic neuropathy: when glia misbehave. *Neuroscientist* 2003 Dec;9(6):485-95.

[76] Shareef S, Sawada A, Neufeld AH. Isoforms of nitric oxide synthase in the optic nerves of rat eyes with chronic moderately elevated intraocular pressure. *Invest Ophthalmol Vis Sci* 1999 Nov;40(12):2884-91.

[77] Liu B, Neufeld AH. Nitric oxide synthase-2 in human optic nerve head astrocytes induced by elevated pressure in vitro. *Arch Ophthalmol* 2001 Feb;119(2):240-5.

[78] Neufeld AH, Sawada A, Becker B. Inhibition of nitric-oxide synthase 2 by aminoguanidine provides neuroprotection of retinal ganglion cells in a rat model of chronic glaucoma. *Proc Natl Acad Sci U S A* 1999 Aug 17;96(17):9944-8.

[79] Neufeld AH. Pharmacologic neuroprotection with an inhibitor of nitric oxide synthase for the treatment of glaucoma. *Brain Res Bull* 2004 Feb 15;62(6):455-9.

[80] Pang IH, Johnson EC, Jia L, Cepurna WO, Shepard AR, Hellberg MR, et al. Evaluation of inducible nitric oxide synthase in glaucomatous optic neuropathy and pressure-induced optic nerve damage. *Invest Ophthalmol Vis Sci* 2005 Apr;46(4):1313-21.

[81] Vorwerk CK, Hyman BT, Miller JW, Husain D, Zurakowski D, Huang PL, et al. The role of neuronal and endothelial nitric oxide synthase in retinal excitotoxicity. *Invest Ophthalmol Vis Sci* 1997 Sep;38(10):2038-44.

[82] El-Remessy AB, Khalil IE, Matragoon S, Abou-Mohamed G, Tsai NJ, Roon P, et al. Neuroprotective effect of (-)Delta9-tetrahydrocannabinol and cannabidiol in N-methyl-D-aspartate-induced retinal neurotoxicity: involvement of peroxynitrite. *Am J Pathol* 2003 Nov;163(5):1997-2008.

[83] Block ER, Herrera H, Couch M. Hypoxia inhibits L-arginine uptake by pulmonary artery endothelial cells. *Am J Physiol* 1995 Nov;269(5 Pt 1):L574-L580.

[84] Kurz S, Harrison DG. Insulin and the arginine paradox. *J Clin Invest* 1997 Feb 1;99(3):369-70.

[85] Grima G, Cuenod M, Pfeiffer S, Mayer B, Do KQ. Arginine availability controls the N-methyl-D-aspartate-induced nitric oxide synthesis: involvement of a glial-neuronal arginine transfer. *J Neurochem* 1998 Nov;71(5):2139-44.

[86] Stevens BR, Kakuda DK, Yu K, Waters M, Vo CB, Raizada MK. Induced nitric oxide synthesis is dependent on induced alternatively spliced CAT-2 encoding L-arginine transport in brain astrocytes. *J Biol Chem* 1996 Sep 27;271(39):24017-22.

[87] do CA, Lopes C, Santos M, Proenca R, Cunha-Vaz J, Carvalho AP. Nitric oxide synthase activity and L-arginine metabolism in the retinas from streptozotocin-induced diabetic rats. *Gen Pharmacol* 1998 Mar;30(3):319-24.

[88] Cossenza M, Cadilhe DV, Coutinho RN, Paes-de-Carvalho R. Inhibition of protein synthesis by activation of NMDA receptors in cultured retinal cells: a new mechanism for the regulation of nitric oxide production. *J Neurochem* 2006 Jun;97(5):1481-93.

[89] Deves R, Boyd CA. Transporters for cationic amino acids in animal cells: discovery, structure, and function. *Physiol Rev* 1998 Apr;78(2):487-545.

[90] Carmo A, Cunha-Vaz JG, Carvalho AP, Lopes MC. L-arginine transport in retinas from streptozotocin diabetic rats: correlation with the level of IL-1 beta and NO synthase activity. *Vision Res* 1999 Nov;39(23):3817-23.

[91] Saenz DA, Cymeryng CB, De NA, Sacca GB, Keller Sarmiento MI, Rosenstein RE. Photic regulation of L-arginine uptake in the golden hamster retina. *J Neurochem* 2002 Feb;80(3):512-9.

[92] Saenz DA, Turjanski AG, Sacca GB, Marti M, Doctorovich F, Sarmiento MI, et al. Physiological concentrations of melatonin inhibit the nitridergic pathway in the Syrian hamster retina. J *Pineal Res* 2002 Aug;33(1):31-6.

[93] Bettahi I, Pozo D, Osuna C, Reiter RJ, Acuna-Castroviejo D, Guerrero JM. Melatonin reduces nitric oxide synthase activity in rat hypothalamus. *J Pineal Res* 1996 May;20(4):205-10.

[94] Leon J, Vives F, Crespo E, Camacho E, Espinosa A, Gallo MA, et al. Modification of nitric oxide synthase activity and neuronal response in rat striatum by melatonin and kynurenine derivatives. *J Neuroendocrinol* 1998 Apr;10(4):297-302.

[95] Pozo D, Reiter RJ, Calvo JR, Guerrero JM. Inhibition of cerebellar nitric oxide synthase and cyclic GMP production by melatonin via complex formation with calmodulin. *J Cell Biochem* 1997 Jun 1;65(3):430-42.

[96] Turjanski A, Chaia ZD, Doctorovich F, Estrin D, Rosenstein R, Piro OE. N-nitrosomelatonin. *Acta Crystallogr C* 2000 Jun;56 (Pt 6):682-3.

[97] Cuzzocrea S, Costantino G, Mazzon E, Micali A, De SA, Caputi AP. Beneficial effects of melatonin in a rat model of splanchnic artery occlusion and reperfusion. *J Pineal Res* 2000 Jan;28(1):52-63.

[98] Siu AW, Reiter RJ, To CH. Pineal indoleamines and vitamin E reduce nitric oxide-induced lipid peroxidation in rat retinal homogenates. *J Pineal Res* 1999 Sep;27(2):122-8.

[99] Louzada-Junior P, Dias JJ, Santos WF, Lachat JJ, Bradford HF, Coutinho-Netto J. Glutamate release in experimental ischaemia of the retina: an approach using microdialysis. *J Neurochem* 1992 Jul;59(1):358-63.

[100] David P, Lusky M, Teichberg VI. Involvement of excitatory neurotransmitters in the damage produced in chick embryo retinas by anoxia and extracellular high potassium. *Exp Eye Res* 1988 May;46(5):657-62.

[101] Mosinger JL, Price MT, Bai HY, Xiao H, Wozniak DF, Olney JW. Blockade of both NMDA and non-NMDA receptors is required for optimal protection against ischemic neuronal degeneration in the in vivo adult mammalian retina. *Exp Neurol* 1991 Jul;113(1):10-7.

[102] Riepe RE, Norenburg MD. Muller cell localisation of glutamine synthetase in rat retina. *Nature* 1977 Aug 18;268(5621):654-5.

[103] Sarthy PV, Lam DM. Biochemical studies of isolated glial (Muller) cells from the turtle retina. *J Cell Biol* 1978 Sep;78(3):675-84.

[104] Thoreson WB, Witkovsky P. Glutamate receptors and circuits in the vertebrate retina. *Prog Retin Eye Res* 1999 Nov;18(6):765-810.

[105] Brooks DE, Garcia GA, Dreyer EB, Zurakowski D, Franco-Bourland RE. Vitreous body glutamate concentration in dogs with glaucoma. *Am J Vet Res* 1997 Aug;58(8):864-7.

[106] Dkhissi O, Chanut E, Wasowicz M, Savoldelli M, Nguyen-Legros J, Minvielle F, et al. Retinal TUNEL-positive cells and high glutamate levels in vitreous humor of mutant quail with a glaucoma-like disorder. *Invest Ophthalmol Vis Sci* 1999 Apr;40(5):990-5.

[107] Shen F, Chen B, Danias J, Lee KC, Lee H, Su Y, et al. Glutamate-induced glutamine synthetase expression in retinal Muller cells after short-term ocular hypertension in the rat. *Invest Ophthalmol Vis Sci* 2004 Sep;45(9):3107-12.

[108] Honkanen RA, Baruah S, Zimmerman MB, Khanna CL, Weaver YK, Narkiewicz J, et al. Vitreous amino acid concentrations in patients with glaucoma undergoing vitrectomy. *Arch Ophthalmol* 2003 Feb;121(2):183-8.

[109] Levkovitch-Verbin H, Martin KR, Quigley HA, Baumrind LA, Pease ME, Valenta D. Measurement of amino acid levels in the vitreous humor of rats after chronic intraocular pressure elevation or optic nerve transection. *J Glaucoma* 2002 Oct;11(5):396-405.

[110] Carter-Dawson L, Crawford ML, Harwerth RS, Smith EL, III, Feldman R, Shen FF, et al. Vitreal glutamate concentration in monkeys with experimental glaucoma. *Invest Ophthalmol Vis Sci* 2002 Aug;43(8):2633-7.

[111] Wamsley S, Gabelt BT, Dahl DB, Case GL, Sherwood RW, May CA, et al. Vitreous glutamate concentration and axon loss in monkeys with experimental glaucoma. *Arch Ophthalmol* 2005 Jan;123(1):64-70.

[112] Martin KR, Levkovitch-Verbin H, Valenta D, Baumrind L, Pease ME, Quigley HA. Retinal glutamate transporter changes in experimental glaucoma and after optic nerve transection in the rat. *Invest Ophthalmol Vis Sci* 2002 Jul;43(7):2236-43.

[113] Naskar R, Vorwerk CK, Dreyer EB. Concurrent downregulation of a glutamate transporter and receptor in glaucoma. *Invest Ophthalmol Vis Sci* 2000 Jun;41(7):1940-4.

[114] Pow DV, Robinson SR. Glutamate in some retinal neurons is derived solely from glia. *Neuroscience* 1994 May;60(2):355-66.

[115] Gegelashvili G, Schousboe A. Cellular distribution and kinetic properties of high-affinity glutamate transporters. *Brain Res Bull* 1998;45(3):233-8.

[116] Tanaka D, Furusawa K, Kameyama K, Okamoto H, Doi M. Melatonin signaling regulates locomotion behavior and homeostatic states through distinct receptor pathways in Caenorhabditis elegans. *Neuropharmacology* 2007 Jul;53(1):157-68.

[117] Tanaka K. Functions of glutamate transporters in the brain. *Neurosci Res* 2000 May;37(1):15-9.

[118] Attwell D, Barbour B, Szatkowski M. Nonvesicular release of neurotransmitter. *Neuron* 1993 Sep;11(3):401-7.

[119] Otis TS, Jahr CE. Anion currents and predicted glutamate flux through a neuronal glutamate transporter. *J Neurosci* 1998 Sep 15;18(18):7099-110.

[120] Vorwerk CK, Naskar R, Schuettauf F, Quinto K, Zurakowski D, Gochenauer G, et al. Depression of retinal glutamate transporter function leads to elevated intravitreal glutamate levels and ganglion cell death. *Invest Ophthalmol Vis Sci* 2000 Oct;41(11):3615-21.

[121] Saenz DA, Goldin AP, Minces L, Chianelli M, Sarmiento MI, Rosenstein RE. Effect of melatonin on the retinal glutamate/glutamine cycle in the golden hamster retina. *FASEB J* 2004 Dec;18(15):1912-3.

[122] Gorovits R, Avidan N, Avisar N, Shaked I, Vardimon L. Glutamine synthetase protects against neuronal degeneration in injured retinal tissue. *Proc Natl Acad Sci U S A* 1997 Jun 24;94(13):7024-9.

[123] Heidinger V, Hicks D, Sahel J, Dreyfus H. Ability of retinal Muller glial cells to protect neurons against excitotoxicity in vitro depends upon maturation and neuron-glial interactions. *Glia* 1999 Feb 1;25(3):229-39.

[124] Patel AJ, Hunt A, Tahourdin CS. Regulation of in vivo glutamine synthetase activity by glucocorticoids in the developing rat brain. *Brain Res* 1983 Oct;312(1):83-91.

[125] Sarkar PK, Chaudhury S. Messenger RNA for glutamine synthetase. Review article. *Mol Cell Biochem* 1983;53-54(1-2):233-44.

[126] Hall ED. High-dose glucocorticoid treatment improves neurological recovery in head-injured mice. *J Neurosurg* 1985 Jun;62(6):882-7.

[127] Rosner M, Lam TT, Tso MO. Therapeutic parameters of methylprednisolone treatment for retinal photic injury in a rat model. *Res Commun Chem Pathol Pharmacol* 1992 Sep;77(3):299-311.

[128] Kalloniatis M, Tomisich G. Amino acid neurochemistry of the vertebrate retina. *Prog Retin Eye Res* 1999 Nov;18(6):811-66.

[129] Yang XL. Characterization of receptors for glutamate and GABA in retinal neurons. *Prog Neurobiol* 2004 Jun;73(2):127-50.

[130] Schwartz EA. Depolarization without calcium can release gamma-aminobutyric acid from a retinal neuron. *Science* 1987 Oct 16;238(4825):350-5.

[131] Andrade da Costa BL, de Mello FG, Hokoc JN. Transporter-mediated GABA release induced by excitatory amino acid agonist is associated with GAD-67 but not GAD-65 immunoreactive cells of the primate retina. *Brain Res* 2000 Apr 28;863(1-2):132-42.

[132] do Nascimento JL, Ventura AL, Paes de CR. Veratridine- and glutamate-induced release of [3H]-GABA from cultured chick retina cells: possible involvement of a GAT-1-like subtype of GABA transporter. *Brain Res* 1998 Jul 6;798(1-2):217-22.

[133] Lopez-Costa JJ, Goldstein J, Pecci-Saavedra J, Della Maggiore VM, De Las Heras MA, Sarmiento MI, et al. GABA release mechanism in the golden hamster retina. *Int J Neurosci* 1999;98(1-2):13-25.

[134] Gadea A, Lopez-Colome AM. Glial transporters for glutamate, glycine, and GABA: II. GABA transporters. *J Neurosci Res* 2001 Mar 15;63(6):461-8.

[135] Honda S, Yamamoto M, Saito N. Immunocytochemical localization of three subtypes of GABA transporter in rat retina. *Brain Res Mol Brain Res* 1995 Nov;33(2):319-25.

[136] Johnson J, Chen TK, Rickman DW, Evans C, Brecha NC. Multiple gamma-Aminobutyric acid plasma membrane transporters (GAT-1, GAT-2, GAT-3) in the rat retina. *J Comp Neurol* 1996 Nov 11;375(2):212-24.

[137] Kawasaki A, Otori Y, Barnstable CJ. Muller cell protection of rat retinal ganglion cells from glutamate and nitric oxide neurotoxicity. *Invest Ophthalmol Vis Sci* 2000 Oct;41(11):3444-50.

[138] Nucci C, Tartaglione R, Rombola L, Morrone LA, Fazzi E, Bagetta G. Neurochemical evidence to implicate elevated glutamate in the mechanisms of high intraocular pressure

(IOP)-induced retinal ganglion cell death in rat. *Neurotoxicology* 2005 Oct;26(5):935-41.

[139] Rosenstein RE, Cardinali DP. Melatonin increases in vivo GABA accumulation in rat hypothalamus, cerebellum, cerebral cortex and pineal gland. *Brain Res* 1986 Nov 29;398(2):403-6.

[140] Rosenstein RE, Estevez AG, Cardinali DP. Time-Dependent Effect of Melatonin on Glutamic Acid Decarboxylase Activity and CI Influx in Rat Hypothalamus. *J Neuroendocrinol* 1989 Dec 1;1(6):443-7.

[141] Osborne NN, Chidlow G, Nash MS, Wood JP. The potential of neuroprotection in glaucoma treatment. *Curr Opin Ophthalmol* 1999 Apr;10(2):82-92.

[142] Sande PH, Fernandez DC, Aldana Marcos HJ, Chianelli MS, Aisemberg J, Silberman DM, et al. Therapeutic effect of melatonin in experimental uveitis. *Am J Pathol* 2008 Dec;173(6):1702-13.

[143] Marcic TS, Belyea DA, Katz B. Neuroprotection in glaucoma: a model for neuroprotection in optic neuropathies. *Curr Opin Ophthalmol* 2003 Dec;14(6):353-6.

[144] Tang Q, Hu Y, Cao Y. Neuroprotective effect of melatonin on retinal ganglion cells in rats4. *J Huazhong Univ Sci Technolog Med Sci* 2006;26(2):235-7, 253.

[145] Weber AJ, Harman CD, Viswanathan S. Effects of optic nerve injury, glaucoma, and neuroprotection on the survival, structure, and function of ganglion cells in the mammalian retina. *J Physiol* 2008 Sep 15;586(Pt 18):4393-400.

[146] Jimenez-Jorge S, Guerrero JM, Jimenez-Caliani AJ, Naranjo MC, Lardone PJ, Carrillo-Vico A, et al. Evidence for melatonin synthesis in the rat brain during development. *J Pineal Res* 2007 Apr;42(3):240-6.

[147] Niles LP, Armstrong KJ, Rincon Castro LM, Dao CV, Sharma R, McMillan CR, et al. Neural stem cells express melatonin receptors and neurotrophic factors: colocalization of the MT1 receptor with neuronal and glial markers. *BMC Neurosci* 2004 Oct 28;5:41.

[148] Kong X, Li X, Cai Z, Yang N, Liu Y, Shu J, et al. Melatonin regulates the viability and differentiation of rat midbrain neural stem cells. *Cell Mol Neurobiol* 2008 Jun;28 (4):569-79.

[149] Imbesi M, Uz T, Manev H. Role of melatonin receptors in the effects of melatonin on BDNF and neuroprotection in mouse cerebellar neurons. *J Neural Transm* 2008 Nov;115(11):1495-9.

[150] Flammer J, Orgul S, Costa VP, Orzalesi N, Krieglstein GK, Serra LM, et al. The impact of ocular blood flow in glaucoma. *Prog Retin Eye Res* 2002 Jul;21(4):359-93.

[151] Fuchsjager-Mayrl G, Wally B, Georgopoulos M, Rainer G, Kircher K, Buehl W, et al. Ocular blood flow and systemic blood pressure in patients with primary open-angle glaucoma and ocular hypertension. *Invest Ophthalmol Vis Sci* 2004 Mar;45(3):834-9.

[152] Galassi F, Sodi A, Ucci F, Renieri G, Pieri B, Baccini M. Ocular hemodynamics and glaucoma prognosis: a color Doppler imaging study. *Arch Ophthalmol* 2003 Dec;121(12):1711-5.

[153] Zink JM, Grunwald JE, Piltz-Seymour J, Staii A, Dupont J. Association between lower optic nerve laser Doppler blood volume measurements and glaucomatous visual field progression 1. *Br J Ophthalmol* 2003 Dec;87(12):1487-91.

[154] Osborne NN, Casson RJ, Wood JP, Chidlow G, Graham M, Melena J. Retinal ischemia: mechanisms of damage and potential therapeutic strategies2. *Prog Retin Eye Res* 2004 Jan;23(1):91-147.

[155] Moore RY, Silver R. Suprachiasmatic nucleus organization. *Chronobiol Int* 1998 Sep;15(5):475-87.

[156] Buijs RM, Kalsbeek A. Hypothalamic integration of central and peripheral clocks. *Nat Rev Neurosci* 2001 Jul;2(7):521-6.

[157] Golombek DA, Rosenstein RE. Physiology of circadian entrainment. *Physiol Rev* 2010 Jul;90(3):1063-102.

[158] Duffy JF, Czeisler CA. Effect of Light on Human Circadian Physiology. *Sleep Med Clin* 2009 Jun;4(2):165-77.

[159] Klerman EB, Rimmer DW, Dijk DJ, Kronauer RE, Rizzo JF, III, Czeisler CA. Nonphotic entrainment of the human circadian pacemaker. *Am J Physiol* 1998 Apr;274(4 Pt 2):R991-R996.

[160] Van Bergen NJ, Crowston JG, Kearns LS, Staffieri SE, Hewitt AW, Cohn AC, et al. Mitochondrial oxidative phosphorylation compensation may preserve vision in patients with OPA1-linked autosomal dominant optic atrophy. *PLoS One* 2011;6(6):e21347.

[161] Freedman MS, Lucas RJ, Soni B, von SM, Munoz M, David-Gray Z, et al. Regulation of mammalian circadian behavior by non-rod, non-cone, ocular photoreceptors. *Science* 1999 Apr 16;284(5413):502-4.

[162] Lucas RJ, Freedman MS, Munoz M, Garcia-Fernandez JM, Foster RG. Regulation of the mammalian pineal by non-rod, non-cone, ocular photoreceptors. *Science* 1999 Apr 16;284(5413):505-7.

[163] Lucas RJ, Douglas RH, Foster RG. Characterization of an ocular photopigment capable of driving pupillary constriction in mice. *Nat Neurosci* 2001 Jun;4(6):621-6.

[164] Wee R, Castrucci AM, Provencio I, Gan L, Van Gelder RN. Loss of photic entrainment and altered free-running circadian rhythms in math5-/- mice. *J Neurosci* 2002 Dec 1;22(23):10427-33.

[165] Berson DM, Dunn FA, Takao M. Phototransduction by retinal ganglion cells that set the circadian clock. *Science* 2002 Feb 8;295(5557):1070-3.

[166] Hattar S, Liao HW, Takao M, Berson DM, Yau KW. Melanopsin-containing retinal ganglion cells: architecture, projections, and intrinsic photosensitivity. *Science* 2002 Feb 8;295(5557):1065-70.

[167] Provencio I, Rollag MD, Castrucci AM. Photoreceptive net in the mammalian retina. This mesh of cells may explain how some blind mice can still tell day from night. *Nature* 2002 Jan 31;415(6871):493.

[168] Mrosovsky N, Hattar S. Impaired masking responses to light in melanopsin-knockout mice. *Chronobiol Int* 2003 Nov;20(6):989-99.

[169] Panda S, Sato TK, Castrucci AM, Rollag MD, DeGrip WJ, Hogenesch JB, et al. Melanopsin (Opn4) requirement for normal light-induced circadian phase shifting. *Science* 2002 Dec 13;298(5601):2213-6.

[170] Ruby NF, Brennan TJ, Xie X, Cao V, Franken P, Heller HC, et al. Role of melanopsin in circadian responses to light. *Science* 2002 Dec 13;298(5601):2211-3.

[171] Hattar S, Kumar M, Park A, Tong P, Tung J, Yau KW, et al. Central projections of melanopsin-expressing retinal ganglion cells in the mouse. *J Comp Neurol* 2006 Jul 20;497(3):326-49.

[172] Kardon R, Anderson SC, Damarjian TG, Grace EM, Stone E, Kawasaki A. Chromatic pupil responses: preferential activation of the melanopsin-mediated versus outer photoreceptor-mediated pupil light reflex. *Ophthalmology* 2009 Aug;116(8):1564-73.

[173] Lucas RJ, Hattar S, Takao M, Berson DM, Foster RG, Yau KW. Diminished pupillary light reflex at high irradiances in melanopsin-knockout mice. *Science* 2003 Jan 10;299(5604):245-7.

[174] Nissen C, Sander B, Lund-Andersen H. The effect of pupil size on stimulation of the melanopsin containing retinal ganglion cells, as evaluated by monochromatic pupillometry. *Front Neurol* 2011;2:92.

[175] Onen SH, Alloui A, Eschalier A, Dubray C. Vocalization thresholds related to noxious paw pressure are decreased by paradoxical sleep deprivation and increased after sleep recovery in rat. *Neurosci Lett* 2000 Sep 8;291(1):25-8.

[176] Perez-Rico C, de l, V, Arribas-Gomez I, Blanco R. Evaluation of functional integrity of the retinohypothalamic tract in advanced glaucoma using multifocal electroretinography and light-induced melatonin suppression. *Exp Eye Res* 2010 Nov;91 (5):578-83.

[177] Kalaboukhova L, Fridhammar V, Lindblom B. Relative afferent pupillary defect in glaucoma: a pupillometric study. *Acta Ophthalmol Scand* 2007 Aug;85(5):519-25.

[178] Kohn AN, Moss AP, Hargett NA, Ritch R, Smith H, Jr., Podos SM. Clinical comparison of dipivalyl epinephrine and epinephrine in the treatment of glaucoma. *Am J Ophthalmol* 1979 Feb;87(2):196-201.

[179] Feigl B, Zele AJ, Fader SM, Howes AN, Hughes CE, Jones KA, et al. The post-illumination pupil response of melanopsin-expressing intrinsically photosensitive retinal ganglion cells in diabetes. *Acta Ophthalmol* 2012 May;90(3):e230-e234.

[180] Drouyer E, Dkhissi-Benyahya O, Chiquet C, WoldeMussie E, Ruiz G, Wheeler LA, et al. Glaucoma alters the circadian timing system. *PLoS One* 2008;3(12):e3931.

[181] Wang HZ, Lu QJ, Wang NL, Liu H, Zhang L, Zhan GL. Loss of melanopsin-containing retinal ganglion cells in a rat glaucoma model. *Chin Med J (Engl)* 2008 Jun 5;121(11): 1015-9.

[182] Jakobs TC, Libby RT, Ben Y, John SW, Masland RH. Retinal ganglion cell degeneration is topological but not cell type specific in DBA/2J mice. *J Cell Biol* 2005 Oct 24;171(2):313-25.

[183] Li RS, Chen BY, Tay DK, Chan HH, Pu ML, So KF. Melanopsin-expressing retinal ganglion cells are more injury-resistant in a chronic ocular hypertension model. *Invest Ophthalmol Vis Sci* 2006 Jul;47(7):2951-8.

[184] Belforte N, Sande P, de ZN, Knepper PA, Rosenstein RE. Effect of chondroitin sulfate on intraocular pressure in rats. *Invest Ophthalmol Vis Sci* 2010 Nov;51(11):5768-75.

[185] de ZN, Plano SA, Fernandez DC, Lanzani MF, Salido E, Belforte N, et al. Effect of experimental glaucoma on the non-image forming visual system. *J Neurochem* 2011 Jun;117(5):904-14.

[186] Kankipati L, Girkin CA, Gamlin PD. The post-illumination pupil response is reduced in glaucoma patients. *Invest Ophthalmol Vis Sci* 2011 Apr;52(5):2287-92.

[187] Kashiwagi K, Tsumura T, Ishii H, Ijiri H, Tamura K, Tsukahara S. Circadian rhythm of autonomic nervous function in patients with normal-tension glaucoma compared with normal subjects using ambulatory electrocardiography. *J Glaucoma* 2000 Jun;9(3):239-46.

[188] La MC, Ross-Cisneros FN, Hannibal J, Montagna P, Sadun AA, Carelli V. Melanopsin-expressing retinal ganglion cells: implications for human diseases. *Vision Res* 2011 Jan 28;51(2):296-302.

[189] Bremner FD, Tomlin EA, Shallo-Hoffmann J, Votruba M, Smith SE. The pupil in dominant optic atrophy. *Invest Ophthalmol Vis Sci* 2001 Mar;42(3):675-8.

[190] Wakakura M, Yokoe J. Evidence for preserved direct pupillary light response in Leber's hereditary optic neuropathy. *Br J Ophthalmol* 1995 May;79(5):442-6.

[191] Cardinali DP, Furio AM, Brusco LI. The use of chronobiotics in the resynchronization of the sleep/wake cycle. Therapeutical application in the early phases of Alzheimer's disease. *Recent Pat Endocr Metab Immune Drug Discov* 2011 May;5(2):80-90.

[192] Carpentieri A, Diaz de BG, Areco V, Peralta LM, Tolosa de TN. New perspectives in melatonin uses. *Pharmacol Res* 2012 Apr;65(4):437-44.

[193] Hardeland R. Melatonin, hormone of darkness and more: occurrence, control mechanisms, actions and bioactive metabolites. *Cell Mol Life Sci* 2008 Jul;65(13):2001-18.

[194] van Geijlswijk IM, Korzilius HP, Smits MG. The use of *exogenous* melatonin in delayed sleep phase disorder: a meta-analysis. Sleep 2010 Dec;33(12):1605-14.

[195] Garzon C, Guerrero JM, Aramburu O, Guzman T. Effect of melatonin administration on sleep, behavioral disorders and hypnotic drug discontinuation in the elderly: a randomized, double-blind, placebo-controlled study. *Aging Clin Exp Res* 2009 Feb;21(1):38-42.

In: New Developments in Melatonin Research ISBN: 978-1-62618-843-3
Editors: D.Acuña-Castroviejo, I.Rusanova, G.Escames © 2013 Nova Science Publishers, Inc.

Chapter 12

Diurnal Expression of Vesicular Glutamate Transporters in the Rat Pineal Gland and its Relationship to Melatonin Secretion

Sachine Yoshida[1,2], Haruo Nogami[1] and Setsuji Hisano[1]
[1] Laboratory of Neuroendocrinology, Graduate School of Comprehensive Human Sciences, University of Tsukuba, Ibaraki, Japan
[2] Unit for Affiliative Social Behavior, RIKEN Brain Science Institute, Saitama, Japan

Abstract

The pineal gland secretes melatonin and expresses three subtypes of vesicular glutamate transporters (VGLUT1, VGLUT2, and VGLUT1v, a VGLUT1 variant) in rats. Although a previous culture study revealed that exogenous glutamate inhibits melatonin production by suppressing activity of melatonin-synthesizing enzyme, the physiological role of endogenous glutamate in pineal function is not fully understood. Our recent study of ontogenetic expression of the VGLUT subtypes reported that only VGLUT2 mRNA expression shows a diurnal rhythm from postnatal day 14 onward, having sensitivity for β-adrenergic stimulation. In the adult, both VGLUT2 mRNA and protein levels increased in the dark phase, with the protein level showing a 6-h delay. The nocturnal elevation of VGLUT2 mRNA level diminished under the constant light condition but maintained under the constant dark condition. These data suggest that VGLUT2-mediated glutamate is involved in some glutamatergic function at the end of dark phase under circadian control. On the other hand, VGLUT1 expression is seen in almost all pinealocytes both in the light and the dark phases. It suggests that VGLUT1 is involved in a certain glutamatergic event occurred in the entire gland throughout the day. VGLUT1v mRNA shows a property to express in cells that possess ribbon synapses, implying that the variant form has some sort of functional merit for such synapses. Here, we will discuss the possible role of glutamate in melatonin secretion, based on a characteristic pattern of VGLUT expression in the pineal gland.

Introduction

Melatonin is secreted by pinealocytes, a parenchymal cell of the pineal gland, as a hormonal message of darkness [1]. Melatonin synthesis shows a diurnal rhythm with a nocturnal increase [2], which is tightly regulated by the master circadian clock in the suprachiasmatic nucleus (SCN) [3]. Information on environmental light conditions via the retinohypothalamic tract reaches the SCN, from which the integrated information is farther conveyed to the pineal gland finally via the superior cervical ganglion along the sympathetic pathway. During the night, norepinephrine (NE) activates adenylate cyclase via β_1-adrenergic receptors on pinealocytes [4], and consequently the elevated level of an intracellular cAMP facilitates the transcription of arylalkylamine *N*-acetyltransferase (AANAT), the rate-limiting enzyme of melatonin synthesis, thereby finally increasing melatonin production [4, 5]. The AANAT activity decreases by the end of night, resulting in the decline of melatonin production [6]. It has been suggested that the pineal gland is a glutamatergic endocrine organ, since this gland contains an abundance of glutamate [7] and expresses not only ionotropic- and metabotropic-glutamate receptors [8-10] but also plasma membrane excitatory amino acid transporters [11]. Moreover, pineal glutamate is secreted by pinealocytes in an exocytotic manner. Within pinealocytes, glutamate is accumulated in synaptic-like microvesicles (SLMV), which are a counterpart of neuronal synaptic vesicles (SV) [12, 13], and is secreted via Ca^{2+}-regulated exocytotic process [14, 15]. A vesicular glutamate transporter (VGLUT), a reliable molecular marker of glutamatergic cells (for reviews see [16, 17]), plays an essential role in the storage of glutamate in SV and SLMV. So far, three distinct subtypes of VGLUT have been identified: VGLUT1 [18-21] that is originally termed brain-specific Na^+-dependent inorganic phosphate cotransporter, BNPI [18] (also referred to as Slc17a7); VGLUT2 [22-27] that is originally termed differentiation-associated inorganic phosphate cotransporter, DNPI [22] (Slc17a6); and VGLUT3 [28-31]. Among these subtypes, VGLUT1 and VGLUT2 have been described to exist in SLMV in pinealocytes [32]. In addition to these subtypes, we reported that VGLUT1v, a VGLUT1 splice variant, is expressed in the rat pineal gland [33]. The VGLUT1v mRNA contains an additional 75-base pair intronic sequence, which suggests that VGLUT1v protein would be 24-amino acid longer than VGLUT1 protein. Our ontogenetic studies have demonstrated that each type of VGLUT shows a unique pattern of expression of its mRNA and protein during early postnatal development of the rat pineal gland, and also even in adulthood [33-35]. Here, we will describe the characteristic patterns of developmental expression of VGLUT subtypes and discuss the possible role of glutamate in the pineal gland, with particular reference to melatonin synthesis.

VGLUT1 Expression

The expression level of VGLUT1 mRNA in the pineal gland is very low at birth but rapidly increases up to adult level during the first two weeks after birth (Figure 1A) [34]. In situ hybridization and immunohistochemical data reveal that the expression mainly occurs in the peripheral part of gland at postnatal day 0 (P0) and then spreads over the entire gland from P7 onward [34]. Double immunostaining for VGLUT1 and synaptophysin, a cytological marker of pinealocyte [36, 37], has reported that VGLUT1 immunoreactivity is localized in synaptophysin-positive cells in both neonatal and the adult rats, showing VGLUT1 expression by pinealocytes. Furthermore, it is interesting that the developmental pattern of VGLUT1 staining is very similar to that of dynamin 1, which also spreads from the pheripheal toward the central area of the gland with development [38].

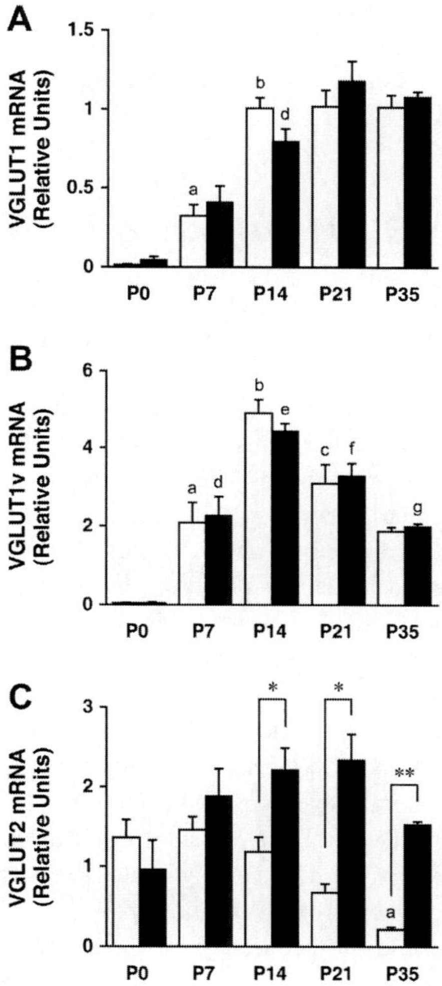

**p < 0.01, *p < 0.05 vs. ZT16 at the same age. Figures are taken from Yoshida et al [35].

Figure 1. Postnatal change in mRNA expressions of VGLUT1, VGLUT1v and VGLUT2. Using quantitative RT-PCR, the VGLUT1 (A), VGLUT1v (B) and VGLUT2 (C) mRNA levels were evaluated at zeitgeber time (ZT) 7 (open bars) and ZT16 (filled bars) of postnatal pups kept under a 12-h light/dark cycle. Values are mean ± SEM. Different alphabetical characters above open (a–c) and filled (d–g) bars show a significant difference against the values of one-week younger ages in the same ZT group.

Dynamin 1 is one of key molecules required for endocytosis and binds to endophilins [39]. Interestingly, endophilin 1 is shown to interact with VGLUT1, but not VGLUT2 or VGLUT3 [40, 41]. Both levels of dynamin 1 and endophilin 1 mRNAs in the rat pineal gland are reported to increase drastically within one week after birth as seen in VGLUT1 [34]. It is noteworthy that VGLUT1 mRNA expression dose not show any diurnal change in both the developing (Figure 1A) and the mature (Figure 2A and C) pineal glands [34, 35]. β-adrenergic stimulation of a dissociated pineal cell population is reported to fail to increase VGLUT1 mRNA level [42]. Histochemical observation reveals that nearly all of pinealocytes express uniformly VGLUT1 in the pineal gland, suggesting that a VGLUT1-related glutamatergic event may occur over the entire gland. Taken together, VGLUT1 seems to act as a dominant vesicular transport system in SLMV of pinealocytes and may be recycled with the aid of a molecular interaction between dynamin 1 and endophilin 1. Moreover, VGLUT1 may be involved in a certain glutamatergic function occurred in mature pinealocytes without relation to day/night transition.

VGLUT1v Expression

VGLUT1v mRNA is expressed almost exclusively in photosensitive organs such as the retina and the pineal gland [33]. The developmental expression of VGLUT1v is differently regulated between pineal gland and retina. In the rat retina, mRNA level increases with age and this variant form becomes the major transcript of the VGLUT1 gene from P14 onward [33]. In contrast, VGLUT1v mRNA expression in the pineal gland continues to sharply increase during two weeks after birth and then decreases with age [33, 34]. As to the structural and functional similarity between these organs, early studies have reported that pinealocytes transiently undergo a retinal photoreceptor-like cell differentiation from P4 to P17 [43], and that the rodent pineal gland is photosensitive only in the neonatal period but not adulthood [44]. The high-level expression of VGLUT1v mRNA in the neonatal period suggests that this variant type is involved in a certain glutamatergic signal transduction which is transiently required for a functional property of photosensitive pineal cells before the complement of pineal organogenesis. Since VGLUT1v mRNA expression shows neither a diurnal change (Figure 1B, 2A and D) [35] nor sensitivity for β-adrenergic stimulation [42], a VGLUT1v-mediated glutamatergic event may be unrelated to photosensitivity of differentiating pineal cells. VGLUT1v mRNA expression is still detectable even after the loss of photosensitivity in pinealocytes [34]. This finding leads at least two hypotheses. One is that VGLUT1v expression may reflect a retinal photoreceptor-like cell differentiation transiently seen in the neonatal period and the persistence of the photoreceptor cell-like property in pinealocytes in adulthood. The other is that VGLUT1v may be engaged in distinct glutamatergic events depending on the age. Previous double labeling data [32, 34] indicates that VGLUT1 is synthesized only in pinealocytes. In this context, it may be speculated that pinealocytes also synthesize VGLUT1v through alternative splicing. In addition, as to the retina we have reported that VGLUT1v mRNA expression occurs in rod photoreceptor cells by organ culture experiment [33]. The pineal and retinal cell types have a morphologically distinctive type of synapses called a ribbon synapse, which is considered to be a specialized structure for continuous exocytotic release of neurotransmitters [45]. Therefore, it is likely that particular cell populations with the ribbon synapse specifically express the VGLUT1v. This variant subtype may have certain favorable characteristics for the function of this special synaptic structure or the formation of a specialized vesicle arrangement.

VGLUT2 Expression

Among pineal VGLUT subtypes, VGLUT2 is the only subtype whose expression shows a diurnal change with the nocturnal elevation in both developing (Figure 1C) and mature rats (Figure 2B and E) kept under normal light/dark condition [34, 35]. Expression level of VGLUT2 mRNA in daytime is already substantial at P0 and then gradually declines after P7 onward, whereas that in nighttime does not reduce with age. Based on the difference in the expression level between daytime and nighttime, we can speculate that a diurnal rhythmicity of VGLUT2 mRNA expression would occur by P14 [35]. The expression of melatonin [46] and some molecules required for melatonin production [47-48] also acquire a diurnal rhythmicity at the second week of the postnatal development. More specifically, activities of AANAT and hydroxyindole-*O*-methyltransferase (an enzyme which catalyzes the final step of melatonin synthesis) as well as the β_1-AR mRNA level are reported to display a diurnal rhythm at the second postnatal week [46-48]. This temporal coincidence of the onset of diurnal rhythm in dynamics of molecules related to melatonin production would suggest some physiological contribution of VGLUT2 to the glutamatergic regulation of rhythmic melatonin production. In adult rats kept in normal light/dark cycle, VGLUT2 mRNA shows a rhythmic pattern of expression which peaks 4 h after light-off and gradually decreases from the end of dark to early light phase [35]. This time course closely resembles that of AANAT mRNA expression [6]. In addition, the time-dependent difference in VGLUT2 expression levels persists even after the entrainment for the constant dark condition but is drastically blocked by the constant exposure to the light, as shown from very low-level VGLUT2 mRNA expression at zeitgeber time (ZT) 16 [35]. This blockage caused by constant light exposure to rats resembles the situation in AANAT, whose activity is under SCN oscillation and no longer detectable 30 days after the onset of constant light exposure [49].

In vitro studies using organotypic [50] or dissociated cell [42] culture experiment have revealed that VGLUT2 mRNA expression is drastically enhanced by stimulation of either β-adrenergic receptor or cAMP synthesis, suggesting that VGLUT2 mRNA expression is under circadian control by the SCN which is related to rhythmic melatonin production as an endogenous oscillator (for a review see [51]). Our previous study using in situ hybridization histochemistry reveals that intense signals of VGLUT2 mRNA are localized in a particular population of pinealocytes [34]. The fact that only the subpopulation expresses a high level of VGLUT2 mRNA may reflect the functional heterogeneity of pinealocytes in intra-pineal glutamatergic signal transduction, suggesting that NE-induced VGLUT2 mRNA expression may be differentially modulated among pinealocytes. However, unlike VGLUT2, AANAT mRNA expression occurs in virtually all pinealocytes [34]. Further analysis will be needed to clarify the biological significance of the inhomogeneous pattern of VGLUT2 mRNA expression. Of particular importance is a finding that the level of VGLUT2 protein is maximally increased at the end of dark phase, 6 h after the mRNA level peaks. In analyses for VGLUT proteins, a previous study has reported that VGLUT1 overexpression in cultured hippocampal neurons facilitates excitatory synaptic transmission by increasing glutamate release per vesicle [52]. In cultured thalamic neurons, miniature EPSC amplitude is reported to reduce in the order of wild-type, VGLUT2 heterozygous, and homozygous knockout mice [53]. These data suggest that the amount of VGLUT proteins determines the amount of glutamate released. Therefore, our results on VGLUT2 protein expression suggest that the intra-pineal VGLUT2-related glutamatergic signal transduction is enhanced at the end of dark phase. AANAT activity is also known to begin to decrease at the end of dark phase, not after the onset of the light phase [6].

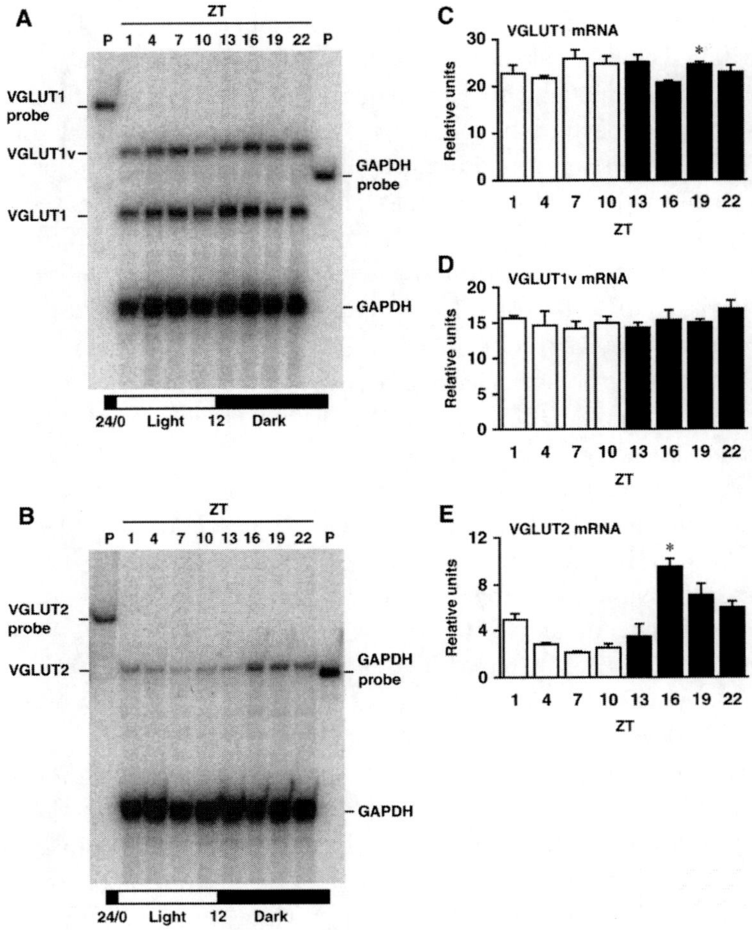

P = probe for VGLUT1 including the variant region, VGLUT2 or GAPDH.
ZT = Zeitgeber time. Values are mean ± SEM.
*p < 0.05 vs. ZT16 in (C),
*p < 0.05 vs. ZT4–ZT10 in (E). Figures are taken from Yoshida et al [35].

Figure 2. mRNA expressions of distinct VGLUT subtypes during a 24-h. VGLUT1 (A), VGLUT1v (A) and VGLUT2 (B) mRNA expressions in the rat pineal gland were analyzed by RNase protection assay. Radioactivity of the fragments was quantified and graphed as the total radioactivity normalized to that of GAPDH (C–E). Open and filled bars show values at light and dark phases, respectively.

A recent study shows that the activity of PDE4B2, a phosphodiesterase, also displays a diurnally rhythmic pattern under SCN control [54]. This enzyme is a candidate of negative regulators for melatonin production by means of cAMP degradation. Similar to the diurnal change in the VGLUT2 protein level, PDE4B2 activity also elevates remarkably during the later half of the dark phase, peaking at the end of this phase when melatonin production is suppressed. Previous studies have demonstrated that exogenous glutamate inhibits NE-enhanced AANAT activity and consequently suppresses melatonin production [55, 56], and that the parasympathetic input suppresses melatonin secretion in the later half of night [57] through the glutamatargic system [55, 56, 58]. Taken together, it is likely that glutamate transported by VGLUT2 operates in an inhibitory mechanism for AANAT activity and melatonin production in subpopulation of pinealocytes.

Conclusion

The pineal gland expresses three distinct VGLUT subtypes (VGLUT1, VGLUT1v and VGLUT2). Each subtype is expressed in a unique manner in the developing and the mature rats. VGLUT1 seems to act as a dominant vesicular transport system in SLMV of pinealocytes and may be involved in a certain glutamatergic function occurred in pinealocytes without relation to day/night transition. VGLUT1v mRNA is expressed in the pineal and the retinal cell types known to possess ribbon synapses, implying that the variant form has some sort of functional merit for such synapses. On the other hand, VGLUT2, unlike VGLUT1 and VGLUT1v, shows a diurnal change in expression. The property of VGLUT2 expression suggests the involvement of VGLUT2-mediated glutamate in the inhibitory mechanism of melatonin production. It is probable that glutamate has diverse functions in the pineal gland via three subtypes of VGLUT.

References

[1] Korf, H.W., Schomerus, C., and Stehle, J.H. (1998). The pineal organ, its hormone melatonin, and the photoneuroendocrine system. *Adv. Anat. Embryol. Cell Biol.* 146, 1-100.

[2] Arendt, J. (1998). Melatonin and the pineal gland: influence on mammalian seasonal and circadian physiology. *Rev. Reprod.* 3, 13-22.

[3] Vanecek, J., Sugden, D., Weller, J., and Klein, D.C. (1985). Atypical synergistic a_1-and b-adrenergic regulation of adenosine 3', 5'-monophosphate and guanosine 3', 5'-monophosphate in rat pinealocytes. *Endocrinology* 116, 2167-2173.

[4] Klein, D.C. (1985). Photoneural regulation of the mammalian pineal gland. In: Everet, D., Clark, D. (Eds.), *Photoperiodism, Melatonin and the Pineal Gland. Ciba Foundation Symposium* 117. Pitman, London, 38-56.

[5] Klein, D.C., Coon, S.L., Roseboom, P.H., Weller, J.L., Bernard, M., Gastel, J.A., Zatz, M., Iuvone, P.M., Rodriguez, I.R., Begay, V., et al. (1997). The melatonin rhythm-generating enzyme: molecular regulation of serotonin N-acetyltransferase in the pineal gland. *Recent Prog. Horm. Res.* 52, 307-357.

[6] Roseboom, P.H., Coon, S.L., Baler, R., McCune, S.K., Weller, J.L., and Klein, D.C. (1996). Melatonin synthesis: analysis of the more than 150-fold nocturnal increase in serotonin N-acetyltransferase messenger ribonucleic acid in the rat pineal gland. *Endocrinology* 137, 3033-3045.

[7] Nir, I., Briel, G., Dames, W., and Neuhoff, V. (1973). Rat pineal free amino acids diurnal rhythm and effect of light. *Arch. Int. Physiol. Biochim.* 81, 617-627.

[8] Pabst, H., and Redecker, P. (1999). Interstitial glial cells of the gerbil pineal gland display immunoreactivity for the metabotropic glutamate receptors mGluR2/3 and mGluR5. *Brain Res.* 838, 60-68.

[9] Yatsushiro, S., Yamada, H., Hayashi, M., Yamamoto, A., and Moriyama, Y. (2000). Ionotropic glutamate receptors trigger microvesicle-mediated exocytosis of L-glutamate in rat pinealocytes. *J. Neurochem.* 75, 288-297.

[10] Kaur, C., Sivakumar, V., and Ling, E.A. (2005). Expression of N-methyl-D-aspartate (NMDA) and alpha-amino-3-hydroxy-5-methyl-4-isoxazolepropionate (AMPA) GluR2/3 receptors in the developing rat pineal gland. *J. Pineal Res.* 39, 294-301.

[11] Berger, U.V., and Hediger, M.A. (2000). Distribution of the glutamate transporters GLAST and GLT-1 in rat circumventricular organs, meninges, and dorsal root ganglia. *J. Comp. Neurol.* 421, 385-399.

[12] Moriyama, Y., and Yamamoto, A. (1995). Microvesicles isolated from bovine pineal gland specifically accumulate-glutamate. *FEBS letters* 367, 233-236.

[13] Moriyama, Y., and Yamamoto, A. (1995). Vesicular L-glutamate transporter in microvesicles from bovine pineal glands. *J. Biol. Chem.* 270, 22314-22320.

[14] Yamada, H., Yamamoto, A., Yodozawa, S., Kozaki, S., Takahashi, M., Morita, M., Michibata, H., Furuichi, T., Mikoshiba, K., and Moriyama, Y. (1996). Microvesicle-mediated exocytosis of glutamate is a novel paracrine-like chemical transduction mechanism and inhibits melatonin secretion in rat pinealocytes. *J. Pineal Res.* 21, 175-191.

[15] Yatsushiro, S., Yamada, H., Kozaki, S., Kumon, H., Michibata, H., Yamamoto, A., and Moriyama, Y. (1997). L-aspartate but not the D form is secreted through microvesicle-mediated exocytosis and is sequestered through Na^+-dependent transporter in rat pinealocytes. *J. Neurochem.* 69, 340-347.

[16] Fremeau, R.T., Jr., Voglmaier, S., Seal, R.P., and Edwards, R.H. (2004). VGLUTs define subsets of excitatory neurons and suggest novel roles for glutamate. *Trends Neurosci.* 27, 98-103.

[17] Moriyama, Y., and Yamamoto, A. (2004). Glutamatergic chemical transmission: look! Here, there, and anywhere. *J. Biochem.* 135, 155-163.

[18] Ni, B., Rosteck, P.R., Nadi, N.S., and Paul, S.M. (1994). Cloning and expression of a cDNA encoding a brain-specific Na^+-dependent inorganic phosphate cotransporter. *Proc. Natl. Acad. Sci. U S A.* 91, 5607-5611.

[19] Bellocchio, E.E., Hu, H., Pohorille, A., Chan, J., Pickel, V.M., and Edwards, R.H. (1998). The localization of the brain-specific inorganic phosphate transporter suggests a specific presynaptic role in glutamatergic transmission. *J. Neurosci.* 18, 8648-8659.

[20] Bellocchio, E.E., Reimer, R.J., Fremeau Jr, R.T., and Edwards, R.H. (2000). Uptake of glutamate into synaptic vesicles by an inorganic phosphate transporter. *Science* 289, 957-960.

[21] Takamori, S., Rhee, J.S., Rosenmund, C., and Jahn, R. (2000). Identification of a vesicular glutamate transporter that defines a glutamatergic phenotype in neurons. *Nature* 407, 189-194.

[22] Aihara, Y., Mashima, H., Onda, H., Hisano, S., Kasuya, H., Hori, T., Yamada, S., Tomura, H., Yamada, Y., and Inoue, I. (2000). Molecular cloning of a novel brain-type Na^+-dependent inorganic phosphate cotransporter. *J. Neurochem.* 74, 2622-2625.

[23] Bai, L., Xu, H., Collins, J.F., and Ghishan, F.K. (2001). Molecular and functional analysis of a novel neuronal vesicular glutamate transporter. *J. Biol. Chem.* 276, 36764-36769.

[24] Hayashi, M., Otsuka, M., Morimoto, R., Hirota, S., Yatsushiro, S., Takeda, J., Yamamoto, A., and Moriyama, Y. (2001). Differentiation-associated Na^+-dependent inorganic phosphate cotransporter (DNPI) is a vesicular glutamate transporter in endocrine glutamatergic systems. *J. Biol. Chem.* 276, 43400.

[25] Herzog, E., Bellenchi, G.C., Gras, C., Bernard, V., Ravassard, P., Bedet, C., Gasnier, B., Giros, B., and El Mestikawy, S. (2001). The existence of a second vesicular glutamate transporter specifies subpopulations of glutamatergic neurons. *J. Neurosci.* 21, RC181.

[26] Takamori, S., Rhee, J.S., Rosenmund, C., and Jahn, R. (2001). Identification of differentiation-associated brain-specific phosphate transporter as a second vesicular glutamate transporter (VGLUT2). *J. Neurosci.* 21, RC182.

[27] Varoqui, H., Schäfer, M.K., Zhu, H., Weihe, E., and Erickson, J.D. (2002). Identification of the differentiation-associated Na^+/PI transporter as a novel vesicular glutamate transporter expressed in a distinct set of glutamatergic synapses. *J. Neurosci.* 22, 142-155.

[28] Fremeau, R.T., Burman, J., Qureshi, T., Tran, C.H., Proctor, J., Johnson, J., Zhang, H., Sulzer, D., Copenhagen, D.R., and Storm-Mathisen, J. (2002). The identification of vesicular glutamate transporter 3 suggests novel modes of signaling by glutamate. *Proc. Natl. Acad. Sci. U S A.* 99, 14488-14493.

[29] Gras, C., Herzog, E., Bellenchi, G.C., Bernard, V., Ravassard, P., Pohl, M., Gasnier, B., Giros, B., and El Mestikawy, S. (2002). A third vesicular glutamate transporter expressed by cholinergic and serotoninergic neurons. *J. Neurosci.* 22, 5442-5451.

[30] Schäfer, M.K., Varoqui, H., Defamie, N., Weihe, E., and Erickson, J.D. (2002). Molecular cloning and functional identification of mouse vesicular glutamate transporter 3 and its expression in subsets of novel excitatory neurons. *J. Biol. Chem.* 277, 50734-50748.

[31] Takamori, S., Malherbe, P., Broger, C., and Jahn, R. (2002). Molecular cloning and functional characterization of human vesicular glutamate transporter 3. *EMBO Reports* 3, 798-803.

[32] Morimoto, R., Hayashi, M., Yatsushiro, S., Otsuka, M., Yamamoto, A., and Moriyama, Y. (2003). Co-expression of vesicular glutamate transporters (VGLUT1 and VGLUT2) and their association with synaptic-like microvesicles in rat pinealocytes. *J. Neurochem.* 84, 382-391.

[33] Nogami, H., Ogasawara, K., Mimura, Y., Mogi, K., Shutoh, F., and Hisano, S. (2006). Developmentally-regulated expression of tissue-specific splice variant of rat vesicular glutamate transporter 1 in retina and pineal gland. *J. Neurochem.* 99, 142-153.

[34] Yoshida, S., Ina, A., Konno, J., Wu, T., Shutoh, F., Nogami, H., and Hisano, S. (2008). The ontogenic expressions of multiple vesicular glutamate transporters during postnatal development of rat pineal gland. *Neuroscience* 152, 407-416.

[35] Yoshida, S., Hira, Y., Ehara, A., Mimura-Yamamoto, Y., Kawano, M., Shutoh, F., Nogami, H., and Hisano, S. (2012). A rhythmic change of vesicular glutamate transporter (VGLUT) 2 expression in the rat pineal gland. *Neurosci. Res.* 72, 16-22.

[36] Jahn, R., Schiebler, W., Ouimet, C., and Greengard, P. (1985). A 38,000-dalton membrane protein (p38) present in synaptic vesicles. *Proc. Natl. Acad. Sci. U S A*. 82, 4137.

[37] Wiedenmann, B., and Franke, W.W. (1985). Identification and localization of synaptophysin, an integral membrane glycoprotein of Mr 38,000 characteristic of presynaptic vesicles. *Cell* 41, 1017.

[38] Redecker, P. (2000). Expression of synaptic vesicle trafficking proteins in the developing rat pineal gland. *Cell Tissue Res*. 301, 255-265.

[39] Ringstad, N., Nemoto, Y., and De Camilli, P. (1997). The SH3p4/Sh3p8/SH3p13 protein family: binding partners for synaptojanin and dynamin via a Grb2-like Src homology 3 domain. *Proc. Natl. Acad. Sci. U S A*. 94, 8569.

[40] De Gois, S., Jeanclos, E., Morris, M., Grewal, S., Varoqui, H., and Erickson, J.D. (2006). Identification of endophilins 1 and 3 as selective binding partners for VGLUT1 and their co-localization in neocortical glutamatergic synapses: implications for vesicular glutamate transporter trafficking and excitatory vesicle formation. *Cell Mol. Neurobiol*. 26, 677-691.

[41] Vinatier, J., Herzog, E., Plamont, M.A., Wojcik, S.M., Schmidt, A., Brose, N., Daviet, L., El Mestikawy, S., and Giros, B. (2006). Interaction between the vesicular glutamate transporter type 1 and endophilin A1, a protein essential for endocytosis. *J. Neurochem*. 97, 1111-1125.

[42] Yoshida, S., and Hisano, S. (2012). Vesicular glutamate transporter 2 expression in the rat pineal gland: detailed analysis of expression pattern and regulatory mechanism. *Kansei Eng. Int. J.* in press.

[43] Zimmerman, B.L., and Tso, M.O.M. (1975). Morphologic evidence of photoreceptor differentiation of pinealocytes in the neonatal rat. *J. Cell Biol*. 66, 60-75.

[44] Zweig, M., Snyder, S.H., and Axelrod, J. (1966). Evidence for a nonretinal pathway of light to the pineal gland of newborn rats. *Proc. Natl. Acad. Sci. U S A*. 56, 515.

[45] Morgans, C.W. (2000). Neurotransmitter release at ribbon synapses in the retina. *Immunol. Cell Biol*. 78, 442-446.

[46] Klein, D.C., Namboodiri, M.A., and Auerbach, D.A. (1981). The melatonin rhythm generating system: developmental aspects. *Life Sci*. 28, 1975-1986.

[47] Ellison, N., Weller, J.L., and Klein, D.C. (1972). Development of a circadian rhythm in the activity of pineal serotonin N-acetyltransferase. *J. Neurochem*. 19, 1335-1341.

[48] Pfeffer, M., Kuhn, R., Krug, L., Korf, H.W., and Stehle, J.H. (1998). Rhythmic variation in b1-adrenergic receptor mRNA levels in the rat pineal gland: circadian and developmental regulation. *Eur. J. Neurosci*. 10, 2896-2904.

[49] Klein, D.C., and Moore, R.Y. (1979). Pineal N-acetyltransferase and hydroxyindole-O-methyl-transferase: control by the retinohypothalamic tract and the suprachiasmatic nucleus. *Brain Res*. 174, 245-262.

[50] Bailey, M.J., Coon, S.L., Carter, D.A., Humphries, A., Kim, J., Shi, Q., Gaildrat, P., Morin, F., Ganguly, S., and Hogenesch, J.B. (2009). Night/Day changes in pineal expression of > 600 genes. *J. Biol. Chem*. 284, 7606-7622.

[51] Meijer, J., and Rietveld, W. (1989). Neurophysiology of the suprachiasmatic circadian pacemaker in rodents. *Physiol. Rev*. 69, 671-707.

[52] Wilson, N.R., Kang, J., Hueske, E.V., Leung, T., Varoqui, H., Murnick, J.G., Erickson, J.D., and Liu, G. (2005). Presynaptic regulation of quantal size by the vesicular glutamate transporter VGLUT1. *J. Neurosci.* 25, 6221-6234.

[53] Moechars, D., Weston, M.C., Leo, S., Callaerts-Vegh, Z., Goris, I., Daneels, G., Buist, A., Cik, M., van der Spek, P., Kass, S., et al. (2006). Vesicular glutamate transporter VGLUT2 expression levels control quantal size and neuropathic pain. *J. Neurosci.* 26, 12055-12066.

[54] Kim, J.S., Bailey, M.J., Ho, A.K., Moller, M., Gaildrat, P., and Klein, D.C. (2007). Daily rhythm in pineal phosphodiesterase (PDE) activity reflects adrenergic/3',5'-cyclic adenosine 5'-monophosphate induction of the PDE4B2 variant. *Endocrinology* 148, 1475-1485.

[55] Yamada, H., Yatsushiro, S., Ishio, S., Hayashi, M., Nishi, T., Yamamoto, A., Futai, M., Yamaguchi, A., and Moriyama, Y. (1998). Metabotropic glutamate receptors negatively regulate melatonin synthesis in rat pinealocytes. *J. Neurosci.* 18, 2056-2062.

[56] Pfeffer, M., Maronde, E., Molina, C.A., Korf, H.W., and Stehle, J.H. (1999). Inducible cyclic AMP early repressor protein in rat pinealocytes: a highly sensitive natural reporter for regulated gene transcription. *Mol. Pharmacol.* 56, 279-289.

[57] Gupta, B.B., Spessert, R., and Vollrath, L. (2005). Molecular components and mechanism of adrenergic signal transduction in mammalian pineal gland: regulation of melatonin synthesis. *Indian J. Exp. Biol.* 43, 115-149.

[58] Govitrapong, P., and Ebadi, M. (1988). The inhibition of pineal arylalkylamine n-acetyltransferase by glutamic acid and its analogues. *Neurochem. Int.* 13, 223-230.

In: New Developments in Melatonin Research ISBN: 978-1-62618-843-3
Editors: D.Acuña-Castroviejo, I.Rusanova, G.Escames © 2013 Nova Science Publishers, Inc.

Chapter 13

Melatonin in Bipolar Disorders

Ana C. García Blanco*[1, 2*]*, Pilar Sierra San Miguel*[1]*,
Lorenzo Livianos Aldana*[1, 2]*, Sergio Arqués Egea*[1,]
***and Luis Rojo Moreno*[1,2]**

[1]Servicio de Psiquiatría, Hospital Universitari i Politècnic la Fe, Valencia, Spain
[2]Universitat de València, Valencia, Spain

Abstract

Biological rhythms research shows that individuals who are born with an arrhythmic clock present an increased risk for developing mood disorders. Evidence points to irregular biological rhythms in bipolar disorder, such as sleep-wake cycles, temperature, melatonin, and cortisol rhythms. The importance of sleep disturbance in bipolar disorder even when mood symptoms are under control between affective episodes has been proved in several studies. During manic episodes, for example, there is a reduced need for sleep, whereas episodes of depression can involve either insomnia or hypersomnia. Sleep disturbances often persist despite treatment, and an important number of euthymic bipolar patients exhibit clinically significant sleep disturbance. Circulating melatonin is a main synchronizer of the sleep/wake cycle control and human mood and behavior. Exogenous melatonin exerts a therapeutic effect in bipolar patients by normalizing the sleep/wake cycle and may improve both sleep duration and quality and, in addition, recent research has shown that exogenous melatonin can have a marked improvement in affective symptoms. Thus, drugs that act on the melatonin receptor, such as ramelteon or agomelatina and exogenous melatonin, may be effective for the management of bipolar, particularly in patients with comorbid substance use, as these agents are not associated with any risk of abuse. In sum, in this review we can conclude that melatonin can be a useful treatment as adjunctive therapy in bipolar patients with sleep alterations and helping in clinical stabilization.

[*] Corresponding author: Ana C. García-Blanco, Universitat de València, Av. Blasco Ibáñez, 21, 46010 Valencia (Spain). Teléfono: +34 963 864547; Fax: +34 963 864697; Email: ana.garcia-blanco@uv.es.

Introduction

In normal subjects, the secretion of melatonin - the pineal hormone that regulates the rhythm of many functions- exhibits a circadian pattern synchronized with the day–night cycle, but as far as some psychiatric disorders are concerned, alterations of the pattern of pineal secretion have been reported. Thus, biological rhythm disturbances have been put forward as relevant factors in the emergence of psychiatric disorders [1;2]. Specifically, several lines of evidence indicate that individuals who are born with an arrhythmic clock, such as sleep-wake cycles, temperature, melatonin, and cortisol rhythms present an increased risk for developing mood disorders [3;4].

Mood disorders comprise a group of psychiatric disorders in which pathological mood are the main feature. The most common mood disorders are major depressive disorder, bipolar disorder and seasonal affective disorder. The episodes are sustained over a period of weeks to months and recur often in a period or in a cyclical trend. Since mood disorders are cyclic in nature, disturbances in circadian rhythms have been often implicated as one of the major precipitating factors for these disorders. However, it is not clear whether this relationship is causal or is only an epiphenomenon of the disease.

This review discusses the role of melatonin in mood disorders with emphasis in bipolar disorder due to the clinical relevance of internal timing in this illness. Periodic episodes of depression and mania are usually linked to disorders of the time-keeping system. In the same way, the cyclic nature of bipolar disorder notices for the diurnal and seasonal variations in its symptomatology and the existence of disturbed sleep-wake and core body temperature rhythms. In fact, the sleep–wake cycle has been a core component of theoretical concept-ualizations of bipolar disorder, and circadian rhythm instability is a frequent complaint in these patients. It has been hypothesized that bipolar disorder patients have a genetic diatheses that may take the form of circadian rhythm instability [5]. Many studies place emphasis on the importance of stable sleep-wake rhythms and proper sleep hygiene for preventing relapses in bipolar disorders [6]. Chronotherapeutic strategies based on controlled exposures to environmental stimuli that act on biological rhythms have shown good efficacy in the treatment of illness episodes. Thus, dysregulation of circadian rhythms and sleep disturbances might be involved in its pathogenesis.

Sleep and Bipolar Disorder

Bipolar disorder is a chronic, severe, and highly disabling psychiatric disorder which affects approximately 1% of the world population. These individuals experience intermittent abnormally elevated [manic] states and, in many cases, abnormally low [depressed] ones – between these extremes, patients can experience symptom-free states of euthymia [7]. Commonly misconceived as a relatively treatment-responsive condition, this illness is characterized by frequent recurrence and incomplete recovery [8], that is, cognitive dysfunction [9], deficits in emotional processing [10], poor functioning [11] and difficulties with social and interpersonal relationships [12] that persist even in euthymic states. During acute episodes, mood and psychotic symptoms possibly explain most of functional impairment. Dysfunction, however, remains in the interepisodic period and mechanisms leading to this state are inadequately comprehended.

Sleep disorders have been proposed to lead to functional impairment and episode recurrence [11;13]. Sleep disorders are a chronic and prevalent problem in patients with bipolar disorder, regardless of their episode [14;15]. It's known that sleep is an active state, critical for our physical, mental and emotional well-being and is favorable for brain plasticity [16-18]. Further, sleep is important for optimal cognitive and overall functioning [19]. In the absence of bipolar disorder, poor sleep is known to have significant negative psychosocial, occupational, health, mood, motivation, cognitive functioning and economic effects [20]. Sleep disorder coexists with a number of physical and psychiatric conditions, including psychoses, anxiety disorders, and mood disorders [19;21;22], with an impact in daytime functioning [23]. Several lines of evidence highlight the importance of sleep disturbance in bipolar disorder. Sleep disturbance is a core symptom of bipolar disorder and is exhibited across mood phases. During manic episodes, for example, there is a reduced need for sleep, whereas episodes of depression can involve either insomnia or hypersomnia. Furthermore, even when their mood symptoms are under control between affective episodes, sleep problems are present [24], which can cause considerable subjective distress, metabolic disorders, impairment in cognition and daytime dysfunction.

Sleep in Eutimia

Harvey et al. [5] examined sleep and actigraphy data from euthymic bipolar patients, patients with insomnia and subjects with good sleep. They found that 70% of the euthymic bipolar patients exhibited a clinically significant sleep disturbance despite treatment and sleep alteration was associated with low daytime activity levels. Moreover, the sleep pattern exhibited by the remitted bipolar group resembles more closely that of an insomnia comparison group than a group of subjects with normal sleep. Thus, the euthymic bipolar patients exhibited diminished sleep efficiency, increased anxiety and fear about poor sleep, decreased daytime activity levels, and a tendency to misperceive sleep, with levels of dysfunctional beliefs about sleep comparable to the insomnia group. Jones et al. [25], using actigraphy, observed that the euthymic bipolar group exhibited more fragmentation of the sleep/wake rhythm and less day-to-day stability relative to comparison subjects. Other study, using sleep diaries and actigraphy, found that euthymic bipolar patients, compared to healthy individuals, exhibited long sleep duration and greater sleep variability [26]. Knowles et al. [27], using polysomnography, observed more shifts to stage I, more frequent arousals in the former and more awake or movement time relative to comparison subjects. Finally, Sitaram et al. [28], using polysomnography, reported higher REM density during the first REM episode and higher percentage of REM sleep in their bipolar group relative to healthy comparison subjects.

Sleep in Bipolar Depression

In spite of their importance, the differences between sleep disorder in bipolar and unipolar depression are not clearly-defined. Some clinicians believe that hypersomnia, rather than insomnia, is more indicative of bipolar than unipolar depression [29-31] with one study reporting insomnia in 100% of depressed bipolar patients [32]. Insomnia, as well as hypersomnia, with prolonged nighttime sleep, difficulty in awakening, and excessive daytime sleepiness is often experienced by depressive bipolar patients [13]. However, bipolar hypersomnolence is more reflective of anergia/fatigue than the true excessive sleepiness seen in other primary sleep disorders [33].

Unfortunately, objective studies of sleep quality in bipolar depression have not been able to clear up this question. Across the polysomnography studies [34-41], a remarkable lack of consensus is evident [42]. This line of research has generally found similar abnormalities in unipolar and bipolar depression, although limited data suggest that bipolar patients may have more early morning awakenings and greater total REM density than unipolar comparison subjects when matched for age, gender, and severity of symptoms [43].

Sleep in Mania

Sleep disturbances are often linked with depression, but a profound alteration of circadian rhythm of sleep is often also a central feature in mania [44]. During episodes of mania, the majority of patients [69%–99%] experience reduced need for sleep or do not sleep at all for even very long periods [3-4 days] [32;45-49]. Only one study was identified that monitored sleep during a mixed episode [46]; reduced need for sleep was the common sleep disturbance. As last note, prior reports have also noted that some patients with rapid cycling bipolar disorder also have irregular sleep wake syndrome or non-24 h sleep–wake cycles [50;51].

Polysomnography as objective measure was conducted in some studies. Despite the fact that the sample sizes for these studies were small, an association between REM sleep and mania in unmedicated patients was evident across most [52-54], indicating shortened total sleep time, increased time awake in bed, and shortened REM latency. This is interesting because REM sleep has been associated with affective functioning [42]. However, we must keep in mind that polysomnographic measures in manic patients may be affected by motor hyperactivity during the day, since sleep architecture can be affected by increased daytime activity in normal subjects [55;56].

Four Reasons for Maintaining Normal Sleep in Bipolar Patients

1. Sleep Disorders Predict Daytime Functioning

Giglio et al. [14] found that sleep complaints have negative influence on general quality of life and global function. On the matter, Gruber et al. [57] reported that short sleep duration in bipolar disorder was associated with a more severe symptom presentation, whereas both short and long sleep duration are associated with poorer function and quality of life compared to normal sleep duration. In concordance with these results, Giglio et al. [58] concluded that biological rhythm dysfunction was a potent predictor of functioning in interepisodic patients with bipolar disorder.

If we consider depressive episode, both sleep disturbance and depressive symptoms are especially related to exhaustion, fatigue, and reports of extra bed time [59]. Individuals with both depressive symptoms and sleep complaints showed lower quality of life and more difficulties in work activities than patients without mood symptoms [23]. Although a body of evidence reported that quality of life was inversely correlated with the level of depression, a comparison study between bipolar and unipolar patients suggested that the level of depression did not fully explain the lower quality of life within patients with bipolar disorder [60;61]. Sleep alteration is a nuclear factor that contributes to low quality of life experience by bipolar patients, unlike patients with unipolar depression. So, interventions for directly addressing sleep and rhythm disturbance may improve both interepisodic and intraepisodic functional outcome in bipolar disorder.

2. Sleep Disturbance Contributes to Relapse in Bipolar Disorder

Primary goals of the treatment of bipolar disorder are to stabilize the patient and prevent the recurrence of episodes [62]. However, despite patients continue the adherence to medication regimens, the risk of relapse over a 5-year period has been estimated to be as high as 73% [63]. For this reason, it is important to enhance our understanding of precipitants of mood episodes and mechanisms that may contribute to inter-episode dysfunction [64].

Impaired sleep may represent vulnerability to relapse into pathological phases of illness. In a systematic review of 11 studies involving 631 patients with bipolar disorder, sleep disturbance was the most common prodrome of mania [reported by 77% of patients] and the sixth most common prodrome of bipolar depression [reported by 24% of patients] [65]. While prodromal symptoms may often be idiosyncratic [66], sleep disturbances were reported to be the most prominent early symptom of mania, and a frequent early symptom of depression [67].

The early identification of prodromal symptoms of mania or depression can allow rapid interventions that mitigate relapses and improve patient functioning. Although this hypothesis is unproven, given the information previously presented connecting both mania and bipolar depression to sleep, sleep disturbance may be a potential therapeutic target in the clinical management of the bipolar patient during the euthymic period.

3. Manipulation of the Circadian Rhythm Can Act as Antidepressive and Antimanic

Alterations to the sleep–wake cycle, whether naturally occurring or manipulated, have been associated repeatedly with strong and immediate changes in mood in patients with bipolar disorder; even these alterations may precipitate mood episodes [68;69]. Besides pharmacological approaches, manipulation of the circadian system has also been used to shorten the manic episode and maintain the antidepressant effects through sleep deprivation in bipolar depression.

For example, prolonged bed rest in darkness has stabilized patients with refractory rapid cycling in two case reports [51;70], and improved the sleep and shortened the episode length in a pilot study of inpatients with mania [71]. Instead, experimentally induced sleep deprivation is associated with reductions in depressive symptoms and the onset of hypomania or mania [72-80]. Bright light in the morning has been shown to sustain antidepressant response to sleep deprivation in bipolar patients and may decrease hospitalization time [81-83]. Furthermore, phase advance [e.g., moving the sleep period several hours earlier than usual] of the sleep period after sleep deprivation has been shown to sustain the antidepressant effects of sleep deprivation in both unipolar and bipolar subjects [84-87].

Interestingly, lower levels of illumination in post-menopausal women have been reported to be associated with more complaints of sleep and depressive symptoms [88] whereas post-partum depression was already suggested as a possible marker/predictor of bipolar depression [89]. Bright light treatment of women suffering from ante-partum depression advanced the rhythm of melatonin secretion and also mitigated depressive symptoms [90].

These studies suggest the possibility that neurobiological substrates underlying bipolar depression might change over the course of the illness, making the depressed phase more amenable to treatment with sleep deprivation [91]. Given that symptoms of depression quickly return after the patient has slept, several approaches are being studied in the hope of extending the therapeutic effects of sleep deprivation by combining it with antidepressant medications, lithium and light therapy, showing promising initial results [84].

4. Sleep is a Critical Factor for Affect Regulation

In healthy participants, Dinges et al. [92] found that mood progressively declined due to sleep deprivation accumulated throughout the week. Drake et al. [93] compared the mood responses of participants across four sleep deprivation conditions. Greater mood impairment was evident in the rapid sleep loss group [0 hours in bed] as opposed to the slow, cumulative sleep loss group [6 hours in bed for 4 nights], who experienced more impairment relative to the control group [no sleep loss for 4 nights]. Zohar et al. [94] found that context is important for determining the direction of the effect of sleep disturbance on affective functioning: sleep loss appears to intensify negative emotions following a goal-thwarting event as well as to diminish positive emotions following a goal-enhancing event.

Although these studies were conducted with healthy volunteers, the observed effects may be greater in patients with bipolar disorder, who presumably have a more vulnerable affect-regulation system. Bauer et al. [68] found that in most patients with bipolar disorder with a significant cross correlation between sleep and/or bed rest and mood, the mood change occurred on the day following the change in sleep and/or bed rest. Sleep changes from a previous pattern, especially those of more than 3 h, may indicate that a large mood change is imminent. This study found too that a decrease in sleep or bed rest was followed by a shift toward hypomania or mania the next day and that an increase in sleep or bed rest was followed by a shift toward depression the next day. The one day latency between the change in sleep and the change in mood is consistent with a marked reduction in sleep during the night immediately before switching from depression to mania [95], with prior reports of sleep loss triggering and intensifying mania at the episode onset [56;96], with one night of total or partial sleep deprivation producing an antidepressant response on the following day [78], and with sleep loss preceding a switch to mania on the following day in patients with rapid cycling [97].

The relationship between mania and sleep loss is particularly apparent at the beginning of a manic episode [98]. At the beginning of a manic episode, clinicians often observe spontaneous sleep deprivation, due to the hyperactivity of the patient, resulting in an increase in manic symptomatology and then in subsequent sleep loss. Thus, sleep loss appears to act not only as a triggering factor of mania, but also as an augmenting factor during the manic episode, with worse symptomatological outcomes following consistent sleep loss [96]. However, Perlman et al. [99], using a prospective, longitudinal design did not find an association between sleep and mania, instead, shorter sleep duration predicted greater depressive symptoms during 6-month follow-up but not manic symptoms. The authors noted several methodological mistakes as possible reason for the lack of this association: manic patients were less likely to complete the sleep measure and self-report of sleep duration were made at monthly intervals, which may not have been frequent enough to detect a relationship between sleep and mania.

These studies all report an association between sleep disturbance and mood, although the nature of the association -particularly whether it is stronger for manic or depressive symptoms- is less consistent. Anyway, Gruber et al. [57] reported that short sleep duration in bipolar disorder was associated with a more severe symptom presentation. Thus, the control of chronic insomnia in patients with bipolar disorder may be a clinically useful therapeutic target because chronic insomnia can cause or exacerbate affective symptoms [56;74;100] and can also increase the risk of suicide [103].

Melatonin as Synchronizer of the Sleep/Wake Cycle

Dysregulation of the sleep–wake cycle and other circadian rhythms may underlie the pathophysiology of bipolar disorder [50;78]. The pattern of periodic recurrence, linked with seasonal or hormonal cycles, characteristic sleep disturbances or diurnal mood fluctuations stimulated specific hypotheses, but the question whether altered biological rhythms in mood disorders reflect an underlying disturbance in “biological clock” is yet unresolved [44].

Several genes known to be important in the generation and regulation of circadian rhythms and the sleep system are associated with bipolar disorder, including Timeless, Clock [311 T to C], and BMal1. These associations are modest, which is consistent with the proposal that bipolar disorder is likely to be associated with multiple genes of small effect [101]. It has been suggested that genetic factors may confer an underlying chronobiological vulnerability for bipolar disorder [102].

The “master clock” is located in the suprachiasmatic nucleus in the anterior hypothalamus. The suprachiasmatic nucleus governs all circadian rhythms and is supplemented by a large number of peripheral clocks across organs and cells. When the system is in harmony, it is fully synchronized by the suprachiasmatic nucleus. But there are many inputs that can influence and contribute to harmony and dysregulation across systems [103]. Theoretically, desynchronization of internal circadian phase and the environment through genetic polymorphism could increase the risk of affective episodes in some bipolar patients. Specifically, the disturbance of circadian rhythms seen in bipolar disorders can be due to disturbance in the function of the suprachiasmatic nucleus – pineal gland – melatonin link.

In this line, melatonin is considered an input which can influence on circadian system and can alter sleep-wake rhythm. Melatonin is an endogenous neurohormone secreted by the pineal gland in a circadian fashion under conditions of darkness, whereas light inhibits its secretion, although the environmental light does not cause the rhythm but only alters its timing. Melatonin secretion reflects signals originating in the suprachiasmatic nucleus [104], the circadian pacemaker, through which photic information from the retina is transmitted to the pineal gland [105], and is also depending upon the genetically determined rhythmic activation of the N-acetyltransferase enzyme in the pinealocyte [106]. The neurotransmitter input to the gland is norepinephrine and the output is melatonin. Melatonin alters the timing of sleep in part by its effect on central circadian pacemaker in the suprachiasmatic nucleus in order to modify the phase of the internal clock [107]. In addition, melatonin action on sleep may also be due to its well known and potent core temperature lowering effect [108].

As a rhythm-regulating factor and as a hormone involved in the physiological regulation of the sleep-wake rhythm, the study of melatonin has gained the attention of investigators interested in bipolar affective disorders. In view of its central role as an internal synchronizer, melatonin meets more appropriately with bipolar illness than with any other type of psychiatric disorder. In fact, significant alterations in levels of melatonin secretion or also in the timing of melatonin secretion have been documented in bipolar patients. These melatonin deficits can be both a "state marker" and a "trait marker" of bipolar disorder.

Melatonin sensitivity to light is one circadian endophenotype proposed as useful in bipolar disorder, particularly in light of evidence that the occurrence of this sensitivity increases in those with high genetic loading for the bipolar affective disorder [109]. It has been observed that bipolar disorder might have a "trait marker" of hypersensitivity of melatonin receptors [110-112]. Anyway, this could be contrasted with drug-free recovered bipolar individuals not showing light hypersensitivity [113]. While methodological differences may account for the variance between studies, more recent research by Nurnberger et al. [114] provides a possible explanation. By comparing euthymic bipolar patients, patients with unipolar depression and non-psychiatrically ill control subjects, these authors did not find differences (a 29.8, 32.2 and 34.6% of light induced melatonin suppression, respectively). However, when bipolar patients were sub-divided into types I and II, patients with bipolar I disorder showed a trend towards increased dark-adjusted melatonin suppression (62.7%) as compared to matched controls [40.0%], reaffirming the evidence for increased suppression of melatonin secretion in bipolar I sub-group patients. Additionally, there are melatonin level studies which support melatonin alterations hypothesis as "trait marker". Kennedy et al. [115], studying bipolar patients during manic, depressed and euthymic stages, found that melatonin levels were lower in bipolar patients than healthy normal controls, regardless of their episode. The authors concluded that the decreased melatonin production is a trait marker and not a state marker of bipolar disorders. Likewise, Wahlund et al. [116] found evidence in favor of this hypothesis: carriers of latent bipolar disease trait are characterized by a cluster of clinical and biochemical variables [melatonin level], which conceivably might have identified this population at the time of the first depressive episode. What is more, studies based on timing of melatonin have supported this hypothesis about possible endophenotype of bipolar disorder. In a more recent study, euthymic bipolar patients exhibited not only lower melatonin levels but a later peak time for melatonin during the night relative to a healthy comparison group [114]. Indeed, the credibility of this hypothesis would increase if we consider the heredability of melatonin secretion. In relation to this, Hallam et al. [117] reported that melatonin secretion is highly heritable with the greatest concordance between monozygotic twins, followed by dizygotic twins and finally low concordance in unrelated individuals.

In contrast, numerous studies have supported the melatonin alterations hypothesis as "state marker", i.e., the level or the phase of melatonin secretion varies systematically with mood changes in bipolar affective disorder. Comparing unipolar and bipolar depressive patients, Beck-Friis et al. [118] noted significantly lower melatonin levels in euthymic bipolar patients. Souetre et al. [119] found less amplitude of melatonin secretion during the depressive episode that returned to normal on remission in bipolar patients. In a longitudinal single-case study, a rise in melatonin secretion was reported during manic phase that was twice that of melatonin levels during the euthymia and depressed states [120]. Timing of melatonin secretion studies reflect that it is also state-dependent. Lewy et al. were the first to note an advance phase position of melatonin levels in manic patients when compared to healthy participants [121]. In a longitudinal study of a single manic patient, Kennedy et al. noted a phase advance of the nocturnal melatonin highest point during the manic phase that preceded that of the euthymic or depressed states by at least 1 h [120].

Both hypotheses, although are not exclusive, need convincing evidence, awaiting future studies. The significance of the association of sleep disturbances and melatonin levels in bipolar patients is still far away from a satisfactory knowledge. Anyway, both hypotheses reflect the importance of melatonin in bipolar disorders.

Melatonin Treatment in Bipolar Disorders

The stabilization of biological rhythms is regarded as an important goal in preventing illness recurrence [1;3], for example, by means of novel therapies targeting biological rhythm pathways, including light therapy [122] or psychosocial interventions such as interpersonal and social rhythm therapy [1;123] or drugs such as agomelatine [124], lithium [125;126] and melatonin [114].

In spite of melatonin having an endogenous origin, it may be altered (according to the chronobiological principles) through exposure to bright light or administration of exogenous melatonin. This manipulation exerts a therapeutic effect by normalizing the sleep / wake cycle due to melatonin is "hands" of the circadian clock that modulate the sleep-wake cycle.

An Indirect Melatonin Treatment: Bright Light Therapy as Regulating Endogenous Melatonin Secretion

Several studies have demonstrated that bipolar patients can be treated with exposure to bright light according to the chronobiological principles. The natural light dark cycle plays an important role in regulating circadian rhythms. Retinal stimulation by light sends a tonic stimulatory signal to the suprachiasmatic nucleus. In turn, the suprachiasmatic nucleus inhibits the firing of neurons in the paraventricular nucleus to regulate melatonin secretion by the pineal gland. During nighttime hours, when the suprachiasmatic nucleus is not stimulated by light, the neurons of the paraventricular nucleus are released from suprachiasmatic nucleus inhibition and pineal melatonin secretion is stimulated.

Lewy et al. [121] were the first to demonstrate that light of intensity higher than 500 lux suppresses melatonin secretion in human beings. More specifically, bright light can shift melatonin levels in humans, with morning light advancing the melatonin rhythm and evening light delaying melatonin rhythm [127].

Subsequently, several studies have demonstrated that inhibition of melatonin by light was greater in bipolar patients than in healthy subjects. An early study showed that suppression of melatonin secretion by 500-lux light caused a 50% suppression of melatonin levels in bipolar patients, but had no effect in controls [128]. In another study, exposure to 500 lux of light at 02:00 and 04:00 h caused suppression of melatonin by 61.5% of euthymic bipolar patients as compared to age- and sex-matched healthy volunteers, in which exposure to light caused only 28% suppression of melatonin secretion [111].

In conclusion, an increased sensitivity to light might be a trait marker for bipolar affective disorder. The fact that some normal subjects also exhibited increased sensitivity to light, pointed to the possibility that those normal individuals which were noted for excessive light-induced suppression of melatonin secretion and may have a risk factor for development of a mood disorder.

Therefore, an increased responsiveness to light in bipolar disorder could explain the circadian rhythm abnormalities (such as phase advances in temperature or REM sleep rhythms). What remains to be established is what mechanism mediates this light-induced suppression response.

In view of the role of light in circadian system, bright light therapy as suppressor of melatonin production may become a well consolidated treatment in bipolar affective disorder. In this line, three meta-analyses published by Cochrane databases support the efficacy of light therapy in mood disorders [129-131].

A Direct Melatonin Treatment: Administration of Exogenous Melatonin

Ingestion of melatonin improves sleep propensity [136] as well as the duration and quality of sleep [132-134]. The effect of the administration of this hormone on daily biological timekeeping is dependent on the hour of the day [107]. When given in the morning, melatonin delays circadian rhythms [135] whilst in the afternoon or early evening melatonin advances circadian rhythms [136].

Several reports from the literature indicate melatonin as a hypnotic [reducing sleep latency] and hypothermic [lowering core body temperature] agent and proposed it as treatment for insomnia [137]. A dose ranging from 2 to 5 mg is described to be effective in elderly subjects with insomnia and in patients with delayed sleep-phase syndrome [138;139]. Liebenluft et al. [140] observed that the administration of 5-10 mg of melatonin in the evening [or midday administration of bright light] stabilized the phase of endogenous melatonin rhythm. Indeed, exogenous melatonin administration can be used to synchronize the sleep-wake cycle in those situations where the normal circadian cycle is altered, e.g., in blind individuals and in subjects with jet lag advanced sleep onset and delayed sleep phase syndrome [141]. Melatonin is a relatively poor hypnotic, but it seems to influence sleep patterns through its effects on phase-shifting the circadian rhythm, which suggests that this result may be mediated through the circadian system rather than the sleep homeostat [142].

In bipolar disorder, a case series of five euthymic rapid-cycling patients suggested that exogenous melatonin had little effect on mood or sleep, although melatonin withdrawal delayed sleep onset time and may have had mild mood-elevating effects [141]. Livianos et al. [143], in a prospective naturalistic study with 14 euthymic bipolar patients that suffered from insomnia, used melatonin as co-adjuvant treatment. They found that all patients experienced a sleep improvement in quantity and quality, and there was a reduction in depressive and manic subsyndromal symptoms. The use of exogenous melatonin is another novel pharmacological approach to improving sleep in manic patients. Bersani and Garavini [144] administered melatonin as a hypnotic in 11 outpatients with mania whose insomnia was resistant to benzodiazepines. No other medication changes were allowed during the 30-day open study. A dramatic improvement in subjective sleep duration was observed, concurrent with a marked improvement in manic symptoms. These results are very motivating because melatonin seems improve sleep disorder as well as mood symptoms.

Similarly, melatonin agonists, such as agomelatine and ramelteon, are particularly interesting in the context of bipolar disorder. Drugs that act on the melatonin receptor are promising because they may be useful in the management of bipolar insomnia, particularly in patients with comorbid substance use, as these agents are not associated with any risk of abuse [65;145]. Agomelatine is promising as overcoat in bipolar depression, as it is both an agonist of the melatonin receptors and an antagonist of the serotonin 5-HT2C receptor [103]. Open-label observations of agomelatine addiction to lithium or valproate in the treatment of bipolar depression showed the efficacy of the melatonergic drug at doses of 25mg/day after 6 weeks of augmentation treatment [124]. A comprehensive review by Gao et al. [146] focused on randomized controlled trials of newly introduced drugs [including agomelatine] for the acute and long-term treatment of bipolar depression. They considered that these results are not conclusive because there are not enough randomized controlled trials for confirming its efficacy. In a more recent review, Fornaro et al. [147] concluded that agomelatine has been reported to be an effective antidepressant therapy. Thus, agomelatine may be an novel option as antidepressant because its pharmacological profile does not induce the side effects related to common antidepressant prescriptions [i.e. gastrointestinal disorders, weight gain, sexual dysfunction, serotonin syndrome, insomnia, discontinuation syndrome, and others] [148]. These outcomes are encouraging because they are imposing a better recognition and management of depressive states associated with bipolar disorders. This is, symptomatic patients with BP-I disorder experience depressive symptoms three to four times more than manic symptoms [149;150] and symptomatic patients with BP-II disorder experience depressive symptoms approximately 39 times more than hypomanic ones [151].

In short, the use of agents that target the melatonin receptor is relatively novel and requires further investigation. Although melatonin and melatonin receptor agonists have shown some promise in treatment-refractory mania in rapid-cycling patients, melatonin has not been carefully studied in maintenance treatment of bipolar disorder. Finally, to what extent the changes in melatonin were related to the pharmacotherapy per se or to the improvement in the mood symptoms remains to be defined yet.

Conclusion

Bipolar disorder is a complex and multifactorial illnesses that is characterized by disruptions in the functioning of a number of physiological, neuroendocrine and behavioral processes. Sleep disturbances and dysregulation of circadian rhythms are core elements of bipolar disorder that might be involved in its pathogenesis. It has been proposed that patients with bipolar disorder have an abnormally shifted or arrhythmic circadian system and that the disturbance of circadian rhythms may be caused by an alteration in the circadian clock machinery. The disturbances in the amplitude and rhythm of melatonin secretion that occur in patients with bipolar disorder resemble those seen in subjects with chronobiological disorders. The finding that insomnia and circadian rhythm abnormalities are prominent features in bipolar illness suggests that a close link exists between melatonin secretion disturbance and mood disorder.

Chronotherapeutic strategies based on controlled exposures to environmental stimuli that act on biological rhythms have shown good efficacy in the treatment of illness episodes, thus confirming the clinical relevance of internal timing in this illness. Super sensitive response to light at night where plasma melatonin levels are suppressed to a greater degree in bipolar I patients than in patients with other affective disorders and healthy control subjects, suggests that its potential usefulness as an endophenotypic marker of the illness is deserving of further research. The use of endophenotypic markers that integrate both clinical and biological observations may provide a powerful tool to target genetic, molecular and behavioral changes in the disorder. Ideally, these observations will inform both aetiological and neurobiological studies of the disorder and ultimately improve clinical treatment of the illness. Interestingly, low doses of both lithium and valproate have been reported to reduce melatonin light sensitivity but not its overall synthesis in healthy volunteers [152;153]. There are no controlled studies with melatonin in patients with bipolar disorder. Case reports and series indicate mixed results [140;143;144]. Anyhow, in patients with vulnerability to develop bipolar disorders, lithium treatment might be considered, both as protective medication and as treatment during the acute stage of the disease episode. In turn, a combination of melatonin with lithium or valproate is reportedly more efficacious than either lithium or valproate alone in the prevention of relapses in patients with a partial or poor response to either monotherapy [89;144;146]. These observations suggest that exogenous melatonin or melatonin agonists are a viable option as co-adjuvant treatment of bipolar disorder due to its effect over sleep and mood.

References

[1] Frank E, Kupfer DJ, Thase ME, Mallinger AG, Swartz HA, Fagiolini AM, et al. Two-year outcomes for interpersonal and social rhythm therapy in individuals with bipolar I disorder. *Arch Gen Psychiatry* 2005 Sep;62(9):996-1004.

[2] McClung CA. Circadian genes, rhythms and the biology of mood disorders. *Pharmacol Ther* 2007 May;114(2):222-32.

[3] Frank E, Swartz HA, Kupfer DJ. Interpersonal and social rhythm therapy: managing the chaos of bipolar disorder. *Biol Psychiatry* 2000 Sep 15;48(6):593-604.

[4] Grandin LD, Alloy LB, Abramson LY. The social zeitgeber theory, circadian rhythms, and mood disorders: review and evaluation. *Clin Psychol Rev* 2006 Oct;26(6):679-94.

[5] Harvey AG, Schmidt DA, Scarna A, Semler CN, Goodwin GM. Sleep-related functioning in euthymic patients with bipolar disorder, patients with insomnia, and subjects without sleep problems. *Am J Psychiatry* 2005 Jan;162(1):50-7.

[6] Frank E, Hlastala S, Ritenour A, Houck P, Tu XM, Monk TH, et al. Inducing lifestyle regularity in recovering bipolar disorder patients: results from the maintenance therapies in bipolar disorder protocol. *Biol Psychiatry* 1997 Jun 15;41(12):1165-73.

[7] Belmaker RH, Bersudsky Y. Bipolar disorder: Mania and depression. *Discov Med* 2004 Oct;4(23):239-45.

[8] Vieta E, Rosa AR. Evolving trends in the long-term treatment of bipolar disorder. *World J Biol Psychiatry* 2007;8(1):4-11.
[9] Kapczinski F, Vieta E, Andreazza AC, Frey BN, Gomes FA, Tramontina J, et al. Allostatic load in bipolar disorder: implications for pathophysiology and treatment. *Neurosci Biobehav Rev* 2008;32(4):675-92.
[10] Harmer CJ, Grayson L, Goodwin GM. Enhanced recognition of disgust in bipolar illness. *Biol Psychiatry* 2002 Feb 15;51(4):298-304.
[11] Huxley N, Baldessarini RJ. Disability and its treatment in bipolar disorder patients. *Bipolar Disord* 2007 Feb;9(1-2):183-96.
[12] Kauer-Sant'Anna M, Tramontina J, Andreazza AC, Cereser K, da CS, Santin A, et al. Traumatic life events in bipolar disorder: impact on BDNF levels and psychopathology. *Bipolar Disord* 2007 Jun;9 Suppl 1:128-35.
[13] Harvey AG. A cognitive model of insomnia. *Behav Res Ther* 2002 Aug;40(8):869-93.
[14] Giglio LM, Andreazza AC, Andersen M, Cereser KM, Walz JC, Sterz L, et al. Sleep in bipolar patients. *Sleep Breath* 2009 May;13(2):169-73.
[15] Giglio LM, Magalhaes PV, Andreazza AC, Walz JC, Jakobson L, Rucci P, et al. Development and use of a biological rhythm interview. *J Affect Disord* 2009 Nov;118(1-3):161-5.
[16] Maquet P. The role of sleep in learning and memory. Science 2001 Nov 2;294(5544):1048-52.
[17] Siegel JM. The REM sleep-memory consolidation hypothesis. *Science* 2001 Nov 2;294(5544):1058-63.
[18] Stickgold R, Hobson JA, Fosse R, Fosse M. Sleep, learning, and dreams: off-line memory reprocessing. *Science* 2001 Nov 2;294(5544):1052-7.
[19] Coleman MP, Reiter RJ. Breast cancer, blindness and melatonin. *Eur J Cancer* 1992;28(2-3):501-3.
[20] Ancoli-Israel S, Roth T. Characteristics of insomnia in the United States: results of the 1991 National Sleep Foundation Survey. I. *Sleep* 1999 May 1;22 Suppl 2:S347-S353.
[21] Ancoli-Israel S. The impact and prevalence of chronic insomnia and other sleep disturbances associated with chronic illness. *Am J Manag Care* 2006 May;12(8 Suppl):S221-S229.
[22] Walsh JK. Clinical and socioeconomic correlates of insomnia. J Clin Psychiatry 2004;65 Suppl 8:13-9.
[23] Phillips B. Sleep-disordered breathing and cardiovascular disease. *Sleep Med Rev* 2005 Apr;9(2):131-40.
[24] Harvey AG. Sleep and circadian rhythms in bipolar disorder: seeking synchrony, harmony, and regulation. *Am J Psychiatry* 2008 Jul;165(7):820-9.
[25] Jones SH, Hare DJ, Evershed K. Actigraphic assessment of circadian activity and sleep patterns in bipolar disorder. *Bipolar Disord* 2005 Apr;7(2):176-86.
[26] Millar A, Espie CA, Scott J. The sleep of remitted bipolar outpatients: a controlled naturalistic study using actigraphy. *J Affect Disord* 2004 Jun;80(2-3):145-53.
[27] Knowles JB, Cairns J, MacLean AW, Delva N, Prowse A, Waldron J, et al. The sleep of remitted bipolar depressives: comparison with sex and age-matched controls. *Can J Psychiatry* 1986 May;31(4):295-8.

[28] Sitaram N, Nurnberger JI, Jr., Gershon ES, Gillin JC. Cholinergic regulation of mood and REM sleep: potential model and marker of vulnerability to affective disorder. *Am J Psychiatry* 1982 May;139(5):571-6.
[29] Bowden CL. A different depression: clinical distinctions between bipolar and unipolar depression. *J Affect Disord* 2005 Feb;84(2-3):117-25.
[30] Casper RC, Redmond DE, Jr., Katz MM, Schaffer CB, Davis JM, Koslow SH. Somatic symptoms in primary affective disorder. Presence and relationship to the classification of depression. *Arch Gen Psychiatry* 1985 Nov;42(11):1098-104.
[31] Detre T, Himmelhoch J, Swartzburg M, Anderson CM, Byck R, Kupfer DJ. Hypersomnia and manic-depressive disease. *Am J Psychiatry* 1972 Apr;128(10):1303-5.
[32] Winokur G, Tanna VL. Possible role of X-linked dominant factor in manic depressive disease. *Dis Nerv Syst* 1969 Feb;30(2):89-94.
[33] Nofzinger EA, Thase ME, Reynolds CF, III, Himmelhoch JM, Mallinger A, Houck P, et al. Hypersomnia in bipolar depression: a comparison with narcolepsy using the multiple sleep latency test. *Am J Psychiatry* 1991 Sep;148(9):1177-81.
[34] de M, V, Hoffman G, Lemaire M, Mendlewicz J. Sleep spindle activity changes in patients with affective disorders. *Sleep* 1987 Oct;10(5):443-51.
[35] Duncan WC, Jr., Pettigrew KD, Gillin JC. REM architecture changes in bipolar and unipolar depression. *Am J Psychiatry* 1979 Nov;136(11):1424-7.
[36] Fossion P, Staner L, Dramaix M, Kempenaers C, Kerkhofs M, Hubain P, et al. Does sleep EEG data distinguish between UP, BPI or BPII major depressions? An age and gender controlled study. *J Affect Disord* 1998 Jun;49(3):181-7.
[37] Giles DE, Rush AJ, Roffwarg HP. Sleep parameters in bipolar I, bipolar II, and unipolar depressions. *Biol Psychiatry* 1986 Nov;21(13):1340-3.
[38] Gillin JC, Duncan W, Pettigrew KD, Frankel BL, Snyder F. Successful separation of depressed, normal, and insomniac subjects by EEG sleep data. *Arch Gen Psychiatry* 1979 Jan;36(1):85-90.
[39] Jernajczyk W. Latency of eye movement and other REM sleep parameters in bipolar depression. *Biol Psychiatry* 1986 May;21(5-6):465-72.
[40] Lauer CJ, Wiegand M, Krieg JC. All-night electroencephalographic sleep and cranial computed tomography in depression. A study of unipolar and bipolar patients. *Eur Arch Psychiatry Clin Neurosci* 1992;242(2-3):59-68.
[41] Thase ME, Himmelhoch JM, Mallinger AG, Jarrett DB, Kupfer DJ. Sleep EEG and DST findings in anergic bipolar depression. *Am J Psychiatry* 1989 Mar;146(3):329-33.
[42] Cartwright R, Baehr E, Kirkby J, Pandi-Perumal SR, Kabat J. REM sleep reduction, mood regulation and remission in untreated depression. *Psychiatry Res* 2003 Dec 1;121(2):159-67.
[43] Riemann D, Voderholzer U, Berger M. Sleep and sleep-wake manipulations in bipolar depression. *Neuropsychobiology* 2002;45 Suppl 1:7-12.
[44] Wirz-Justice A, Graw P, Krauchi K, Sarrafzadeh A, English J, Arendt J, et al. 'Natural' light treatment of seasonal affective disorder. *J Affect Disord* 1996 Apr 12;37(2-3):109-20.
[45] Carlson GA, Strober M. Affective disorder in adolescence: issues in misdiagnosis. *J Clin Psychiatry* 1978 Jan;39(1):59-66.

[46] Cassidy F, Murry E, Forest K, Carroll BJ. Signs and symptoms of mania in pure and mixed episodes. *J Affect Disord* 1998 Sep;50(2-3):187-201.

[47] Clayton PJ, Pitts FN, Jr. Affect disorder. IV. Mania. *Compr Psychiatry* 1965 Oct;6(5):313-22.

[48] Loudon JB, Blackburn IM, Ashworth CM. A study of the symptomatology and course of manic illness using a new scale. *Psychol Med* 1977 Nov;7(4):723-9.

[49] Serretti A, Olgiati P. Profiles of "manic" symptoms in bipolar I, bipolar II and major depressive disorders. *J Affect Disord* 2005 Feb;84(2-3):159-66.

[50] Wehr TA, Sack D, Rosenthal N, Duncan W, Gillin JC. Circadian rhythm disturbances in manic-depressive illness. *Fed Proc* 1983 Aug;42(11):2809-14.

[51] Wehr TA, Turner EH, Shimada JM, Lowe CH, Barker C, Leibenluft E. Treatment of rapidly cycling bipolar patient by using extended bed rest and darkness to stabilize the timing and duration of sleep. *Biol Psychiatry* 1998 Jun 1;43(11):822-8.

[52] Hudson JI, Lipinski JF, Frankenburg FR, Grochocinski VJ, Kupfer DJ. Electroencephalographic sleep in mania. *Arch Gen Psychiatry* 1988 Mar;45(3):267-73.

[53] Hudson JI, Lipinski JF, Keck PE, Jr., Aizley HG, Lukas SE, Rothschild AJ, et al. Polysomnographic characteristics of young manic patients. Comparison with unipolar depressed patients and normal control subjects. *Arch Gen Psychiatry* 1992 May;49(5):378-83.

[54] Linkowski P, Kerkhofs M, Van CE. Sleep and biological rhythms in man: a twin study. *Clin Neuropharmacol* 1992;15 Suppl 1 Pt A:42A-3A.

[55] Horne JA, Moore VJ. Sleep EEG effects of exercise with and without additional body cooling. *Electroencephalogr Clin Neurophysiol* 1985 Jan;60(1):33-8.

[56] Wehr TA, Sack DA, Rosenthal NE. Sleep reduction as a final common pathway in the genesis of mania. *Am J Psychiatry* 1987 Feb;144(2):201-4.

[57] Gruber J, Harvey AG, Wang PW, Brooks JO, III, Thase ME, Sachs GS, et al. Sleep functioning in relation to mood, function, and quality of life at entry to the Systematic Treatment Enhancement Program for Bipolar Disorder (STEP-BD). *J Affect Disord* 2009 Apr;114(1-3):41-9.

[58] Giglio LM, Magalhaes PV, Kapczinski NS, Walz JC, Kapczinski F. Functional impact of biological rhythm disturbance in bipolar disorder. *J Psychiatr Res* 2010 Mar;44(4):220-3.

[59] Theorell-Haglow J, Lindberg E, Janson C. What are the important risk factors for daytime sleepiness and fatigue in women?. *Sleep* 2006 Jun;29(6):751-7.

[60] Berlim MT, Pargendler J, Caldieraro MA, Almeida EA, Fleck MP, Joiner TE. Quality of life in unipolar and bipolar depression: are there significant differences?. *J Nerv Ment Dis* 2004 Nov;192(11):792-5.

[61] Yatham LN, Lecrubier Y, Fieve RR, Davis KH, Harris SD, Krishnan AA. Quality of life in patients with bipolar I depression: data from 920 patients. *Bipolar Disord* 2004 Oct;6(5):379-85.

[62] Practice guideline for the treatment of patients with bipolar disorder (revision). *Am J Psychiatry* 2002 Apr;159(4 Suppl):1-50.

[63] Gitlin MJ, Swendsen J, Heller TL, Hammen C. Relapse and impairment in bipolar disorder. *Am J Psychiatry* 1995 Nov;152(11):1635-40.

[64] Johnson SL. Mania and dysregulation in goal pursuit: a review. *Clin Psychol Rev* 2005 Feb;25(2):241-62.
[65] Johnson MW, Suess PE, Griffiths RR. Ramelteon: a novel hypnotic lacking abuse liability and sedative adverse effects. *Arch Gen Psychiatry* 2006 Oct;63(10):1149-57.
[66] Keitner GI, Solomon DA, Ryan CE, Miller IW, Mallinger A, Kupfer DJ, et al. Prodromal and residual symptoms in bipolar I disorder. *Compr Psychiatry* 1996 Sep;37(5):362-7.
[67] Jackson A, Cavanagh J, Scott J. A systematic review of manic and depressive prodromes. *J Affect Disord* 2003 May;74(3):209-17.
[68] Bauer M, Grof P, Rasgon N, Bschor T, Glenn T, Whybrow PC. Temporal relation between sleep and mood in patients with bipolar disorder. *Bipolar Disord* 2006 Apr;8(2):160-7.
[69] Leibenluft E, Suppes T. Treating bipolar illness: focus on treatment algorithms and management of the sleep-wake cycle. *Am J Psychiatry* 1999 Dec;156(12):1976-81.
[70] Wirz-Justice A, Quinto C, Cajochen C, Werth E, Hock C. A rapid-cycling bipolar patient treated with long nights, bedrest, and light. *Biol Psychiatry* 1999 Apr 15;45(8):1075-7.
[71] Barbini B, Benedetti F, Colombo C, Dotoli D, Bernasconi A, Cigala-Fulgosi M, et al. Dark therapy for mania: a pilot study. *Bipolar Disord* 2005 Feb;7(1):98-101.
[72] Benedetti F, Barbini B, Colombo C, Smeraldi E. Chronotherapeutics in a psychiatric ward. *Sleep Med Rev* 2007 Dec;11(6):509-22.
[73] Benedetti F, Fresi F, Maccioni P, Smeraldi E. Behavioural sensitization to repeated sleep deprivation in a mice model of mania. *Behav Brain Res* 2008 Mar 5;187(2):221-7.
[74] Colombo C, Benedetti F, Barbini B, Campori E, Smeraldi E. Rate of switch from depression into mania after therapeutic sleep deprivation in bipolar depression. *Psychiatry Res* 1999 Jun 30;86(3):267-70.
[75] Feldman-Naim S, Turner EH, Leibenluft E. Diurnal variation in the direction of mood switches in patients with rapid-cycling bipolar disorder. *J Clin Psychiatry* 1997 Feb;58(2):79-84.
[76] Kasper S, Wehr TA. The role of sleep and wakefulness in the genesis of depression and mania. *Encephale* 1992 Jan;18 Spec No 1:45-50.
[77] Szuba MP, Baxter LR, Jr., Fairbanks LA, Guze BH, Schwartz JM. Effects of partial sleep deprivation on the diurnal variation of mood and motor activity in major depression. *Biol Psychiatry* 1991 Oct 15;30(8):817-29.
[78] Wirz-Justice A, Van den Hoofdakker RH. Sleep deprivation in depression: what do we know, where do we go?. *Biol Psychiatry* 1999 Aug 15;46(4):445-53.
[79] Wirz-Justice A, Benedetti F, Berger M, Lam RW, Martiny K, Terman M, et al. Chronotherapeutics (light and wake therapy) in affective disorders. *Psychol Med* 2005 Jul;35(7):939-44.
[80] Wu JC, Bunney WE. The biological basis of an antidepressant response to sleep deprivation and relapse: review and hypothesis, *Am J Psychiatry* 1990 Jan;147(1):14-21.
[81] Benedetti F, Colombo C, Barbini B, Campori E, Smeraldi E. Morning sunlight reduces length of hospitalization in bipolar depression. *J Affect Disord* 2001 Feb;62(3):221-3.

[82] Benedetti F, Barbini B, Fulgosi MC, Colombo C, Dallaspezia S, Pontiggia A, et al. Combined total sleep deprivation and light therapy in the treatment of drug-resistant bipolar depression: acute response and long-term remission rates, J *Clin Psychiatry* 2005 Dec;66(12):1535-40.

[83] Colombo C, Lucca A, Benedetti F, Barbini B, Campori E, Smeraldi E. Total sleep deprivation combined with lithium and light therapy in the treatment of bipolar depression: replication of main effects and interaction. *Psychiatry Res* 2000 Jul 24;95(1):43-53.

[84] Benedetti F, Barbini B, Campori E, Fulgosi MC, Pontiggia A, Colombo C. Sleep phase advance and lithium to sustain the antidepressant effect of total sleep deprivation in bipolar depression: new findings supporting the internal coincidence model?. *J Psychiatr Res* 2001 Nov;35(6):323-9.

[85] Berger M, Vollmann J, Hohagen F, Konig A, Lohner H, Voderholzer U, et al. Sleep deprivation combined with consecutive sleep phase advance as a fast-acting therapy in depression: an open pilot trial in medicated and unmedicated patients. *Am J Psychiatry* 1997 Jun;154(6):870-2.

[86] Neumeister A, Goessler R, Lucht M, Kapitany T, Bamas C, Kasper S. Bright light therapy stabilizes the antidepressant effect of partial sleep deprivation. *Biol Psychiatry* 1996 Jan 1;39(1):16-21.

[87] Riemann D, Konig A, Hohagen F, Kiemen A, Voderholzer U, Backhaus J, et al. How to preserve the antidepressive effect of sleep deprivation: A comparison of sleep phase advance and sleep phase delay. *Eur Arch Psychiatry Clin Neurosci* 1999;249(5):231-7.

[88] Kripke DF, Jean-Louis G, Elliott JA, Klauber MR, Rex KM, Tuunainen A, et al. Ethnicity, sleep, mood, and illumination in postmenopausal women. *BMC Psychiatry* 2004 Apr 7;4:8.

[89] Robertson E, Jones I, Haque S, Holder R, Craddock N. Risk of puerperal and non-puerperal recurrence of illness following bipolar affective puerperal (post-partum) psychosis. *Br J Psychiatry* 2005 Mar;186:258-9.

[90] Srinivasan V, Pandi-Perumal SR, Trakht I, Spence DW, Hardeland R, Poeggeler B, et al. Pathophysiology of depression: role of sleep and the melatonergic system. *Psychiatry Res* 2009 Feb 28;165(3):201-14.

[91] Gill DS, Ketter TA, Post RM. Antidepressant response to sleep deprivation as a function of time into depressive episode in rapidly cycling bipolar patients. *Acta Psychiatr Scand* 1993 Feb;87(2):102-9.

[92] Dinges DF, Pack F, Williams K, Gillen KA, Powell JW, Ott GE, et al. Cumulative sleepiness, mood disturbance, and psychomotor vigilance performance decrements during a week of sleep restricted to 4-5 hours per night. *Sleep* 1997 Apr;20(4):267-77.

[93] Drake CL, Roehrs TA, Burduvali E, Bonahoom A, Rosekind M, Roth T. Effects of rapid versus slow accumulation of eight hours of sleep loss. *Psychophysiology* 2001 Nov;38(6):979-87.

[94] Zohar D, Tzischinsky O, Epstein R, Lavie P. The effects of sleep loss on medical residents' emotional reactions to work events: a cognitive-energy model. *Sleep* 2005 Jan;28(1):47-54.

[95] Bunney WE, Jr., Murphy DL, Goodwin FK, Borge GF. The switch process from depression to mania: relationship to drugs which alter brain amines. *Lancet* 1970 May 16;1(7655):1022-7.

[96] Barbini B, Bertelli S, Colombo C, Smeraldi E. Sleep loss, a possible factor in augmenting manic episode. *Psychiatry Res* 1996 Nov 15;65(2):121-5.

[97] Leibenluft E, Albert PS, Rosenthal NE, Wehr TA. Relationship between sleep and mood in patients with rapid-cycling bipolar disorder. *Psychiatry Res* 1996 Jul 31;63(2-3):161-8.

[98] Carlson GA, Goodwin FK. The stages of mania. A longitudinal analysis of the manic episode. *Arch Gen Psychiatry* 1973 Feb;28(2):221-8.

[99] Perlman CA, Johnson SL, Mellman TA. The prospective impact of sleep duration on depression and mania. *Bipolar Disord* 2006 Jun;8(3):271-4.

[100] Wehr TA, Goodwin FK, Wirz-Justice A, Breitmaier J, Craig C. 48-hour sleep-wake cycles in manic-depressive illness: naturalistic observations and sleep deprivation experiments. *Arch Gen Psychiatry* 1982 May;39(5):559-65.

[101] Mansour HA, Monk TH, Nimgaonkar VL. Circadian genes and bipolar disorder. *Ann Med* 2005;37(3):196-205.

[102] Wirz-Justice A. Biological rhythm disturbances in mood disorders. *Int Clin Psychopharmacol* 2006 Feb;21 Suppl 1:S11-S15.

[103] Wirz-Justice A. Chronobiology and mood disorders. *Dialogues Clin Neurosci* 2003 Dec;5(4):315-25.

[104] Reppert SM, Weaver DR, Rivkees SA, Stopa EG. Putative melatonin receptors in a human biological clock. *Science* 1988 Oct 7;242(4875):78-81.

[105] Brzezinski A. Melatonin in humans. *N Engl J Med* 1997 Jan 16;336(3):186-95.

[106] Sassone-Corsi P. Molecular clocks: mastering time by gene regulation. *Nature* 1998 Apr 30;392(6679):871-4.

[107] Dawson D, Encel N. Melatonin and sleep in humans. *J Pineal Res* 1993 Aug;15(1):1-12.

[108] Cagnacci A, Elliott JA, Yen SS. Melatonin: a major regulator of the circadian rhythm of core temperature in humans. *J Clin Endocrinol Metab* 1992 Aug;75(2):447-52.

[109] Nurnberger JI, Jr., Berrettini W, Tamarkin L, Hamovit J, Norton J, Gershon E. Supersensitivity to melatonin suppression by light in young people at high risk for affective disorder. A preliminary report. *Neuropsychopharmacology* 1988 Sep;1(3): 217-23.

[110] Hallam KT, Begg DP, Olver JS, Norman TR. An investigation of the effect of immediate and extended release venlafaxine on nocturnal melatonin and cortisol release in healthy adult volunteers. *Hum Psychopharmacol* 2008 Mar;23(2):129-37.

[111] Lewy AJ, Nurnberger JI, Jr., Wehr TA, Pack D, Becker LE, Powell RL, et al. Supersensitivity to light: possible trait marker for manic-depressive illness. *Am J Psychiatry* 1985 Jun;142(6):725-7.

[112] Nathan PJ, Burrows GD, Norman TR. Melatonin sensitivity to dim white light in affective disorders. *Neuropsychopharmacology* 1999 Sep;21(3):408-13.

[113] Whalley LJ, Perini T, Shering A, Bennie J. Melatonin response to bright light in recovered, drug-free, bipolar patients. *Psychiatry Res* 1991 Jul;38(1):13-9.

[114] Nurnberger JI, Jr., Adkins S, Lahiri DK, Mayeda A, Hu K, Lewy A, et al. Melatonin suppression by light in euthymic bipolar and unipolar patients. *Arch Gen Psychiatry* 2000 Jun;57(6):572-9.

[115] Kennedy SH, Kutcher SP, Ralevski E, Brown GM. Nocturnal melatonin and 24-hour 6-sulphatoxymelatonin levels in various phases of bipolar affective disorder. *Psychiatry Res* 1996 Jul 31;63(2-3):219-22.

[116] Wahlund B, Grahn H, Saaf J, Wetterberg L. Affective disorder subtyped by psychomotor symptoms, monoamine oxidase, melatonin and cortisol: identification of patients with latent bipolar disorder. *Eur Arch Psychiatry Clin Neurosci* 1998;248(5):215-24.

[117] Hallam KT, Olver JS, Chambers V, Begg DP, McGrath C, Norman TR. The heritability of melatonin secretion and sensitivity to bright nocturnal light in twins. *Psychoneuroendocrinology* 2006 Aug;31(7):867-75.

[118] Beck-Friis J, Ljunggren JG, Thoren M, von RD, Kjellman BF, Wetterberg L. Melatonin, cortisol and ACTH in patients with major depressive disorder and healthy humans with special reference to the outcome of the dexamethasone suppression test. *Psychoneuroendocrinology* 1985;10(2):173-86.

[119] Souetre E, Salvati E, Belugou JL, Pringuey D, Candito M, Krebs B, et al. Circadian rhythms in depression and recovery: evidence for blunted amplitude as the main chronobiological abnormality. *Psychiatry Res* 1989 Jun;28(3):263-78.

[120] Kennedy SH, Tighe S, McVey G, Brown GM. Melatonin and cortisol "switches" during mania, depression, and euthymia in a drug-free bipolar patient. *J Nerv Ment Dis* 1989 May;177(5):300-3.

[121] Lewy AJ, Wehr TA, Goodwin FK, Newsome DA, Markey SP. Light suppresses melatonin secretion in humans. *Science* 1980 Dec 12;210(4475):1267-9.

[122] Sit D, Wisner KL, Hanusa BH, Stull S, Terman M. Light therapy for bipolar disorder: a case series in women. *Bipolar Disord* 2007 Dec;9(8):918-27.

[123] Vieta E, Colom F. Psychological interventions in bipolar disorder: From wishful thinking to an evidence-based approach. *Acta Psychiatr Scand Suppl* 2004;(422):34-8.

[124] Calabrese JR, Guelfi JD, Perdrizet-Chevallier C. Agomelatine adjunctive therapy for acute bipolar depression: preliminary open data. *Bipolar Disord* 2007 Sep;9(6):628-35.

[125] Abe M, Herzog ED, Block GD. Lithium lengthens the circadian period of individual suprachiasmatic nucleus neurons. *Neuroreport* 2000 Sep 28;11(14):3261-4.

[126] Kripke DF, Mullaney DJ, Atkinson M, Wolf S. Circadian rhythm disorders in manic-depressives. *Biol Psychiatry* 1978 Jun;13(3):335-51.

[127] Minors DS, Waterhouse JM, Wirz-Justice A. A human phase-response curve to light. *Neurosci Lett* 1991 Nov 25;133(1):36-40.

[128] Lewy AJ, Wehr TA, Goodwin FK, Newsome DA, Rosenthal NE. Manic-depressive patients may be supersensitive to light. *Lancet* 1981 Feb 14;1(8216):383-4.

[129] Forbes D, Morgan DG, Bangma J, Peacock S, Pelletier N, Adamson J. Light therapy for managing sleep, behaviour, and mood disturbances in dementia. *Cochrane Database Syst Rev* 2004;(2):CD003946.

[130] Montgomery P, Dennis J. Bright light therapy for sleep problems in adults aged 60+. *Cochrane Database Syst Rev* 2002;(2):CD003403.

[131] Tuunainen A, Kripke DF, Endo T. Light therapy for non-seasonal depression. *Cochrane Database Syst Rev* 2004;(2):CD004050.

[132] Chase JE, Gidal BE. Melatonin: therapeutic use in sleep disorders. *Ann Pharmacother* 1997 Oct;31(10):1218-26.

[133] Lieberman HR, Waldhauser F, Garfield G, Lynch HJ, Wurtman RJ. Effects of melatonin on human mood and performance. *Brain Res* 1984 Dec 10;323(2):201-7.

[134] Semm P, Demaine C, Vollrath L. Electrical responses of pineal cells to melatonin and putative transmitters. Evidence for circadian changes in sensitivity. *Exp Brain Res* 1981;43(3-4):361-70.

[135] Lewy AJ, Ahmed S, Jackson JM, Sack RL. Melatonin shifts human circadian rhythms according to a phase-response curve. *Chronobiol Int* 1992 Oct;9(5):380-92.

[136] Sack RL, Lewy AJ, Blood ML, Stevenson J, Keith LD. Melatonin administration to blind people: phase advances and entrainment. *J Biol Rhythms* 1991;6(3):249-61.

[137] Lushington K, Pollard K, Lack L, Kennaway DJ, Dawson D. Daytime melatonin administration in elderly good and poor sleepers: effects on core body temperature and sleep latency. *Sleep* 1997 Dec;20(12):1135-44.

[138] Garfinkel D, Laudon M, Nof D, Zisapel N. Improvement of sleep quality in elderly people by controlled-release melatonin. *Lancet* 1995 Aug 26;346(8974):541-4.

[139] Oldani A, Ferini-Strambi L, Zucconi M, Stankov B, Fraschini F, Smirne S. Melatonin and delayed sleep phase syndrome: ambulatory polygraphic evaluation. *Neuroreport* 1994 Dec 30;6(1):132-4.

[140] Leibenluft E, Feldman-Naim S, Turner EH, Wehr TA, Rosenthal NE. Effects of exogenous melatonin administration and withdrawal in five patients with rapid-cycling bipolar disorder. *J Clin Psychiatry* 1997 Sep;58(9):383-8.

[141] Zisapel N. The use of melatonin for the treatment of insomnia. *Biol Signals Recept* 1999 Jan;8(1-2):84-9.

[142] Turek FW, Gillette MU. Melatonin, sleep, and circadian rhythms: rationale for development of specific melatonin agonists. *Sleep Med* 2004 Nov;5(6):523-32.

[143] Livianos L, Sierra P, Arques S, Garcia A, Rojo L. Is melatonin an adjunctive stabilizer?. *Psychiatry Clin Neurosci* 2012 Feb;66(1):82-3.

[144] Bersani G, Garavini A. Melatonin add-on in manic patients with treatment resistant insomnia. Prog Neuropsychopharmacol *Biol Psychiatry* 2000 Feb;24(2):185-91.

[145] Griffiths RR, Johnson MW. Relative abuse liability of hypnotic drugs: a conceptual framework and algorithm for differentiating among compounds. *J Clin Psychiatry* 2005;66 Suppl 9:31-41.

[146] Gao K, Calabrese JR. Newer treatment studies for bipolar depression. *Bipolar Disord* 2005;7 Suppl 5:13-23.

[147] Fornaro M, Prestia D, Colicchio S, Perugi G. A systematic, updated review on the antidepressant agomelatine focusing on its melatonergic modulation. *Curr Neuropharmacol* 2010 Sep;8(3):287-304.

[148] Rouillon F. Efficacy and tolerance profile of agomelatine and practical use in depressed patients. *Int Clin Psychopharmacol* 2006 Feb;21 Suppl 1:S31-S35.

[149] Judd LL, Akiskal HS, Schettler PJ, Endicott J, Maser J, Solomon DA, et al. The long-term natural history of the weekly symptomatic status of bipolar I disorder. *Arch Gen Psychiatry* 2002 Jun;59(6):530-7.

[150] Post RM, Denicoff KD, Leverich GS, Altshuler LL, Frye MA, Suppes TM, et al. Morbidity in 258 bipolar outpatients followed for 1 year with daily prospective ratings on the NIMH life chart method. J Clin Psychiatry 2003 Jun;64(6):680-90.

[151] Judd LL, Akiskal HS, Schettler PJ, Coryell W, Endicott J, Maser JD, et al. A prospective investigation of the natural history of the long-term weekly symptomatic status of bipolar II disorder. *Arch Gen Psychiatry* 2003 Mar;60(3):261-9.

[152] Hallam KT, Olver JS, Horgan JE, McGrath C, Norman TR. Low doses of lithium carbonate reduce melatonin light sensitivity in healthy volunteers. *Int J Neuropsychopharmacol* 2005 Jun;8(2):255-9.

[153] Hallam KT, Olver JS, Norman TR. Effect of sodium valproate on nocturnal melatonin sensitivity to light in healthy volunteers. *Neuropsychopharmacology* 2005 Jul;30(7):1400-4.

In: New Developments in Melatonin Research ISBN: 978-1-62618-843-3
Editors: D.Acuña-Castroviejo, I.Rusanova, G.Escames © 2013 Nova Science Publishers, Inc.

Chapter 14

Nanoemulsion Technology for Sublingual Delivery of Melatonin: Characterization and Preliminary Data of Absorption

***A. Fratter*[1]*, A. Semenzato*[2]*, A. Casiraghi*[3] *and P. Minghetti*[3]**

[1]Innovation Technology- R&D Department, Labomar Srl, Istrana (TV), Italy
[2]Department of Pharmaceutical and Pharmacological Sciences, Università degli Studi di Padova, Italy
[3]Department of Pharmaceutical Sciences, Università degli Studi di Milano, Italy

Abstract

Melatonin (5-methoxytryptamine) is a natural occurring molecule which exerts physiologic role of circadian sleep-wake cycle in humans. Melatonin is secreted from the pineal gland placed in the center of the brain, far from blood-brain barrier. Thanks to its ascertained safety in humans and low cost, melatonin is widely employed in the market of drugs and nutritional supplements mainly claiming its effectiveness in sleep-wake cycle regularization, anxiolytic and antioxidant activity. Over the last decades, melatonin bioavailability has been investigated in humans and animal models. Literature data pointed out a limited bioavailability of melatonin after oral intake, together with a high variability from subject to subject.

This chapter describes, characterizes and preliminary assesses the effectiveness of a new nanoemulsified system for the sublingual administration of melatonin. The very small droplet size which characterizes this system, potentially allows melatonin to be delivered from a sublingual spray formulation which promotes its absorption through the lingual epithelium so reaching venous systemic circulation avoiding first liver passage through the portal circulation. It seems, in fact, that liver first passage express the main biochemical phenomena involved in the high clearance and relative low bioavailability of melatonin after oral assumption.

Keywords: Melatonin, nanoemulsion, ascorbyl palmitate, bioavailability

Introduction

Several new topical delivery nanosystems have been developed in recent years in order to improve the membrane permeation of active molecules [1-3]. Generally speaking, nanosystems are expected to improve the efficacy of drugs, cosmetics, functional food or nutriceuticals by means of an enhancement of the flux of active molecules through skin and mucosae. Moreover, it has been demonstrated that these formulations provide a significant improvement in terms of the stability of active ingredients, for example from oxidation [4], and concentration, leading to an enhanced safety and a better product compliance [5-9]. The success of nanoemulsified systems intended for skin and mucosal delivery can be related to their capability to entrap medium-high concentrations of active molecules, both hydrophilic and lipophilic, the mild processing conditions and the possibility of stabilizing the formulations for the required product shelf life [5;10;11].

Depending on the processing method adopted and the physicochemical properties of the ingredients, the droplet sizes of nanoemulsions can vary from 20 to 500 nm, much smaller than the range 1-100 μm of conventional emulsions. These differences are due to the production method. Indeed, high energy emulsification procedures (i.e. high pressure homogenization) often lead to smaller size globules, while when a low-energy emulsification process (Phase Inversion Temperature technique) is used the droplet size is governed by the formulation parameters. Usually the average droplet size of nanoemulsions ranges from 100 and 500 nm and they generally show narrow size distribution with low polydispersity [12]. The small droplet size guarantees the enhanced physical stability of nanoemulsions vs macroemulsions, reducing flocculation and coalescence. The creaming process is inhibited because the droplet's Brownian motion is enough to overcome the gravitational separation force [13;14].

In this study a new nanoemulsified system (nanoemulsion) was proposed as a novel approach to sublingually administer melatonin. Because of the short half-life and poor oral bioavailability, melatonin is not a good candidate for oral immediate-release technology, when a physiologic-like plasma level profile is desired. Indeed, the administration of 2 and 4 mg oral tablets in dosages a showed poor absolute bioavailability, either due to the poor oral absorption, large first-pass metabolism, or a combination of both [15]. To mimic the normal endogenous plasma melatonin profile, sustained- or controlled-release (CR) delivery systems with rapid onset and rapid offset may be necessary. Nevertheless, after administration of oral sustained-release or CR formulations in human volunteers, a large intersubject variability in the plasma level profiles and poor bioavailability were reported along with nutritional status effects on oral bioavailability [16-18].

The feasibility of transdermal delivery systems was also investigated because of the potential to avoid first-pass metabolism and more closely mimic the physiologic endogenous plasma profile of melatonin. A preliminary data on a transdermal delivery system applied to four volunteers suggested that melatonin can be delivered transdermally in human subjects, even if an intersubject variability in both plasma melatonin concentration and urinary excretion rate of its major metabolite, namely 6-sulphatoxymelatonin, was evidenced [17]. These results were recently confirmed by Aeschbach and coworkers: the transdermal delivery of melatonin during the daytime in healthy subjects could elevate the melatonin plasma levels and reduce waking after sleep onset, by promoting sleep in the latter part of an 8-h sleep opportunity [19]. The feasibility of conventional semisolid formulations [20] and transdermal patches [21] was investigated by several authors. Due to the inadequate transdermal absorption, lag time and depot-effect, the transdermal permeation of melatonin was improved by using of ethanolic vehicles [22;23] and chemical skin penetration enhancers [24;25]. The results suggested that some enhancers, i.e. oleic acid in a suitable vehicle, could improve the skin permeation and shorten the lag time (26), even if oleic acid in a mixture of diethylene glycol monoethyl ether and propylene glycol laurate failed to shorten the melatonin lag time [27]. In recent years, the attention has been also focused on nanoparticles and liposomes have been also studied. Lecithin/chitosan nanoparticles provided 1.3-2.3-fold higher flux compared to melatonin solution [28]. The loading of melatonin in elastic liposomal formulations [29] and ethosomal carriers [30] provided an enhanced transdermal flux and decreased lag time of 0.9 h across human cadaver skin in comparison to liposomal formulation and hydroethanolic melatonin solution.

To overcome issues reported for the aforementioned routes of administration, the oral mucosae is considered a promising alternative to overcome issues reported for the aforementioned routes of administration. Benes and coworkers developed a transmucosal delivery system (TMD) consisting of a small, flexible mucoadhesive patch that can be comfortably applied to the gum or to the mucosal side of the lip or cheek. The transmucosal administration of melatonin in twelve male Caucasian volunteers allowed to closely mimicking the physiological, nocturnal plasma profile of the endogenous hormone. Relatively steady plasma melatonin levels were quickly achieved, and plasma melatonin concentration abruptly fell after removal of the TMD patch. No tissue depot effect was noted [31].

Thermodynamic Topics of Nanoemulsions and Microemulsions

The main difference between nanoemulsion and microemulsion under a thermodynamic point of view is that the former one can be considered a kinetically stable physical form but thermodynamically metastable according to Gibbs law and the latter a kinetically and thermodynamically stable form. The main reason of this difference is that in a microemulsion, thanks to the highly efficient synergy and high amount of the emulsifying agents bulk, micellar surfaces become hugely elastic and capable of better adapt surface itself to the diameter reduction in opposition to the internal droplet high pressure, even though a very low energy is imparted to the system. This fact can be explained according to Gibbs law [14;32] as the very high entropic state achieved after small droplets dispersion in the medium permits to balance the enthalpy energy rate (few mN/m^2) of the system: the physical consequence is the reaching of a thermodynamic balance or in some cases a spontaneous emulsification process with negative values of ΔG (eq. 1):

$$\Delta G_f = \gamma \Delta A - T\Delta S \quad \text{(eq. 1)}$$

where ΔG is the free energy of formation, γ is the surface tension of the oil–water interface, ΔA represents the dimensional change of interfacial micellar area, ΔS is the variation of entropy of the system which is induced by the dispersion, and T is the temperature. It should be realized that when a microemulsion is achieved, the variation of ΔA is very large because of the large number of very small droplets formed [14;33].

Synergy between Ascorbyl Palmitate and Polysorbate in the Production of Nanoemulsion

We aim herewith to describe a new very peculiar association of active surface agents capable of creating very stable nanoemulsions with an average micellar diameter of about 100–150 nm.

This technology has been developed to solve the bioavailability impairment of several pharmaceutics and especially nutraceutics which are poorly absorbed through intestinal mucosae or massively metabolized in liver microsomes in order to reduce their biological activity. Some examples are trans-resveratrol, melatonin and others. Resveratrol, for instance, is well absorbed from intestinal mucosa, but massively destroyed in the liver microsomes [34]. Of great interest, melatonin is metastable in both aqueous and alcoholic media [35;36] even though the most of the nutritional supplements markedly available are hydroalcoholic solutions.

This new projected nanoemulsifing system is capable of effectively encapsulate lipophilic, oily soluble or poorly water soluble molecules, e.g. trans-resveratrol, melatonin, l-tryptophan, polyunsaturated fatty acids (PUFA) and others in a final water-based nanoemulsion to be administered as oral liquid or spray.

The main innovation of the proposed technology consists in the use of peculiar association of emulsifying agents allowing the micellar dimension reduction under the 100 nm, notoriously the dimensional limit under which a real nanoemulsion is recognizable even though several authors claim that an emulsion is nanosized under 500 nm [37]. Generally speaking in the nanoemulsion formulation, very performing emulsifying systems allow the reduction of the micelle diameter.

To create a nanoemulsion it is necessary the use of a binary or ternary emulsifying system in which the synergy of the surfactants efficiently decreases the interfacial tension between the continuous water phase and the oily droplets. Moreover, the emulsifying system make the micellar surface more flexible and able to overcome the very high interface energy produced when a droplet of internal phase is forced to reduce its dimension according to Laplace's law (eq. 2).

$$\Delta P = 2\gamma / r \quad \text{(eq. 2),}$$

where ΔP is the gradient of pressure between out and inside the micelle; γ is the surface tension, and $\boldsymbol{r}$ is the radius of the micelle assumed spherical.

The smaller the radius of the micelle, the higher the surface tension to overcome and, therefore, the energy required to reduce it.

The micellar diameter can be reduced by decreasing the high difference between internal and external pressure according to the following strategies:

- Applying a very high force on the external micellar surface to reduce the ratio between internal and external pressure (high pressure emulsification device), according to (eq. 2 and 3);
- Reducing the ratio between 2γ and r (effective surfactants association), according to (eq. 2).

$$W = Pext*\Delta V \qquad \text{(eq. 3)},$$

where *W* is the energy to oppose to the internal pressure to reduce micellar volume; P_{ext} is the pressure to apply; and *ΔV* is the volume reduction to achieve assuming that the micellar geometry is a sphere.

The difference between internal and external pressure of the micelle is the ratio between 2γ and r (Laplace's Law).

This study describes for the first time the use of ascorbyl palmitate (ASP), the lipophilic ester of l-ascorbic acid and palmitic acid (Figure 1), as co-emulsifying agent to produce stable nanoemulsion in association with polysorbate 80 (PS 80). ASP is a well-known excipient in pharmaceutical, cosmetic and nutritional industries, and it is widely used as antioxidant agent to decrease the peroxidation of unsaturated lipids peroxidation.

Thanks to the palmitic moiety, in fact, ASP can be easily solubilized in both solid and liquid lipid/fat-based preparation, reducing oxidation and peroxidation in force of the effective reducing ascorbic radical. Some papers describe also its use as lipophilic form of l-ascorbic acid potentially capable of improving skin bioavailability of l-ascorbic acid, but reliable scientific data are far to be convincing [38]. Because of its amphiphilic structure consisting of very hydrophilic ascorbic moiety and very lipophilic palmitic moiety, ASP perfectly complies with the definition of surfactant: in fact, there are some papers describing chemical-physico behaviour of ASP previously ionized in alkaline water to self-assembly and form micellar structures called ASPASOMES (39) (Figure 2), investigated for the capability to form vesicles potentially involved in the improvement of the bioavailability of some drugs [40].

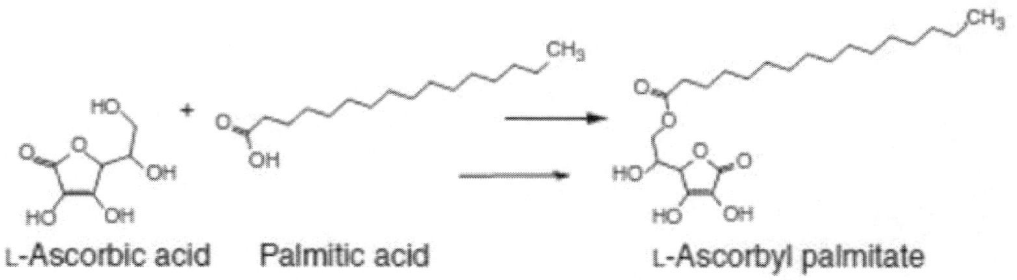

Figure 1. ascorbyl palmitate structure.

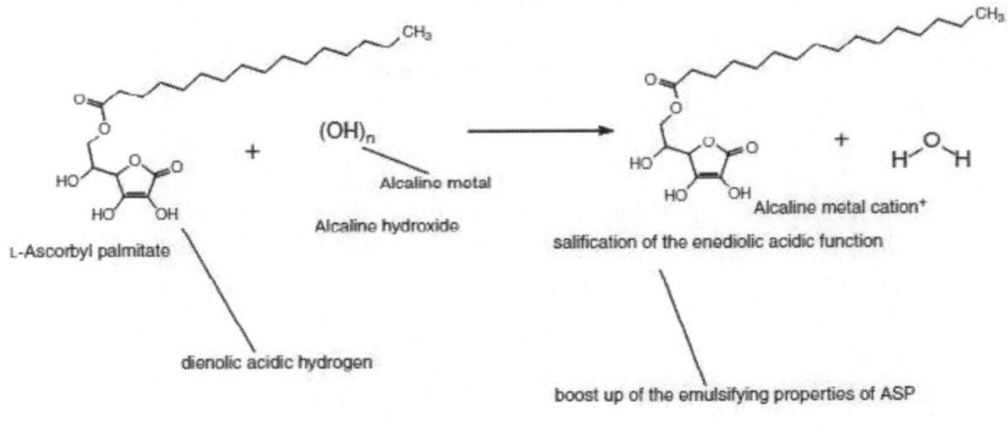

Figure 2. Boosting up of the emulsifying features of ascorbyl palmitate, by means of salification of enediolic acidic function.

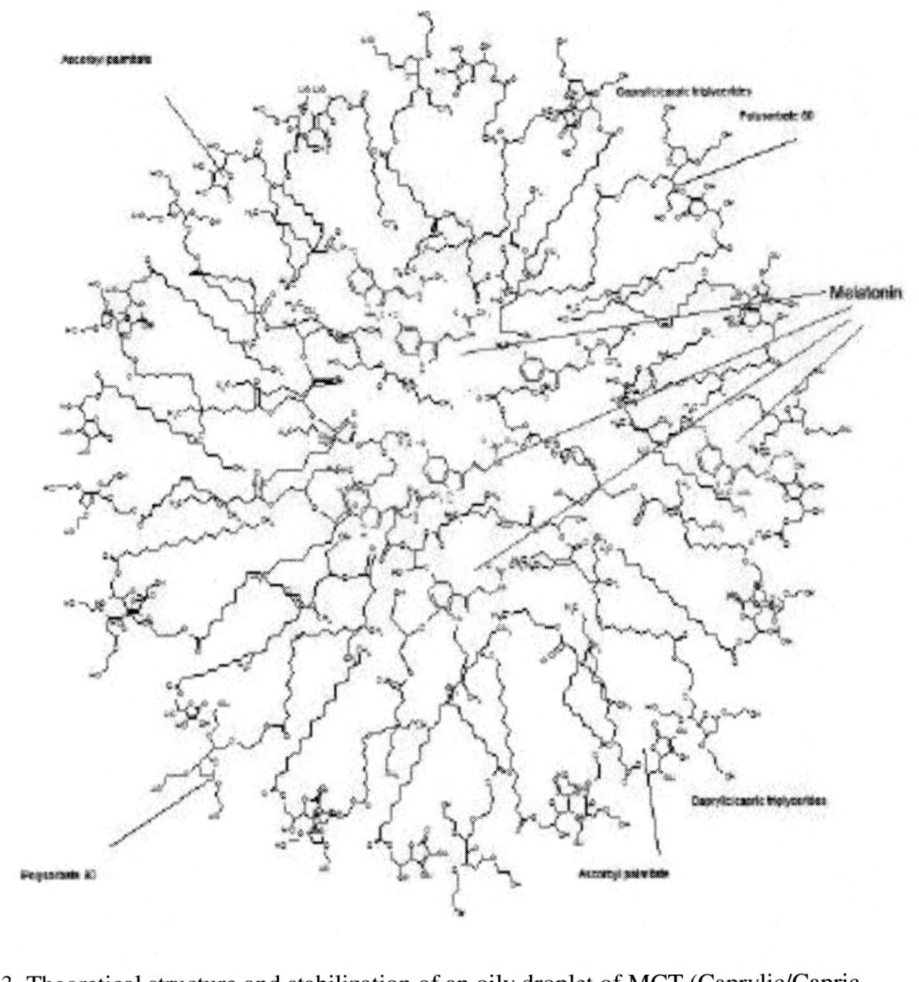

Figure 3. Theoretical structure and stabilization of an oily droplet of MCT (Caprylic/Capric Trigliceride) nanoemulsion surrounded by a monolayer of polysorbate 80 and ascorbyl palmitate.

For the aforementioned reasons, ASP is clearly a surfactant molecule capable of reducing water–oil interface tension, so favouring the emulsification process. This feature is referable to its amphiphilic structure as above-mentioned and described.

The synergy between ASP and PS 80 seems to find its rational of effectiveness in reducing the droplet surface tension, thanks to a regular geometric disposition of the surfactant molecules taking place to in an elastic monolayer surrounding oily droplet surface (Figure 3).

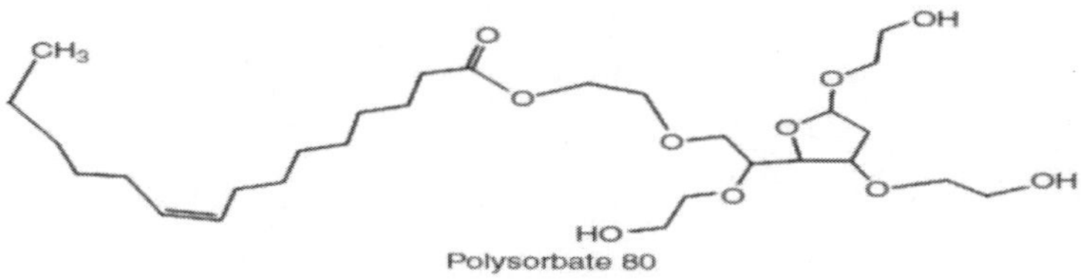

Figure 4. Structure of polysorbate 80.

Particularly, the high structure affinity between carbon chains of both emulsifiers and triglycerides could favour molecules packing and box up. On the other hand, it can be speculated that double bond in the centre of PS 80 carbon chain (Figure 4) could improve flexibility and elasticity of the oily droplet surface, so promoting an easier diameter reduction in the micelles. This fact is partially, but not completely confirmed, by the evidence that other similar polysorbate molecules such as polysorbate 20, 40 and 60, which are not equipped with a double bound of insaturation in the alkylic chain, are less performing in association with ASP in the production of very thin nanoemulsion and above all less effective in ensuring its stability over time. Further evaluations must be anyway carried out to prove the real chemico-physical behaviour and inter-phase phenomena of this emulsification process.

Nanoemulsion Characterization

Dynamic Light Scattering

Nanoemulsions were characterized by dynamic light scattering (DLS) using a Malvern Zetasizer Nano ZS at 25°C. Firstly, the decisive role of ASP in the nanoemulsion system development was verified comparing the DLS patterns of the same formulation prepared with and without ASP.

The results confirmed the significant interface effects of ASP that is able to reduce the mean diameter droplet size of about ten times, in respect to the sample prepared using only PS 80 as surfactant agent, even if an increase of polidispersity index value was detected.

The addition of melatonin (0.5% w/v) to the nanoemulsion did not affect its formation, as confirmed by the GRAPH 3. DLS results met the instrumental quality criteria in terms of correlation data, but the presence of different droplet populations in the samples could represent a point of criticism in terms of stability over time. During storage at 25 °C for 6 months and 40 °C for 2 months nanoemulsion, showed a good stability of both reference and melatonin nanoemulsions. The DLS patterns (GRAPHS 4-5) of the reference nanoemulsion stored for 6 months at 25 °C, and the nanoemulsion loaded with the active ingredient stored at 40 °C for 2 months, put out the shift of the Z average value in the range 100-200 nm. The increase of the mean diameter size was analogous in all samples stored at different temperatures, indicating that the system stability was slightly affected by thermal stresses. In contrast, temperature seems to have such a positive effect on the polydispersity index. The Z average diameter of the stored samples remained within the nanoemulsion range, confirming the good stability of the formulation.

			Size (d.n...	% Intensity	Width (d.n...
Z-Average (d.nm):	32.55	Peak 1:	43.91	87.5	31.60
PdI:	0.503	Peak 2:	3408	7.2	1292
Intercept:	0.878	Peak 3:	845.3	5.3	338.0
Result quality	Good				

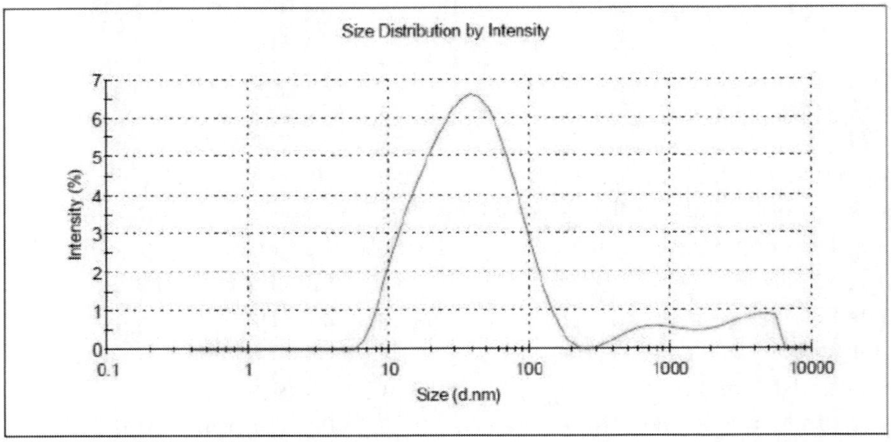

Graph 1. Formulation with ASP.

			Size (d.nm...	% Intensity	Width (d.n...
Z-Average (d.nm):	371.0	Peak 1:	415.0	100.0	125.4
PdI:	0.105	Peak 2:	0.000	0.0	0.000
Intercept:	0.930	Peak 3:	0.000	0.0	0.000
Result quality	Good				

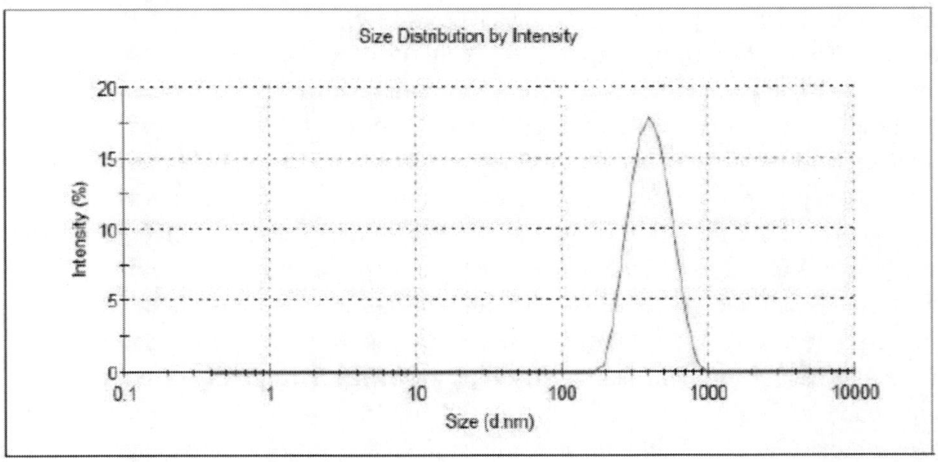

Graph 2. Formulation without ASP.

			Size (d.nm...	% Intensity	Width (d.n...
Z-Average (d.nm):	34.59	Peak 1:	52.01	100.0	33.33
PdI:	0.288	Peak 2:	0.000	0.0	0.000
Intercept:	0.968	Peak 3:	0.000	0.0	0.000
Result quality	Good				

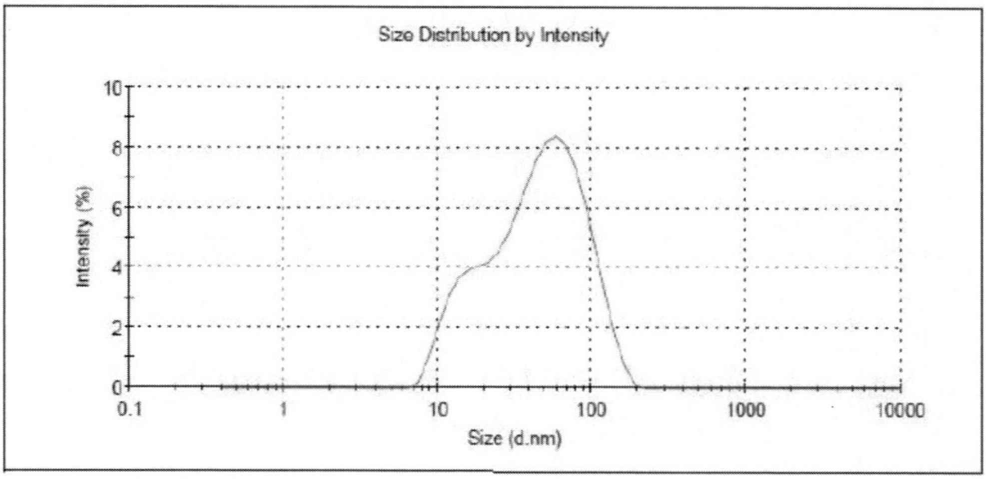

Graph 3. Nanoemulsion sample added with melatonin (Time=0).

			Size (d.nm...	% Intensity	Width (d.n...
Z-Average (d.nm):	98.52	Peak 1:	115.7	96.8	42.33
PdI:	0.300	Peak 2:	4940	3.2	643.5
Intercept:	0.967	Peak 3:	0.000	0.0	0.000
Result quality	Good				

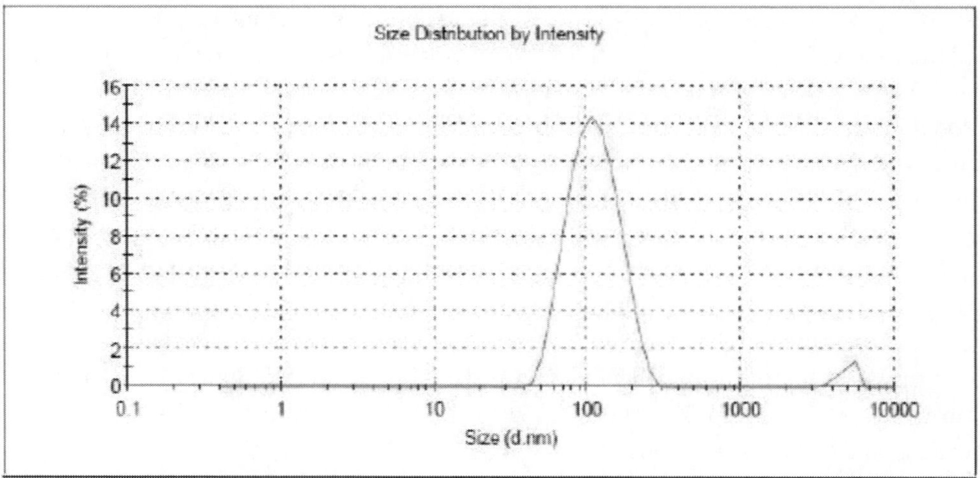

Graph 4. Nanoemulsion after 6 months of storage at 25°C.

			Size (d.nm...	% Intensity	Width (d.n...
Z-Average (d.nm):	181.2	Peak 1:	200.0	100.0	59.06
PdI:	0.099	Peak 2:	0.000	0.0	0.000
Intercept:	0.946	Peak 3:	0.000	0.0	0.000
Result quality	Good				

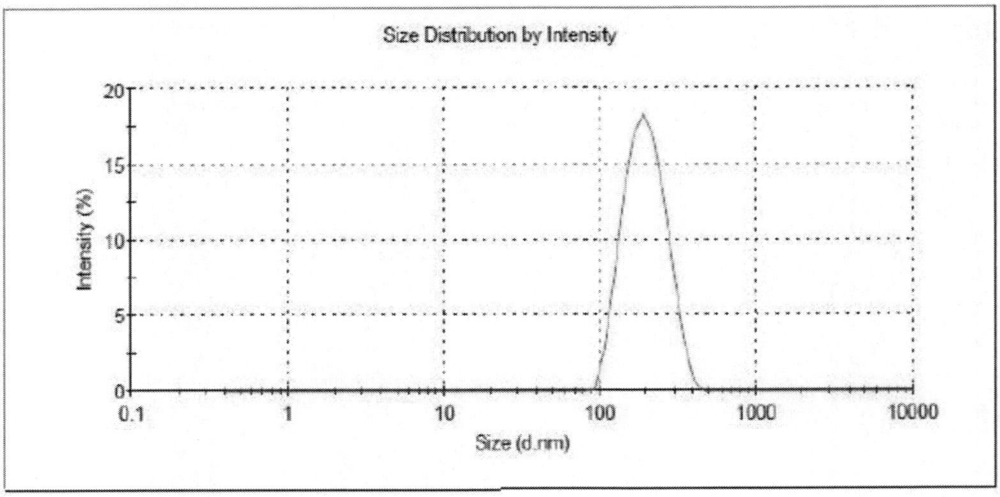

Graph 5. Nanoemulsion with melatonin after 2 months of storage at 40°C.

The analytical evaluation with Dynamic Back Scattering Laser device of the afore described nanoemulsions shows a substantially stable nanostructured system with an average droplet size of about 100–200 nm. The interesting consideration is that this system seems to be poorly affected by thermal stress over 60 days at 40°C. It can speculate that a prolonged thermal stress condition paradoxically improves stability and homogeneity of the dispersed system, thanks to a process of solubilization of the small oily droplets inside the continuous water phase. A deeper study is required to better assess the role of the prolonged thermal stress on the stability and chemico-physical features of this nanoemulsion.

After emulsification processes, the nucleus of the emulsion showed a slight acidic pH of about 4.2–4.5, indicating that ascorbic moiety of ASP surrounds the oily droplet exposing the hydrophilic and acidic portion to the external water phase so producing an acidic environment. As there are no other molecules of both lipophilic and hydrophilic nature capable of conferring an acidic character to the nanoemulsion, it is possible to speculate the correct orientation of ASP at the surface area of the oily droplets and so drawing a reliable structural model of nanoemulsion. Another interesting consideration is that after the adding of potassium sorbate to the nanostructured system nucleus, an improving in clearness of the system occurs because of the salification of ASP which improves its capability to emulsify. The experimental proof of this phenomenon is that after the addition of potassium sorbate the pH of the system raises up from 4.2 to about 5.2. At this pH value, ASP is ionized at one of its two enediolic acidic function (ASP pKa: 4.2).

After further acidification of the system with citric acid, the previous achieved clearness of the system did not change, remaining stable over time and thermal stress.

Bioavailability Assessment

Porcine Cheek Epithelium Preparation

The permeation study was performed by using porcine cheek epithelium that was prepared following standard procedures. The porcine cheek mucosa was frozen at –20°C within 24 h after removal. Prior to preparation, the mucosa was thawed to room temperature and then dipped for 1 min in pH 7.4 saline isotonic solution at 70°C. Then the epithelium was peeled from the edges of the mucosa. A circular epithelium membrane of 4.91 cm^2 area was stored in the refrigerator overnight until use. Prior to experimental use the membrane was hydrated at room temperature by immersion in pH 7.4 saline isotonic solution for 1 h and then carefully inspected visually for any defects before mounting it on a Franz diffusion cell.

Permeation Study through Porcine Cheek Epithelium

The circular epithelium membrane was placed between the donor and the receptor chamber of a modified Franz diffusion cell [41]. The upper and lower parts of the Franz cell were sealed with Teflon and Parafilm® to avoid the evaporation of receiver medium.

Melatonin, 5 mg, nanoemulsion, and Melatonin, 3 mg, sublingual tablet were used as donor phase and the melatonin content was 0.5% w/v in both experiments. Therefore, about 920 µl of nanoemulsion (volume equivalent to a single sprayed dose) or 600 µl of a melatonin tablet suspended in pH 6.4 phosphate buffer (corresponding to melatonin 0.5% w/v) were applied to the surface of the epithelium membrane. The receiver compartments were filled with a pH 7.4 phosphate buffer solution filtered through a filter membrane with pore size 0.2 µm. Special care was taken to avoid air bubbles between the receiver solution and the membrane. The prepared Franz cells, containing the receiver medium, was continuously stirred with a small magnetic bar and were kept at 37±1°C with a circulating water bath, throughout the experiment, so that the membrane surface temperature was 32±1°C. Only the receptor compartment was in contact with the circulating water at 37±1°C. At predetermined times (1, 3, 5, 7 and 24 h) 200µl samples were withdrawn from the receiver compartment and immediately replaced with fresh receiver medium. Sink conditions were maintained throughout the experiment. The withdrawn samples were assayed directly by HPLC to determine the concentrations of the compounds that had permeated through the porcine cheek epithelium. All values represent the mean ± standard deviation of five parallel experiments, at least.

Melatonin Retention into Porcine Cheek Epithelium

Modified Franz diffusion cells were disassembled; after 24 h following application of the formulations and the porcine cheek epithelium samples were carefully removed from the cells. Residuals of solution or tablet suspension were removed from the epithelium surface. Then, the epithelium was washed with 10 ml pH 7.4 phosphate buffer solution and 10 ml methanol to remove the excess of substance that was not permeated through the epithelium.

The membranes were cut into small pieces and collected in different Eppendorf microtubes containing 5 ml methanol. The samples were sonicated for 5 hours and left to stand for 12 h. Afterwards, the supernatant was filtered through a filter membrane with pore size 0.45 μm and the amount of melatonin retained in the mucosae was quantified by the HPLC method reported below.

Analysis of Melatonin

Melatonin assay was performed on a C18 reverse phase column (Hypersil Gold, 5μm, 250 x 4.6 mm, Thermo Fisher Scientific). The mobile phase, consisting of water and methanol 40:60 v:v, was eluted at 1 ml/min for about 8 minutes. The sample volume injected was 20 μl. The absorbance was measured at 223 nm. Quantification was performed based on a standard calibration curve. The standard calibration curve was represented by five known concentrations of the melatonin ranging from 0.01 to 5 μg/ml (r^2=0.9997) from 5 to 50 μg/ml (r^2=0.9998).

Results

We verified the performance of this system by measuring the *in vitro* permeation through porcine cheek epithelium and the retained amount of melatonin using modified Franz diffusion cells. The obtained results were compared to those obtained by using a commercial sublingual tablet.

By using the placebo nanoemulsion, it was preliminary verified that both cheek epithelium and the formulation components did not interfere with the determination of melatonin concentrations in the receiver medium. The melatonin permeation profiles through porcine cheek epithelium of the nanoemulsion and sublingual tablet are reported in *Figure 5.* In both cases, the melatonin permeation profiles were linear over the considered period of time. The measured lag time was very short for the nanoemulsion (0.7 h), while it was doubled in case of tablets (1.66 h).

The nanoemulsion showed better performances also in terms of the permeated amount after 24 h and the flux (*Table 1)* given that both values were statistically different (t-test, p=0.02). Differences between formulations were more evident within the first hours of the permeation study. As expected, the permeated amount after 24 h and the flux measured through the buccal mucosa were higher than those reported through the skin, with the only exception of the elastic liposome or ethosomes [29;30]. As far as the retained amount into porcine cheek epithelium is concerned, no statistical differences were found using both dosage forms.

Taking into account that no tissue depot effect was reported in vivo after transmucosal administration [36;37], the measured values should be due to the prolonged contact between the formulation and mucosae in the in vitro experiment. Hence, the proposed nanoemulsion seemed suitable for the sublingual administration of melatonin.

Table 1. Permeation parameters measured through porcine cheek epithelium by using nanoemulsion and sublingual tablet (n≥5; mean ± std. dev.)

	Permeated amount after 24 h (µg/cm2)	Flux (µg/cm2/h)	Retained amount after 24 h (µg/g mucosa)
Nanoemulsion	659.21 ± 178.69	29.72 ± 7.53	588.28 ± 85.17
Sublingual tablet	400.75 ± 171.37	17.72 ± 7.70	581.64 ± 210.69

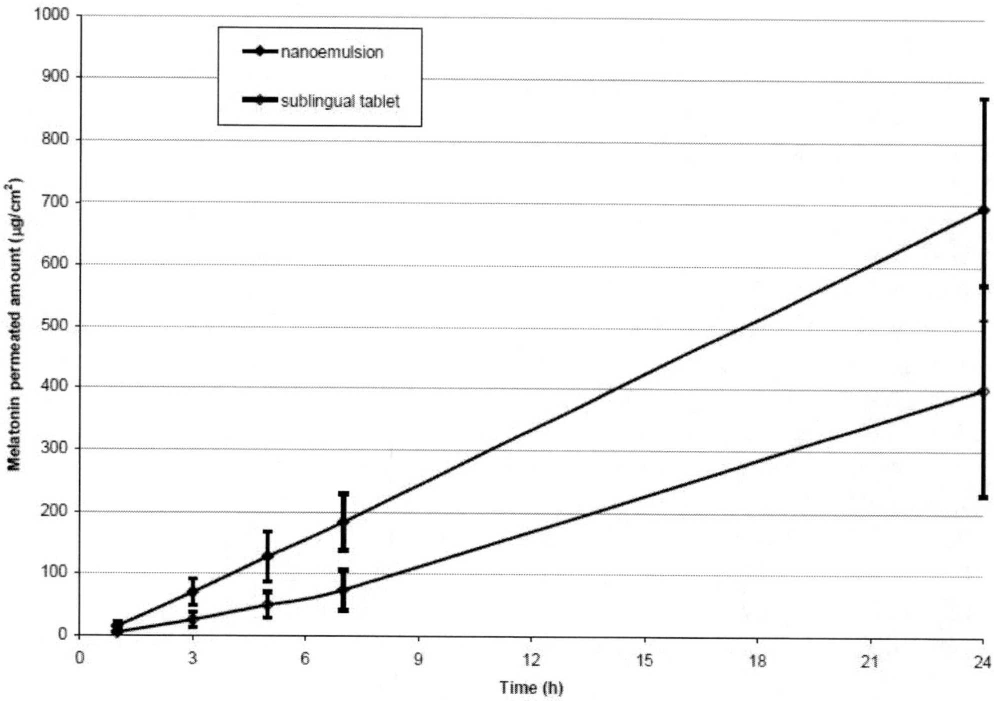

Figure 5. Melatonin permeation profiles through porcine cheek epithelium by using nanoemulsion (black diamonds) and sublingual tablet (white diamonds) (n≥5; mean ± std. dev.)

Conclusion

A new emulsification technology was developed to the delivery of melatonin. Preliminary data on the physical-chemical stability of the system and in vitro the performance of melatonin absorption through sublingual mucosal indicates a promising path to improve bioavailability of poorly absorbed active ingredients, particularly in the field of nutritional supplement formulations, not often answering to the minimal bioavailability requirements according to human pharmacology and physiology principles.

The inedited association of ASP and PS 80 can guarantee a good stability, namely clearness, no occurring of coalescence and Ostwald ripening macroscopic phenomena over time and under thermal stress conditions, and maintain the organoleptic features necessary for the oral administration.

This technology seems to be particularly promising to encapsulate water unstable molecules, poorly absorbed through the intestinal mucosa or hugely metabolized in the liver microsomes and to improve their absorption through the lingual mucosal so to avoid first-pass effect. Further investigations should be carried out to evaluate the effectiveness of the ASP/PS80 association to improve the stability under oxidative stress conditions of melatonin and other substrates, such as fish oils and other molecules, very susceptible to oxidation.

References

[1] Azeem A, Talegaonkar S, Negi LM, Ahmad FJ, Khar RK, Iqbal Z. Oil based nanocarrier system for transdermal delivery of ropinirole: a mechanistic, pharmacokinetic and biochemical investigation. *Int. J. Pharm.* 2012 Jan 17;422(1-2):436-44.

[2] Rizwan M, Aqil M, Talegaonkar S, Azeem A, Sultana Y, Ali A. Enhanced transdermal drug delivery techniques: an extensive review of patents. *Recent Pat. Drug Deliv. Formul.* 2009 Jun;3(2):105-24.

[3] Talegaonkar S, Azeem A, Ahmad FJ, Khar RK, Pathan SA, Khan ZI. Microemulsions: a novel approach to enhanced drug delivery. *Recent Pat. Drug Deliv. Formul.* 2008;2(3):238-57.

[4] Schaffazick SR, Pohlmann AR, de Cordova CA, Creczynski-Pasa TB, Guterres SS. Protective properties of melatonin-loaded nanoparticles against lipid peroxidation. *Int. J. Pharm.* 2005 Jan 31;289(1-2):209-13.

[5] Bernardi DS, Pereira TA, Maciel NR, Bortoloto J, Viera GS, Oliveira GC, et al. Formation and stability of oil-in-water nanoemulsions containing rice bran oil: in vitro and in vivo assessments. *J. Nanobiotechnology* 2011;9:44.

[6] Gershanik T, Benita S. Self-dispersing lipid formulations for improving oral absorption of lipophilic drugs. *Eur. J. Pharm. Biopharm.* 2000 Jul;50(1):179-88.

[7] Klang S, Abdulrazik M, Benita S. Influence of emulsion droplet surface charge on indomethacin ocular tissue distribution. *Pharm. Dev. Technol.* 2000;5(4):521-32.

[8] Klang SH, Siganos CS, Benita S, Frucht-Pery J. Evaluation of a positively charged submicron emulsion of piroxicam on the rabbit corneum healing process following alkali burn. *J. Control Release* 1999 Jan 4;57(1):19-27.

[9] Solans C, Kunieda H. *Industrial applications of microemulsions*. 1997.

[10] Huang Q, Yu H, Ru Q. Bioavailability and delivery of nutraceuticals using nanotechnology. *J. Food Sci.* 2010 Jan;75(1):R50-R57.

[11] McClements DJ, Li Y. Structured emulsion-based delivery systems: controlling the digestion and release of lipophilic food components. *Adv. Colloid Interface Sci.* 2010 Sep 15;159(2):213-28.

[12] Izquierdo P, Esquena J, Tadros TF, Dederen JC, Feng J, Garcia-Celma MJ, et al. Phase behavior and nano-emulsion formation by the phase inversion temperature method. *Langmuir* 2004 Aug 3;20(16):6594-8.

[13] Esquena J, Solans C, Llorens J. Nitrogen Sorption Studies of Silica Particles Obtained in Emulsion and Microemulsion Media. *J. Colloid Interface Sci.* 2000 May 15;225(2):291-8.

[14] Tadros T, Izquierdo P, Esquena J, Solans C. Formation and stability of nano-emulsions. *Adv. Colloid Interface Sci.* 2004 May 20;108-109:303-18.
[15] DeMuro RL, Nafziger AN, Blask DE, Menhinick AM, Bertino JS, Jr. The absolute bioavailability of oral melatonin. *J. Clin. Pharmacol.* 2000 Jul;40(7):781-4.
[16] Aldhous M, Franey C, Wright J, Arendt J. Plasma concentrations of melatonin in man following oral absorption of different preparations. *Br. J. Clin. Pharmacol.* 1985 Apr;19(4):517-21.
[17] Lee BJ, Parrott KA, Ayres JW, Sack RL. Preliminary evaluation of transdermal delivery of melatonin in human subjects. *Res. Commun. Mol. Pathol. Pharmacol.* 1994 Sep;85(3):337-46.
[18] Lee BJ, Ryu SG, Choi HG, Kim CK, Parrott KA, Ayres JW, et al. Batch variation and pharmacokinetics of oral sustained release melatonin-loaded sugar spheres in human subjects. *Arch. Pharm. Res.* 1997 Dec;20(6):555-9.
[19] Aeschbach D, Lockyer BJ, Dijk DJ, Lockley SW, Nuwayser ES, Nichols LD, et al. Use of transdermal melatonin delivery to improve sleep maintenance during daytime. *Clin. Pharmacol. Ther.* 2009 Oct;86(4):378-82.
[20] Fischer TW, Greif C, Fluhr JW, Wigger-Alberti W, Elsner P. Percutaneous penetration of topically applied melatonin in a cream and an alcoholic solution. *Skin Pharmacol. Physiol.* 2004 Jul;17(4):190-4.
[21] Kanikkannan N, Andega S, Burton S, Babu RJ, Singh M. Formulation and in vitro evaluation of transdermal patches of melatonin. *Drug Dev. Ind. Pharm.* 2004 Feb;30(2):205-12.
[22] Kandimalla KK, Kanikkannan N, Singh M. Optimization of a vehicle mixture for the transdermal delivery of melatonin using artificial neural networks and response surface method. *J. Control. Release* 1999 Aug 27;61(1-2):71-82.
[23] Kikwai L, Kanikkannan N, Babu RJ, Singh M. Effect of vehicles on the transdermal delivery of melatonin across porcine skin in vitro. *J. Control Release* 2002 Oct 4;83(2):307-11.
[24] Kandimalla KK, Babu RJ, Singh M. Biphasic flux profiles of melatonin: the Yin-Yang of transdermal permeation enhancement mediated by fatty alcohol enhancers. *J. Pharm. Sci.* 2010 Jan;99(1):209-18.
[25] Kanikkannan N, Singh M. Skin permeation enhancement effect and skin irritation of saturated fatty alcohols. *Int. J. Pharm.* 2002 Nov 6;248(1-2):219-28.
[26] Oh HJ, Oh YK, Kim CK. Effects of vehicles and enhancers on transdermal delivery of melatonin. *Int. J. Pharm.* 2001 Jan 5;212(1):63-71.
[27] Gwak HS, Kim SU, Chun IK. Effect of vehicles and enhancers on the in vitro permeation of melatonin through hairless mouse skin. *Arch. Pharm. Res.* 2002 Jun;25(3):392-6.
[28] Hafner A, Lovric J, Pepic I, Filipovic-Grcic J. Lecithin/chitosan nanoparticles for transdermal delivery of melatonin. *J. Microencapsul.* 2011;28(8):807-15.
[29] Dubey V, Mishra D, Asthana A, Jain NK. Transdermal delivery of a pineal hormone: melatonin via elastic liposomes. *Biomaterials* 2006 Jun;27(18):3491-6.
[30] Dubey V, Mishra D, Jain NK. Melatonin loaded ethanolic liposomes: physicochemical characterization and enhanced transdermal delivery. *Eur. J. Pharm. Biopharm.* 2007 Sep;67(2):398-405.

[31] Benes L, Claustrat B, Horriere F, Geoffriau M, Konsil J, Parrott KA, et al. Transmucosal, oral controlled-release, and transdermal drug administration in human subjects: a crossover study with melatonin. *J. Pharm. Sci.* 1997 Oct;86(10):1115-9.

[32] Kittelmann M, Rahe P, Kuhnle A. Molecular self-assembly on an insulating surface: interplay between substrate templating and intermolecular interactions. *J. Phys. Condens. Matter.* 2012 Sep 5;24(35):354007.

[33] Miller CA, Abbott NL, de Pablo JJ. Surface activity of amphiphilic helical beta-peptides from molecular dynamics simulation. *Langmuir* 2009 Mar 3;25(5):2811-23.

[34] Walle T, Hsieh F, DeLegge MH, Oatis JE, Jr., Walle UK. High absorption but very low bioavailability of oral resveratrol in humans. *Drug. Metab. Dispos.* 2004 Dec;32(12):1377-82.

[35] Bouchemal K, Briancon S, Perrier E, Fessi H. Nano-emulsion formulation using spontaneous emulsification: solvent, oil and surfactant optimisation. *Int. J. Pharm.* 2004 Aug 6;280(1-2):241-51.

[36] Cavallo A, Hassan M. Stability of melatonin in aqueous solution. *J. Pineal. Res.* 1995 Mar;18(2):90-2.

[37] Windholz M. The Merck index an encyclopedia of chemicals, drugs, and biologicals. 1983;10th ed.

[38] Pinnell SR, Yang H, Omar M, Monteiro-Riviere N, DeBuys HV, Walker LC, et al. Topical L-ascorbic acid: percutaneous absorption studies. *Dermatol. Surg.* 2001 Feb;27(2):137-42.

[39] Gopinath D, Ravi D, Rao BR, Apte SS, Renuka D, Rambhau D. Ascorbyl palmitate vesicles (Aspasomes): formation, characterization and applications. *Int. J. Pharm.* 2004 Mar 1;271(1-2):95-113.

[40] Date AA, Naik B, Nagarsenker MS. Novel drug delivery systems: potential in improving topical delivery of antiacne agents. *Skin Pharmacol. Physiol.* 2006;19(1):2-16.

[41] Minghetti P, Casiraghi A, Cilurzo F, Montanari L, Marazzi M, Falcone L, et al. Comparison of different membranes with cultures of keratinocytes from man for percutaneous absorption of nitroglycerine. *J. Pharm. Pharmacol.* 1999 Jun;51(6):673-8.

In: New Developments in Melatonin Research ISBN: 978-1-62618-843-3
Editors: D.Acuña-Castroviejo, I.Rusanova, G.Escames © 2013 Nova Science Publishers, Inc.

Chapter 15

Therapeutic Potential of Melatonin Associated with Other Drugs

Alejandro Romero[1*], Eva Ramos[1], Esther Parada[2,3] and Javier Egea[2,3]
[1]Department of Toxicology and Pharmacology, Faculty of Veterinary Medicine, Complutense University of Madrid, Madrid, Spain
[2]Instituto Teófilo Hernando,
[3]Departamento de Farmacología y Terapéutica, Facultad de Medicina, Universidad Autónoma de Madrid, Madrid, Spain

Abstract

Melatonin is a well-known potent antioxidant synthesized mainly in the pineal gland. The therapeutic value by itself is well known in several diseases, but is in the last decade when several studies report that the coadministration of melatonin with other drugs, enhances melatonin´s protective effect as well as the own effect of the drug. Even when the drug itself induces damage melatonin is capable to minimize the side effects. This is reinforced by the low cost of melatonin and its very low toxic hazard. Combined action with melatonin can be of critical importance for the development of novel therapeutic strategies. Finally, this chapter collates evidence from many research laboratories with special emphasis on the clinical aspects and potential uses of melatonin in several diseases.

Introduction

It is known that melatonin is a versatile and ubiquitous molecule, originally discovered as a hormone synthesized mainly in the pineal gland, is also produced by immune system cells

* Corresponding author: Alejandro Romero PhD. Department of Toxicology and Pharmacology, Faculty of Veterinary Medicine, Complutense University of Madrid. Avda. Puerta de Hierro s/n 28040 Madrid. Spain Phone: +34-913943834 Fax: +34-913943840; email: manarome@ucm.es.

and in many peripheral tissues including brain, airway epithelium, bone marrow, gut, ovary, testes, skin and likely other tissues [1]. In mammals, three major melatoninergic membrane receptors have been identified. Among them, MT1 and MT2 are considered to represent the melatonin receptor system and their physiological functions and pharmacological properties are well documented [2]. MT3 receptor also has been identified as quinone reductase 2 [3]. However, nuclear binding sites/receptors also exist for this indole and have been identified as a further class of melatonin receptors [4]. The distribution of receptors and other binding sites indicates a remarkable pleiotropy of melatonin, which may potentially affect most of the cells, in addition to other receptor-independent mechanisms may contribute to explain the different and tissue-specific functions of melatonin [5-7]. The antioxidant abilities of this neurohormone may derive either from direct scavenging of free radicals at high (millimolar) concentrations or by increasing the activity and expression of antioxidant enzymes, a response observed at low (nanomolar) concentrations. Thus, deficiencies in melatonin production or melatonin receptor expression and decreases in melatonin levels are likely to cause numerous dysfunctions associated with a multitude of pathophysiological changes [8]. The toxicity and tissue damage induced by a large number of drugs is consequence of free radical generation and related reactants [9]. Recent advances in melatonin knowledge have suggested the possibility of enhancing the therapeutic activity of different drugs and/or to reduce the possible side effects when they are administered [9]. Melatonin has been administered in both physiological and pharmacological amounts to humans and animals, and there is widespread agreement that it is a non-toxic molecule. Considering its diverse actions via both receptor and receptor-independent actions and given melatonin's high lipophilicity and the ease with which it cross morphophysiological barriers, its use as a combination therapy with a wide variety of currently used drugs suggests interesting therapeutic perspectives.

In this chapter, we summarize the studies that show the diverse effects of the multifunctional indole, melatonin, alone or in combination with pharmaceutical agents used for the treatment against mental disorders and neurodegenerative diseases, autoimmune diseases, cancer, gastrointestinal tract diseases, endocrine diseases, cardiovascular and infectious diseases.

Mental Disorders and Neurodegenerative Diseases

Increasing evidence suggests that melatonin rhythmicity plays by itself a key role in several metabolic functions as antioxidant, anti-inflammatory chronobiotic and epigenetic regulator, through mechanisms which include nuclear receptors, histone acetylating and DNA methylating enzymes [10]. In neurodegenerative diseases, there are three frequently interrelated processes (glutamate excitotoxicity, free radical-mediated damage and mitochondrial dysfunction), identified as common pathophysiological mechanisms leading to neuronal death [11]. Neuroprotective properties of melatonin against these three processes, added to its regulatory effects on circadian disturbances, point to melatonin as a therapeutic substance in the symptomatic treatment of neurodegenerative diseases.

Epilepsy is one of the most common chronic neurologic disorders. Evidence suggesting a possible relationship between melatonin and epilepsy was found in the 1970s when pinealectomy of previously parathyroidectomiced rats induced violent convulsions [12]. Reviewing the literature, we found many *in vivo* studies showing the anticonvulsant properties of melatonin. Hence, melatonin applied at doses 75 mg/kg or higher, significantly increased the after discharge threshold, and suppressed generalized seizures in amygdala kindled rats, which is a model for temporal lobe human epilepsy [13]. The pinealectomy exerted a significant influence on amygdala kindling development by reducing the number of stimulations needed to reach stage 5, suggesting that endogenous melatonin may act as a neuroprotective factor [14]. In mice, melatonin (50 mg/kg) significantly raised the electroconvulsive threshold, and when administered at a subprotective dose of 25 mg/kg, it enhanced the antielectroshock activity of carbamazepine and phenobarbital. In this work, the authors show that the anti-electroshock efficacy of melatonin depends on purinergic and GABA-ergic neurotransmission [15]. In other model, a combination of melatonin, applied at subprotective doses (10 and 20 mg/kg), with L-arginine also resulted in a potent anticonvulsant action. These findings may imply involvement of the L-arginine/nitric oxide (NO) pathway in the melatonin-induced modulation of seizure susceptibility in mice [16]. However, there are few studies showing proconvulsant effects of melatonin [17, 18]. In clinical studies, only a few small scale trials of adjunctive melatonin administration in humans have indicated that melatonin may decrease the incidence of seizures. A double-blind, placebo-controlled study in epileptic children assessed the effects of add-on melatonin administration on their quality of life. Improved physical function, emotional well-being, cognitive function, social function, and behavior suggested that melatonin might be an advantageous adjunctive drug in epileptic patients [19]. Most of the data indicate anticonvulsant properties of melatonin when applied at pharmacological doses in both animal models and clinical investigations.

Accumulating evidence suggests that melatonin plays a role in the pathophysiology of schizophrenia. Decreased nocturnal secretion of melatonin has been detected in drug-free paranoid schizophrenic patients [20]. Moreover, there is evidence of pineal calcification in schizophrenia, associated with cortical atrophy [21]. Two recent meta-analyses showed that schizophrenia is accompanied by monocytic activation including increased levels of proinflammatory cytokines and altered T cell activation [22, 23]. There is also evidence for increased neuroinflammation in schizophrenic patients. Melatonin is not only a hypnotic and circadian rhythm resynchronizing compound, it is also a strong antioxidant and anti-inflammatory agent [24, 25]. Melatonin plays a role in the pathophysiology, developmental etiology, course and treatment of schizophrenia. Melatonin decreases anti-psychotic side effects, hypertension [26], sleep disorders, glucose dysregulation [27], obesity [28] and tardive dyskinesia as well as increasing the longevity of a population of people.

Alzheimer Disease (AD) is an age-associated neurodegenerative disease characterized by progressive and cognitive function, loss of cholinergic neurons, impaired memory and other neurological manifestations. Genetic factors, chronic inflammation associated with cytokine release, oxidative stress, and trace element neurotoxicity have been suggested as possible causes of the disease [29]. Reviewing the literature, we found many *in vitro* and *in vivo* studies showing the neuroprotective effect of melatonin alone or in combination with other drugs. In neuroblastoma models using Aβ peptides or okadaic acid as model of AD, melatonin inhibits free radical production measured as lipid peroxidation by scavenging free radicals generated by these two neurotoxic agents [30, 31]. In this study, either melatonin or vitamin C administration prevented the effects of okadaic acid. The reduction of free radical damage was greater with melatonin, due to the fact that melatonin increases glutathione S-transferase and glutathione reductase levels. In another work, melatonin also reversed glycogen synthase kinase-3 (GSK-3) activation produced by calyculin-A, supporting that melatonin´s actions are not only based on its scavenging effect [32]. In AD patients, a 20 - 50% reduction of α7 nicotinic acetylcholine receptors (nAChRs) has been observed in specific brain areas [33]. Hence, it is important to maintain an intact cholinergic function to avoid cognitive impairments. Melatonin is a modulator of nAChRs as demonstrated in studies in vas deferens contraction by acetylcholine in rats [34, 35]. Recently, it has been proposed that melatonin should be administered at night to increase the number of α7 nAChRs and allow a reduction in anti-cholinesterase dose [36]. In this sense, it has been demonstrated that combination of sub-effective concentrations of melatonin and galantamine protects against oxidative stress in neuroblastoma cells [37].

In several experiments transgenic (Tg) murine models of AD have been used to assess a possible therapeutical beneficial effect of melatonin. Melatonin was found to be effective, inhibiting Aβ deposition in APP 695 Tg mice alleviating behavioral impairments and memory deficits deficiencies following long-term administration of melatonin at a daily dose of 10 mg/kg [38]. In APP/PS1 Tg mice melatonin from 2 to 2.5 months reduced cognitive impairments, decreasing Aβ deposition and inflammatory cytokines in hippocampus and entorhinal cortex [39]. APP/PS1 Tg mice were also used to assess the efficacy of a tacrine-melatonin hybrid to inhibit amyloid-induced cell death. The efficacy of the tacrine-melatonin hybrid to reduce Aβ toxicity suggested the possibility for a new potential therapeutic strategy in AD [40].

Several clinical trials have been focused on the possible application of melatonin to improve some of the symptoms of AD, such as sleep difficulties and cognitive impairment. Melatonin (3mg/day; 9 patients *vs* placebo; 11 patients) for 4 weeks significantly prolonged the sleep time and decreased locomotor activity at night, in a double-blind study. Melatonin treatment also caused an improvement in cognition [41]. Melatonin, in earlier stages of the AD in patients with mild cognitive impairment, also showed significantly better performance concomitantly with an improvement in wakefulness and sleep quality [42]. However, in two multicenter, randomized, placebo-controlled clinical trials, melatonin (2.5 or 10 mg slow-release; 8.5 mg immediate release and 1.5 mg sustained release) did not show significant differences compared to placebo in objective sleep measures and circadian rhythmicity [43, 44].

Parkinson Disease (PD) is the second most common neurodegenerative disease after AD. PD is characterized by the progressive degeneration of DA-containing neurons in the substantia nigra pars compacta. Biochemical studies suggest that reactive oxygen/nitrogen species are important mediators in the pathogenesis of PD. Hence, the antioxidant properties of melatonin may be useful in PD patients. There are many *in vitro* and *in vivo* studies showing the neuroprotective effect of melatonin against toxicity induced by 1-methyl-4-phenyl-1,2,3,6-tetrahydropyridine (MPTP) [45, 46] and 6-hydroxydopamine [47, 48]. In these models, melatonin significantly prevented the increased lipid peroxidation and also increased the levels of antioxidant enzymes, such as Cu/Zn- superoxide dismutase and glutathione peroxidase (GSH-Px). Moreover, MPTP was able to inhibit mitochondrial complex I of the electronic transport chain (ETC). It has been suggested that melatonin by increasing the activity of complex I and IV of the ETC, exerts a beneficial effect on MPTP-induced damage [49].

Studies carried out in patients with PD assess the possible role of melatonin in the modification of symptoms associated with this disease, such as sleep difficulties, cognitive impairment or motor dysfunctions. A double-blind, placebo-controlled cross-over trial enrolled 40 subjects with PD who complained of sleep disturbances. A significant improvement in total nighttime sleep duration was observed during the 50 mg melatonin treatment. Furthermore, there was also a significant improvement in subjective sleep quality and quantity, and daytime sleepiness during the 5 mg melatonin treatment compared to placebo [50]. In another study 18 PD patients were randomized to receive melatonin (3 mg) or placebo 1 h before bedtime for 4 weeks [51]. Sleep fragmentation tended to be more severe in patients on lower doses of levodopa although melatonin significantly improved subjective quality of sleep. Melatonin was not able to improve motor dysfunction.

As in the case of AD and PD, in Huntington's disease (HD) patients sleep disturbances are very prevalent and can substantially impair their quality of life. Moreover, it has been observed an abnormal secretion of melatonin in early stage HD patients [52]. Furthermore, diurnal melatonin levels strongly correlated with both motor and functional impairment, indicating that melatonin levels in HD may progressively decline with advanced disease [52]. Melatonin administration was reported to defer the clinical signs of the disease in an animal model of HD [53]. More recently, Melatonin delayed disease onset and prolongs lifespan in the R6/2 transgenic mouse HD model. The authors demonstrated the importance of the MT1 receptors in the protective effect of melatonin in this genetic model of HD [54].

Amyotrophic lateral sclerosis (ALS) is the most common form of motor neuron disease. It is typically characterized by adult-onset degeneration of the upper and lower motor neurons, and is usually fatal within a few years of onset. There are a limited number of studies with melatonin in ALS. In a mouse genetic model of ALS, orally administered melatonin delayed disease progression by 25% and extended survival. In 31 ALS patients, melatonin (5 mg/kg) was applied nightly as a suppository during 2 to 24 months. Melatonin was well tolerated with some patients reporting improved sleep quality and reduced protein carbonyls in blood, for up to 4 months, compared to levels before treatment onset [55].

Melatonin and Cancer

The possible role of melatonin in preventing tumor initiation, promotion, and progression was hypothesized by numerous scientists during the latter half of the last century, and different studies have been carried out to assess the oncostatic properties of melatonin against different neoplasias including breast cancer, leukemia, colorectal cancer, melanoma, prostate cancer, pancreatic cancer etc. [56]. Thus, the multiple modes of action of melatonin (antiproliferative, antimetastatic and prodifferentiation) within the cell make it an excellent candidate molecule for the prevention of cancer in risk individuals or for the treatment of cancer in combination with other conventional therapies. Furthermore, the decline in the biosynthesis of melatonin with age has been suggested as one of the major contributors to immunosenescence and development of neoplastic diseases. Reviewing the literature, we found many *in vitro* and *in vivo* studies exploring the possible mechanism of melatonin anticancer action. In both *in vitro* and *in vivo* investigations, melatonin protected healthy cells from radiation-induced and chemotherapeutic drug-induced toxicity due to its antioxidant property. Radiotherapy induces the formation of reactive oxygen species (ROS) including free radicals, which, in many cases, are sources of the negative side effects of these therapies. Melatonin, considered as an antioxidant radioprotector, may delay the saturation of the repair enzymes, thus allowing the repair of induced damage and applying higher doses of radiation may provide better therapeutic value [57]. Chemotherapy is the treatment of choice for patients with disease unresponsive to endocrine agents or with rapidly progressive visceral disease. Chemotherapeutic agents inhibit tumour growth by mechanisms that are drug specific. These therapies prolonged survival of patients. Additionally, however, they generate free radicals that cause extensive molecular damage or dysfunction that can lead to organ pathology, and produce important side effects such as cardiotoxicity, neuropathy, hematological toxicity, skin necrosis, gastric effects (nausea and vomiting), etc.[58]. Melatonin as an adjuvant therapy protects against side effects of different chemotherapeutic drugs and, in some cases, potentiates their oncostatic effects. Thus, doxorubicin (Adriamycin) belongs to group of antineoplastic agents, widely used in the treatment of breast cancer and it has also been successfully used to treat a variety of soft and solid tumours. But its use is complicated by significant acute and chronic side effects and the development of cardiomyopathy [59]. Studies performed in rats treated with doxorubicin alone or in combination with melatonin reported beneficial effects against doxorubicin cardiotoxicity [60]. In this line, melatonin, compared with a classical antioxidant, vitamin E, were found to protect, equally effectively against doxorubicin-induced cardiomyopathy. In this study, melatonin at a 50-fold lower dose than vitamin E, improved the antitumour activity more than the vitamin antioxidant [61]. It should be pointed out that melatonin does not interfere with the action of doxorubicin on tumour cells, rather, actually enhances the effect of anticancer drug [62]. Because of its combined actions as an antioxidant and tumour suppressor, melatonin may exaggerate the anticancer efficacy of doxorubicin [63]. Cisplatin (*cis*-diamminedichloroplatinum), like doxorubicin, is a widely used chemotherapy agent, the dose and use is limited by its toxicity. The biochemical basis of cisplatin toxicity is believed to relate to free radicals generated in kidney, peripheral nerves and structures of the inner ear [64]. Several antioxidants have been tested, with limited success, as potential agents to ameliorate the destructive actions of this chemotherapeutic drug [65]. Thus, some investigators have also used melatonin as a potential mitigating agent against the collateral damage caused by cisplatin. The beneficial effects of melatonin, in reducing cisplatin toxicity, has been shown at the level or the inner ear [66], attenuating a severe oxidative stress on renal tissue [67] and ameliorative cytotoxicity effects in peripheral blood mononuclear cells[68]. Also, it is worth mentioning that, in reference to relationship of melatonin and cisplatin to cancer-cell proliferation, the study of Futagami et al.[69] proposed that melatonin may improve the efficacy of cisplatin as a treatment for ovarian cancer. The protective action of melatonin in these studies was again presumed to be due to melatonin´s scavenging of free radicals that resulted from cisplatin-induced toxicity. Another commonly used cancer chemotherapeutic agent, bleomycin, dose-dependently induces interstitial pulmonary fibrosis, as well as, changing the activity of antioxidative enzymes in broncho-alveolar fluid and lung tissues. Administration of melatonin (10 mg/kg i.p twice weekly), after 25 days of treatment of rats with bleomycin (10 mg/kg i.p twice daily), markedly reduced all parameters indicative of oxidative stress, with which, based on the outcome of this study, melatonin is a good candidate as an agent to reduce bleomycin toxicity and prevent the associated interstitial pulmonary fibrosis [70]. Melatonin had also been reported to protect against the cytotoxicity of cytarabine [71], a mylosuppressive cytotoxic drug used in the treatment of cancer. The authors showed that each of the changes associated with cytarabine administration (bone-marrow damage, including lowered total leucocyte counts and a reduced number of platelets) were prevented in the rats given melatonin after the injection of the drug. In reference to taxanes, melatonin (1nM) enhances the antitumor effects of paclitaxel in the estrogen receptor positive endometrial cancer cell line [72].

Table 1. Clinical trials on melatonin application in combination with other drugs for the treatment of different types of cancer

Pathology	Melatonin combined with other drugs or therapies	Effect	Melatonin dose used
Metastatic colorectal cancer patients.	IL-2.	Effective as a second-line therapy to induce tumour regression [145].	20 mg/day
Untreatable endocrine tumours (thyroid cancers and endocrine pancreatic tumours).	IL-2.	Well-tolerated and potentially active therapy of untreatable advanced endocrine tumours [146].	40 mg/day
Different advanced solid tumours.	IL-2 or TNF	Prevent hypotension occurred during cancer immunotherapy [147].	40 mg/day
Metastatic prostate cancer	Triptorelin	PSA mean concentrations significantly decreased [148].	20 mg/day
Advanced small cell lung cancer	Chemotherapy	Percent of 1-year survival was significantly higher in patients treated with combined therapy [149].	20 mg/day
Metastatic breast cancer in woman	Epirubicin	Platelets number was normalized and tumor regression was achieved in 41% patients [150].	20 mg/day
Metastatic solid tumours.	Chemotherapy	Higher tumour regression rate with combined administration of melatonin was observed. Furthermore, in patients concomitantly treated with melatonin reduced thrombocytopenia, neurotoxicity, cardiotoxicity, stomatitis and asthenia [151].	20 mg/day
Metastatic colorectal cancer	Irinotecan	The efficacy of Irinotecan may be enhanced by melatonin.[152]	20 mg/day
Metastatic non-small cell lung cancer or gastrointestinal tumours	Different combinations of cisplatin, etoposide, gemcitabine, oxaliplatin, 5-fluorouracil, Epirubicin and folates	Melatonin increased 2-year survival rate [153]	20 mg/day

In other experimental study, a model of chemically induced hamster pancreatic tumour, the combined administration of capecitabine and melatonin improved the antitumour effect of the cytostatic. Thus, only 10% of the animals treated with melatonin plus capecitabine developed moderately differentiated pancreatic adenocarcinomas [73].

The ability of melatonin to decrease the toxicity and increase the efficacy of cancer chemotherapeutic agents has been exploited at clinical level as well [74]. Of the few studies in humans, most were carried out in patients with advanced metastatic cancer, essentially at the terminal state, and some were unblinded or were not placebo controlled. In most cases, melatonin was used as an adjuvant therapy, associated with other drugs or radiation, to reduce the side effects of the usual treatments. These studies are summarized in *Table 1*. In most of the studies, the dose of melatonin was 20 mg orally, once a day. The 20-mg dosage of melatonin shown to be effective in reducing the risk of cancer, which is much higher than the 1.5-5 mg regularly used for the treatment of insomnia and jet-lag. Generally, melatonin is considered relatively safe even at high doses, and the trials included in this chapter reported no significant side effects. Thus, probably the most important property of melatonin administration in humans, and the one that may eventually allow it to proceed to treatment, is its lack of toxicity.

The objective tumour regression rate, as well as the 1-year survival rate, was improved by melatonin co-treatment and, moreover, melatonin significantly reduced the frequency of thrombocytopenia, neurotoxicity, cardiotoxicity, stomatitis and asthenia. When melatonin (in combination with other therapies) has been initiated at an early stage, it seems to be more effective in terms of clinical status and survival of the patients.

Melatonin and Gastrointestinal Tract

Melatonin was initially considered to be exclusively derived from pineal gland. But, as shown originally by Raikhlin and Kvetnoy [75], the gastrointestinal tract (GIT) produces melatonin mainly in serotonin-rich entero-endocrine (EE) cells. The amount of melatonin in the gastrointestinal tissues is about 400 times larger than the content of melatonin in the pineal gland [76]. The function of GIT melatonin is not clear yet because the intestine is not only source but also sink of melatonin, brought by the circulation. It has been also demonstrated that luminal melatonin stimulates duodenal HCO_3^- secretion, which suggests that this indole may be a mediator of acid-induced secretion [77]. Furthermore its antioxidant properties, some of the melatonin effects on the GIT seem to be mediated by MT2 receptors [77]. However, the presence of MT1 receptor has been also demonstrated in human gallbladder epithelium from patients with cholelithiasis and gallbladder carcinoma [78].

Indometacin, a nonsteroideal anti-inflammatory drug (NSAID), presents an important side effect producing ulcerative lesions of the gastrointestinal tract. The mechanism by which indometacin induces ulcers seems to involve inhibition of prostaglandin synthesis and oxygen radical generation[79]. In an experimental rat model of indometacin toxicity, melatonin induced a protective effect against lesions to the gastric mucosa caused by a single oral dose of indometacin (20 mg/kg) [80]. Additionally, melatonin reduced the ulcer index (total mm^2 of damaged mucosa), lowered the level of thiobarbituric acid reactive substances (TBARS or lipid peroxidation products) and restored the depressed levels of GSH-Px [80]. Authors attributed melatonin´s protective actions to the indole´s radical scavenging activity and possibly to other unidentified mechanism.

In other similar study in which indometacin was used to induce both gastric damage and testicular oxidative stress, melatonin co-treatment would seem to be a reasonable treatment when using indometacin as well as other free-radical-generating drugs[81].

However, melatonin heals indometacin-induced stomach damage in rats, indeed, this effect was completely abolished when a melatonin receptor antagonist, luzindole, was administered [82]. Thus, melatonin seems to induce a protective effect on indometacin-induced stomach damage through antioxidative processes and mechanisms of melatonin receptor binding.

Melatonin may also be useful in the protection of gastric mucosa against noxious agents as salicylates. The gastric mucosal injury induced by acetylsalicylic acid is associated not only with their detrimental effect on prostaglandins biosynthesis but also with increased oxidative stress resulting from the neutrophil activation polymorphonuclear leukocytes (PMN). Despite these side effects, acetylsalicylic acid is among the most widely used medications in the world because of its high efficacy in reducing pain, inflammation, protection against stroke, and myocardial infarction.

A study on 21 (20-50 years) healthy male volunteers, with intact gastro-duodenal mucosa, concluded that pre-treatment with melatonin (5 mg 30 min prior to aspirin 2g) significantly decrease the gastric mucosal lesion induced by salicylate [83]. Two well-known anti-ulcer drugs, omeprazole and famotidine, were compared with melatonin, in terms of their ability to protect against acetylsalicylic-acid-induced gastric mucosal damage [84]. In this *in vivo* study, melatonin was more effective than either omeprazole or famotidine in preventing acetylsalicylic acid induced damage in the stomach. The authors of this study justify this indole protective mechanism due to its antioxidant properties.

Several studies have compared melatonin's efficacy in protecting against stress-induced gastric ulceration with widely used anti-ulcer medication such as ranitidine and omeprazole [85-87]. Ranitidine blocks histamine stimulated acid secretion in the stomach while omeprazole, completely interrupts acid secretion.

Both drugs however, have side effects including, among others, headache, dizziness, diarrhea and skin rashes. In these studies, Melatonin was found to dose-dependently reduce gastric mucosal damage in these ulcerative models and to be more effective than ranitidine but less efficient than omeprazole in lowering the incidence of ulcers. It is noteworthy that when melatonin treatment was combined with either ranitidine or omeprazole the drugs were much more efficient in reducing stress-mediated mucosal breakdown in the stomach. Thus, in rats co-treated with melatonin and ranitidine or omeprazole the gastric mucosa was protected from ulcers at doses where either drug alone had no protective effect. This is important since by reducing the dose of either ranitidine or omeprazole, the side effects also would likely be eliminated or significantly suppressed. However, it seems that, in addition to its direct scavenging actions, melatonin has other indirect (antioxidative and otherwise) means by which it reduces damage to the lining of the stomach.

Infection with *Helicobacter pylori* (*H. pylori*) is a substantial public health problem that affects 20-50% of people in industrialized nations. *H. pylori* is associated with many gastro-duodenal disorders, including peptic ulcer disease, gastric carcinoma and gastric mucosa-associated lymphoid tissue (MALT) lymphoma. All international guidelines recommend eradication of *H. pylori* using the proton pump inhibitors, such as omeprazole, as well as the combinations of amoxicillin and clarithromycin. In a recent report by Celinski et al. [88] concluded that melatonin or L-tryptophan added to omeprazole treatment, significantly accelerates the healing rate of *H. pylori* infected chronic gastroduodenal ulcers compared to the healing rate obtained with omeprazole alone. In this line, in functional dyspepsia, especially when coexisting with *H. pylori* infection, melatonin significantly reduces the oxidative DNA damage of gastric mucosa [89].

Inflammatory bowel disease (IBD) encompass several chronic inflammatory conditions, most significantly ulcerative colitis (UC) and Crohn's disease (CD). The etiology of IBD is believed to involve several factors, including inflammation and oxidative stress [90]. Experimental data from *in vivo* and *in vitro* studies suggest that melatonin is an important regulator of both inflammation and motility in the GIT, thus suggesting that supplemental melatonin may have positive effects on colitis [91].

To date, there are only limited clinical data available (three published case reports) of on the therapeutic role of melatonin in IBD (Table 2). In one case report, after the self-administered use of melatonin, the patient observed that his ulcerative colitis (UC) symptoms were virtually absent [92]. In contrast, there are at least two descriptions of cases in which melatonin showed exacerbated symptoms associated with UC or Crohn's disease [93, 94], perhaps as consequence of the immunostimulatory role of this indoleamine [93]. However, Clinical trials should be performed to evaluate a possible beneficial or detrimental effect of melatonin in IBD; presently available literature is inconclusive, though basic studies strongly suggest beneficial effects.

The antioxidant effects of melatonin, with the subsequent protective effects on GIT mucosa, would makes melatonin an excellent treatment choice when associated with drugs that cause mucosa damage. Thus, melatonin should be also taken into consideration for the treatment of GIT problems.

Table 2. Case reports of melatonin self-administration in patients with ulcerative colitis and Crohn's disease

Autor	Age, gender, disease	Treatment	Dose	Result
Maldonado et al.[93]	56, male, UC	Added melatonin to the otherwise unchanged drug treatment (salazosulfapyridine, corticosteroids)	3 mg/od	Two months later, the patient started to experience the symptoms of active UC, including bloody diarrhea.
Mann et al.[92]	47, male, UC	Added melatonin to an existing medication of mesalamine due to ongoing bloody diarrhea	3 mg/od	Symptoms resolved fast (2–3 d) and the beneficial effect was long lasting.
Calvo et al.[94]	35, female, UC	After becoming pregnant, the patient interrupted the treatment with melatonin, corticoids and salazosulfapyridine and symptoms of CD emerged again	3 mg/od	Recurrence of diarrhea and abdominal cramps within 4 days.

Melatonin and Endocrine Diseases

Diabetes mellitus is a chronic metabolic disorder characterized by hyperglycemia and caused by a deficiency of insulin, often combined with insulin resistance. Like melatonin, insulin levels show a circadian rhythm in humans that changes in an opposite manner to melatonin [95]. A decrease in melatonin secretion has been linked to many diseases, including diabetes [96]. It is known that melatonin mediates signal transduction in pancreatic β-cells by MT1 and MT2 receptors, leading to an increase or a decrease in the production of insulin [96]. Interestingly, a combination therapy of insulin plus melatonin has been postulated to decrease oxidative stress that originates exacerbated diabetic pathology. In this line of research, the combination of insulin (6 U/kg, subcutaneously (s.c.) and melatonin (10 mg/kg, i.p.) administered for 8 weeks, reduces hyperglycemia, oxidative stress and restores endothelial function completely in diabetic rats induced by streptozotocin injection [97]. In this context, it has been recently discovered that co-administration of nicotinamide, a Poly (ADP-ribose) polymerase inhibitor (100 and 300 mg/kg) and melatonin (3 and 10 mg/kg) for two weeks has larger neuroprotective effects against diabetic neuropathy than the two drugs separately [98].

Another example of the combination therapy benefits is a novel study in patients poorly controlled with metformin. Treatment with melatonin (10 mg) and zinc acetate (50 mg), in a single daily dose, significantly reduced total cholesterol (TC), triglycerides (TG), and low-density lipoprotein cholesterol (LDL-C) plasma levels. In addition, melatonin and zinc treatment acetate significantly reduced MAU after 30 and 90 days of treatment in type 2 diabetic patients [99]. The combined use of melatonin with other drugs could be an adjuvant in the antidiabetic therapy. However, much more research investigations and clinical trials are required to turn this into an actual therapy in patients.

Metabolic syndrome is a combination of several risk factors that increase the chance of developing heart disease and diabetes mellitus. These are: Obesity, elevated plasma levels of TG and low of HDL, hypertension and hyperglycemia. It is well known that melatonin supplementation significantly reduces the body weight and the mass of white adipose tissue in animal models of diet-induced obesity [100]. Furthermore, body weight was increased in pinealectomized rats, and this was reversed by melatonin administration (30 mg/kg day for 3 weeks). In addition melatonin treatment for 8-12 weeks (4-10 mg/kg) also reduced plasma glucose, leptin, TG and TC levels of the rat models of high fat diet-induced obesity [101, 102]. Another example of the beneficial effects of melatonin are research conducted in Zucker diabetic fatty (ZDF) rats in which melatonin treatment (10 mg/kg/day) for 6 weeks significantly reduced the levels of TG, low-density-lipoprotein (LDL) cholesterol and serum free fatty acids in ZDF rats. Also, melatonin lowered insulinemia, hyperglycemia and HbA1c [103, 104]. Despite these beneficial effects, no clinical trials have evaluated the weight lowering potential of melatonin in humans. Hyperthyroidism is another of the most common metabolic disorders. It produces an excess of thyroid gland function that leads to hypersecretion of thyroid hormones (thyroxin (T4) free triiodothyronine (T3) free, or both) and subsequently abnormally high plasma levels of these hormones. In this hypermetabolic state, the increase of free radicals as well as lipid peroxidation is patent [105, 106]. That is why melatonin may be useful in this disease, because it has scavenger properties and also protective effects against different models of oxidative stress [38, 107, 108]. The studies carried out on patients with hypo- and hyperthyroidism concludes that the circadian rhythm of melatonin secretion is not altered [109]. However, this does not mean that no relationship exists between them, since pinealectomy together with hyperthyroidism further increased the levels of malondialdehyde (MDA), a marker of oxidative damage, while reducing levels of glutathione (GSH), a marker of antioxidant systems [110]. Interestingly, melatonin treatment (3 mg/kg/day intraperitoneal) for three weeks restored the levels of MDA and GSH (brain, liver and heart tissues) in hypertensive rats induced by L-thyroxin. In addition, high-dose melatonin treatment may decrease the hyperthyroidism-induced disturbances of lipid peroxidation and anti-oxidant enzyme activity and oxidative damage by restoring blood malondialdehyde, glutathione and superoxide dismutase levels in the same experimental model of hyperthyroidism [111, 112]. Although these studies are promising, much more research is needed to know whether melatonin can be established as an adjuvant treatment in hyperthyroidism, to improve the oxidative stress and lipid oxidation, currently there are not enough trials which combine melatonin and antithyroid drugs such as methimazole or propylthiouracil.

Melatonin and Autoimmune Diseases

Immune mechanisms are regulated by a complex neuro-endocrine network [113]. Since melatonin is produced not only by the pineal gland, but also in the retina and in other parts of the body, this indole would be able to modulate immune functions through its neuro-endocrine action [114]. Although many studies involve melatonin as a positive regulator of immune system, other reports have also suggested that melatonin may act as an anti-inflammatory agent through inhibition of immune responses. The potential use of melatonin as a pharmaceutical agent derives from numerous *in vitro* studies where melatonin doses exceeding the nocturnal plasma levels are required to exert clear effects. Thus, considering melatonin as an immune modulatory agent with multiple anti-inflammatory and antioxidant effects [74] generally would seemingly favour its clinical application in some of these conditions. However, its immunostimulatory and antiapoptotic actions can theoretically promote autoimmune diseases. Which use is discouraged. It seems that melatonin may differentially modulate the immune responses in a dose-dependent manner *in vitro* and *in vivo*. Low-dose melatonin may restore attenuated T-cell activity and increase Th1 cytokine levels [115]. In contrast, high-dose melatonin significantly reduced the humoral response in rats. This may partially explain why the dosage of melatonin used to study autoimmune diseases.

The protective role of melatonin has also been demonstrated reducing significant side effects caused by immunosuppressive agents as cyclosporine. While the mechanisms that account for the toxicity of this drug are unknown, the experimental data suggest that free radical generation at these sites may be responsible for the liver and kidney damage [116]. Considering this, nephropathy and ciclosporin-induced morphological damage to the renal cortex may be prevented by melatonin administration due to its antioxidative capacity [117]. The liver also exhibits damage after ciclosporin treatment, however melatonin provides a significant protection in this organ when is functionally and biochemically injured by ciclosporin [118].

In the context of autoimmune diseases, given that melatonin is generally considered to be immunoenhancing, the question whether it should be taken by individuals with an autoimmune disease has been raised. On the other hand, melatonin exhibits both anti-inflammatory and immunomodulatory activities by regulating cytokine production of immunocompetent cells. From these considerations, could be melatonin considered effective in improving the clinical course of autoimmune inflammatory diseases?

For individuals with chronic sarcoidosis who do not respond to corticosteroids, melatonin may be an effective alternative therapy [119]. But, nocturnal asthma is associated with elevation and phase delay of peak serum melatonin levels. Elevated melatonin levels might contribute to the pathogenesis of nocturnal asthma [120].

Multiple sclerosis (MS) is an autoimmune demyelinating disease of the central nervous system (CNS) that develops in genetically susceptible individuals and may require additional environmental triggers causing immune dysregulation leading to neuroinflammation and degeneration [121]. Prior reports have documented melatonin levels to be inversely correlated with MS disease activity [122]. IFN-β, which is an approved disease modifying drug for relapsing MS, was also found to increase melatonin levels [123]. These findings may be explained by recent evidence suggesting that melatonin has anti-inflammatory effects, anti-oxidative properties and it may exert favorable effects in diseases such as MS, where axonal loss is part of the pathogenesis and seems to be induced, at least partially, by oxidative stress.

Due it´s antioxidant activity, melatonin could be beneficial in rheumatoid arthritis (RA) However; most of the studies addressing the effect of melatonin on the immune system report an immunoenhancing effect. Melatonin is recognized to increase the production of Th1-type and inflammatory cytokines in RA and to enhance both cell mediated and humoral responses [124]. In this situation, addition of exogenous melatonin would hardly exert any significant therapeutic effect in RA.

Melatonin and Infectious Diseases

Melatonin, in addition to its antioxidative and immunostimulatory properties, also possesses antibacterial and antiviral activity [125]. Melatonin participates in various functions of the body, among which its immunomodulatory role has assumed considerable significance in recent years. Melatonin receptors and signaling mechanisms are detectable in immune system cells [126]. Since it was demonstrated that inhibition of melatonin synthesis causes inhibition of cellular and humoral immune responses in mice [127], many studies have shown that melatonin affects both cellular and humoral of the immune response [128]. Its immunoregulatory role has a cyclicity which shows both circadian and seasonally dependent characteristics [129]. In humans, proinflammatory cytokines such as IFN-α and IFN-γ are increased during winter compared to the summer season [130]. Increases in IFN-γ and decreases in IL-10 were reported in a study undertaken in Antarctica during the winter season [131]. Melatonin significantly prevents liver injury in mice during malaria, reducing the levels of serum transaminases, alkaline phosphatase and bilirubin content, which are indices of hepatic cell damage. This hepatoprotective effect is due to the antiapoptotic actions of melatonin [132]. Furthermore, the combined actions of zinc and melatonin have beneficial effects in counteracting parasite-induced immune dysregulation, protecting animals against the harmful actions of chronic *Trypanosoma cruzi* infection, protozoan parasite which produce Chagas' disease [133].

In humans, Gitto et al. [134] used melatonin to treat newborns who were suffering with severe sepsis. Melatonin (two doses of 10 mg with a 1-h interval) significantly reduced several parameters of sepsis such as lipid peroxidation products and death in the treated neonates compared with controls. In this study, 30% of septic children who were not treated with melatonin died within 72 h after diagnosis of sepsis and, none of the 10 septic newborns treated with melatonin died. Melatonin treatment, in combination with magnesium, phosphate and fatty acids, was tested in a single blind, randomized study in which 70 patients showing symptoms of infection with Herpes virus; another 75 patients received treatment of 200 mg Acyclovir. 95.7% of patients treated with melatonin reported a complete regression of symptoms after 7 days, whereas only 85.3% of those treated with Acyclovir reported regression of symptoms in the same period [135].

Melatonin in Cardiovascular Diseases

Cardiovascular diseases (coronary heart disease, hypertension, ischemia/reperfusion (I/R), etc.) are the major cause of disability and mortality in most developed countries.

Hypertension is recognized as a multi-factorial situation resulting from the effect of a combination of environmental and genetic factors. Early data demonstrated that hypertension is the major factor in the development of heart failure. The use of melatonin as an antihypertensive, antioxidant and anti-ischemic drug has been explored and opens new opportunities for the management of cardiovascular dysfunction and disease. The hypotheses to explain the hypotensive effects of melatonin include its endothelium-relaxing effects, a lowering of catecholamine levels, its function as a potent scavenger of free radicals (which negatively influence blood Pressure), or epigenetic mechanisms at the level of the area postrema [136]; to date, the precise mechanisms of melatonin's hypotensive effects remain unknown.

There are numerous pharmaceutical agents in use to reduce hypertension. Moreover, the majority of these drugs have recognized negative side-effects. One infrequently mentioned side-effect of the use of beta-adrenergic blocking agents is the inhibition of the night-time rise in endogenous melatonin production and secretion [137]. This may be of special importance given that experimental findings have identified melatonin itself as an antihypertensive agent [136, 138].

The use of melatonin either alone or in combination with other antihypertensive drugs was assessed in three different randomized trials [139-141]. In the first of these [139] administration of melatonin alone (6 mg at 22.00h) or in combination with inhibitors of the angiotensin-converting enzyme (ACE) had hypotensive and vasodilating effects.

The second study [140] was focused on the antihypertensive effects of the association of melatonin with moxonidine (MOX) (a centrally acting antihypertensive drug similar to clonidine). In this case, MOX had a pronounced antihypertensive effect; however, addition of melatonin to MOX resulted in a greater antihypertensive effects and normalization of circadian rhythms of BP and heart rate. In the third clinical trial [141] patients treated with caposide-50 (C-50) (combination of a diuretic such as hydrochlorothiazide plus captopril, an

ACE inhibitor) combined with melatonin showed a more pronounced decline of systolic, diastolic and mean BP than those patients receiving C-50 alone.

I/R occurs when the blood supply to an organ or region is temporarily interrupted and then restored. Much of the tissue destruction that occurs during I/R injury in the heart is a result of derivatives of oxygen; these include free radicals and their by-products. But, the mechanism for the enhanced ROS generation as well as cellular and subcellular targets of ROS attack is not totally known. The initial studies related to the ability of melatonin to limit cardiac damage and restore function of the ischemic/reperfused heart are summarized in an interesting review performed by Reiter and Tan [142]. However, despite some clinical trials, still in progress, to study whether melatonin confers cardio-protection against I/R injury [143], the role of melatonin in the treatment of patients with ischemic heart disease has not been widely investigated.

Stroke (hypoxia/ischemia or ischemia) is the second leading cause of death throughout the world. Nowadays, limited therapeutic treatments are available clinically and these treatments are only applicable to highly selected groups. Tissue plasminogen activator (t-PA), which is the only US Food and Drug Administration (FDA)-approved drug for acute stroke treatment, and prourokinase used for thrombolysis and modified viper venom used for defibrinogenation need to be applied to patients within three to six hours, and it has been noted that these agents increase incidence of intracerebral hemorrhage.

Abundant literature demonstrated that administering melatonin significantly reduces brain infarction and neurological deficits. Thus, when melatonin administered in combination with t-PA, ameliorates brain damage caused for the thrombolytic agent in animal stroke models [144]. Cumulatively, in an acute stage of cerebral hypoxia/ischemia melatonin shows a capacity to reduce brain damage by I) reducing oxidative stress, II) promoting mitochondrial functions, III) decreasing excitotoxicity, IV) suppressing inflammation and V) diminishing apoptosis.

Conclusion

Almost daily, publications appear which examine the efficiency of melatonin to counteract the toxic reactions of drugs and other processes that generate free radicals and associated reactants. It is not possible to summarize herein all the data which document the clinically relevant aspects of melatonin about several diseases. In many occasions we have heard the ironic comment that ''melatonin helps against everything'', perhaps in reference to the exceptional pleiotropy of this neurohormone and its beneficial effects in several diseases. Mechanistically, melatonin has a variety of actions such as a direct free radical scavenger activity, its indirect antioxidant properties, it anti-inflammatory and neuromodulatory effects. As we described in this review, for example, melatonin´s cognitive benefits have been demonstrated either in AD patients or in AD mice, its potential role in immune regulation, and the action of melatonin alone or in combination with other drugs may be used to prevent tumor initiation, promotion, and progression. Another possible use of melatonin alone or combined with other drugs would be for the treatment of several psychiatric disorders due to its anxiolytic, sedative, anticonvulsant and anti-hypertensive properties.

Considering melatonin's low toxicity and high efficacy in reducing oxidative damage in animals, it spectrum of uses seems to be wide and its marked potential for improving human health, it should be earnestly considered for use in clinical trials, either as a single molecule and/or in combination with other drugs.

References

[1] Reiter, R. J.,Paredes, S. D.,Manchester, L. C.,Tan, D. X. Reducing oxidative/nitrosative stress: a newly-discovered genre for melatonin. *Critical reviews in biochemistry and molecular biology*, 2009 44,175-200.

[2] Dubocovich, M. L.,Markowska, M. Functional MT1 and MT2 melatonin receptors in mammals. *Endocrine,* 2005 27,101-110.

[3] Nosjean, O.,Ferro, M.,Coge, F.,Beauverger, P.,Henlin, J. M.,Lefoulon, F.,Fauchere, J. L.,Delagrange, P.,Canet, E.,Boutin, J. A. Identification of the melatonin-binding site MT3 as the quinone reductase 2. *The Journal of biological chemistry,* 2000 275,31311-31317.

[4] Rafii-El-Idrissi, M.,Calvo, J. R.,Harmouch, A.,Garcia-Maurino, S.,Guerrero, J. M. Specific binding of melatonin by purified cell nuclei from spleen and thymus of the rat. *Journal of neuroimmunology*, 1998 86,190-197.

[5] Hardeland, R. Antioxidative protection by melatonin: multiplicity of mechanisms from radical detoxification to radical avoidance. *Endocrine*, 2005 27,119-130.

[6] Reiter, R. J. Interactions of the pineal hormone melatonin with oxygen-centered free radicals: a brief review. Brazilian journal of medical and biological research = Revista brasileira de pesquisas medicas e biologicas / *Sociedade Brasileira de Biofisica* [et al], 1993 26,1141-1155.

[7] Tan, D. X.,Manchester, L. C.,Terron, M. P.,Flores, L. J.,Reiter, R. J. One molecule, many derivatives: a never-ending interaction of melatonin with reactive oxygen and nitrogen species? *Journal of pineal research, 2007 42,28-42.*

[8] Hardeland, R.,Cardinali, D. P.,Srinivasan, V.,Spence, D. W.,Brown, G. M.,Pandi-Perumal, S. R. Melatonin--a pleiotropic, orchestrating regulator molecule. *Progress in neurobiology*, 2011 93,350-384.

[9] Reiter, R. J.,Tan, D. X.,Sainz, R. M.,Mayo, J. C.,Lopez-Burillo, S. Melatonin: reducing the toxicity and increasing the efficacy of drugs. *The Journal of pharmacy and pharmacology,* 2002 54,1299-1321.

[10] Korkmaz, A.,Reiter, R. J. Epigenetic regulation: a new research area for melatonin? *Journal of pineal research*, 2008 44,41-44.

[11] Reiter, R. J. Oxidative damage in the central nervous system: protection by melatonin. Progress in neurobiology, 1998 56,359-384.

[12] Reiter, R. J.,Blask, D. E.,Talbot, J. A.,Barnett, M. P. Nature and the time course of seizures associated with surgical removal of the pineal gland from parathyroidectomized rats. *Experimental neurology*, 1973 38,386-397.

[13] Mevissen, M.,Ebert, U. Anticonvulsant effects of melatonin in amygdala-kindled rats. *Neuroscience letters*, 1998 257,13-16.

[14] Janjoppi, L.,Silva De Lacerda, A. F.,Scorza, F. A.,Amado, D.,Cavalheiro, E. A.,Arida, R. M. Influence of pinealectomy on the amygdala kindling development in rats. *Neuroscience letters*, 2006 392,150-153.

[15] Borowicz, K. K.,Kaminski, R.,Gasior, M.,Kleinrok, Z.,Czuczwar, S. J. Influence of melatonin upon the protective action of conventional anti-epileptic drugs against maximal electroshock in mice. *Eur. Neuropsychopharmacol.*, 1999 9,185-190.

[16] Yahyavi-Firouz-Abadi, N.,Tahsili-Fahadan, P.,Riazi, K.,Ghahremani, M. H.,Dehpour, A. R. Involvement of nitric oxide pathway in the acute anticonvulsant effect of melatonin in mice. *Epilepsy Res.*, 2006 68,103-113.

[17] Musshoff, U.,Speckmann, E. J. Diurnal actions of melatonin on epileptic activity in hippocampal slices of rats. Life sciences, 2003 73,2603-2610.

[18] Stewart, L. S.,Leung, L. S. Hippocampal melatonin receptors modulate seizure threshold. *Epilepsia,* 2005 46,473-480.

[19] Gupta, M.,Aneja, S.,Kohli, K. Add-on melatonin improves quality of life in epileptic children on valproate monotherapy: a randomized, double-blind, placebo-controlled trial. *Epilepsy and behavior* : EandB, 2004 5,316-321.

[20] Monteleone, P.,Natale, M.,La Rocca, A.,Maj, M. Decreased nocturnal secretion of melatonin in drug-free schizophrenics: no change after subchronic treatment with antipsychotics. *Neuropsychobiology*, 1997 36,159-163.

[21] Sandyk, R.,Kay, S. R. The relationship of pineal calcification to cortical atrophy in schizophrenia. *The International journal of neuroscience*, 1991 57,179-191.

[22] Potvin, S.,Stip, E.,Sepehry, A. A.,Gendron, A.,Bah, R.,Kouassi, E. Inflammatory cytokine alterations in schizophrenia: a systematic quantitative review. *Biol. Psychiatry*, 2008 63,801-808.

[23] Miller, B. J.,Buckley, P.,Seabolt, W.,Mellor, A.,Kirkpatrick, B. Meta-analysis of cytokine alterations in schizophrenia: clinical status and antipsychotic effects. *Biol. Psychiatry,* 70,663-671.

[24] Maldonado, M. D.,Reiter, R. J.,Perez-San-Gregorio, M. A. Melatonin as a potential therapeutic agent in psychiatric illness. *Hum. Psychopharmacol.*, 2009 24,391-400.

[25] Maldonado, M. D.,Perez-San-Gregorio, M. A.,Reiter, R. J. The role of melatonin in the immuno-neuro-psychology of mental disorders. *Recent Pat. CNS Drug Discov.*, 2009 4,61-69.

[26] Chang, H. M.,Wu, U. I.,Lan, C. T. Melatonin preserves longevity protein (sirtuin 1) expression in the hippocampus of total sleep-deprived rats. *Journal of pineal research*, 2009 47,211-220.

[27] Shieh, J. M.,Wu, H. T.,Cheng, K. C.,Cheng, J. T. Melatonin ameliorates high fat diet-induced diabetes and stimulates glycogen synthesis via a PKCzeta-Akt-GSK3beta pathway in hepatic cells. *Journal of pineal research,* 2009 47,339-344.

[28] Martin, M.,Macias, M.,Leon, J.,Escames, G.,Khaldy, H.,Acuna-Castroviejo, D. Melatonin increases the activity of the oxidative phosphorylation enzymes and the production of ATP in rat brain and liver mitochondria. *The international journal of biochemistry and cell biology*, 2002 34,348-357.

[29] Ehrnhoefer, D. E.,Wong, B. K.,Hayden, M. R. Convergent pathogenic pathways in Alzheimer's and Huntington's diseases: shared targets for drug development. *Nat. Rev. Drug Discov.,* 10,853-867.

[30] He, H.,Dong, W.,Huang, F. Anti-amyloidogenic and anti-apoptotic role of melatonin in Alzheimer disease. *Current neuropharmacology,* 8,211-217.

[31] Benitez-King, G.,Tunez, I.,Bellon, A.,Ortiz, G. G.,Anton-Tay, F. Melatonin prevents cytoskeletal alterations and oxidative stress induced by okadaic acid in N1E-115 cells. *Experimental neurology*, 2003 182,151-159.

[32] Li, X. C.,Wang, Z. F.,Zhang, J. X.,Wang, Q.,Wang, J. Z. Effect of melatonin on calyculin A-induced tau hyperphosphorylation. *European journal of pharmacology*, 2005 510,25-30.

[33] Perry, E. K.,Morris, C. M.,Court, J. A.,Cheng, A.,Fairbairn, A. F.,Mckeith, I. G.,Irving, D.,Brown, A.,Perry, R. H. Alteration in nicotine binding sites in Parkinson's disease, Lewy body dementia and Alzheimer's disease: possible index of early neuropathology. *Neuroscience*, 1995 64,385-395.

[34] Carneiro, R. C.,Cipolla-Neto, J.,Markus, R. P. Diurnal variation of the rat vas deferens contraction induced by stimulation of presynaptic nicotinic receptors and pineal function. *The Journal of pharmacology and experimental therapeutics*, 1991 259,614-619.

[35] Markus, R. P.,Zago, W. M.,Carneiro, R. C. Melatonin modulation of presynaptic nicotinic acetylcholine receptors in the rat vas deferens. *The Journal of pharmacology and experimental therapeutics*, 1996 279,18-22.

[36] Cecon, E.,Markus, R. P. Relevance of the chronobiological and non-chronobiological actions of melatonin for enhancing therapeutic efficacy in neurodegenerative disorders. *Recent patents on endocrine, metabolic and immune drug discovery*, 5,91-99.

[37] Romero, A.,Egea, J.,Garcia, A. G.,Lopez, M. G. Synergistic neuroprotective effect of combined low concentrations of galantamine and melatonin against oxidative stress in SH-SY5Y neuroblastoma cells. *Journal of pineal research*, 49,141-148.

[38] Feng, Z.,Qin, C.,Chang, Y.,Zhang, J. T. Early melatonin supplementation alleviates oxidative stress in a transgenic mouse model of Alzheimer's disease. *Free radical biology and medicine*, 2006 40,101-109.

[39] Olcese, J. M.,Cao, C.,Mori, T.,Mamcarz, M. B.,Maxwell, A.,Runfeldt, M. J.,Wang, L.,Zhang, C.,Lin, X.,Zhang, G.,Arendash, G. W. Protection against cognitive deficits and markers of neurodegeneration by long-term oral administration of melatonin in a transgenic model of Alzheimer disease. *Journal of pineal research*, 2009 47,82-96.

[40] Spuch, C.,Antequera, D.,Isabel Fernandez-Bachiller, M.,Isabel Rodriguez-Franco, M.,Carro, E. A new tacrine-melatonin hybrid reduces amyloid burden and behavioral deficits in a mouse model of Alzheimer's disease. *Neurotoxicity research*, 17,421-431.

[41] Asayama, K.,Yamadera, H.,Ito, T.,Suzuki, H.,Kudo, Y.,Endo, S. Double blind study of melatonin effects on the sleep-wake rhythm, cognitive and non-cognitive functions in Alzheimer type dementia. *J. Nippon Med. Sch.*, 2003 70,334-341.

[42] Furio, A. M.,Brusco, L. I.,Cardinali, D. P. Possible therapeutic value of melatonin in mild cognitive impairment: a retrospective study. *Journal of pineal research*, 2007 43,404-409.

[43] Singer, C.,Tractenberg, R. E.,Kaye, J.,Schafer, K.,Gamst, A.,Grundman, M.,Thomas, R.,Thal, L. J. A multicenter, placebo-controlled trial of melatonin for sleep disturbance in Alzheimer's disease. *Sleep*, 2003 26,893-901.

[44] Gehrman, P. R.,Connor, D. J.,Martin, J. L.,Shochat, T.,Corey-Bloom, J.,Ancoli-Israel, S. Melatonin fails to improve sleep or agitation in double-blind randomized placebo-

controlled trial of institutionalized patients with Alzheimer disease. *Am. J. Geriatr. Psychiatry*, 2009 17,166-169.

[45] Acuna-Castroviejo, D.,Coto-Montes, A.,Gaia Monti, M.,Ortiz, G. G.,Reiter, R. J. Melatonin is protective against MPTP-induced striatal and hippocampal lesions. *Life sciences*, 1997 60,PL23-29.

[46] Thomas, B.,Mohanakumar, K. P. Melatonin protects against oxidative stress caused by 1-methyl-4-phenyl-1,2,3,6-tetrahydropyridine in the mouse nigrostriatum. *Journal of pineal research,* 2004 36,25-32.

[47] Mayo, J. C.,Sainz, R. M.,Uria, H.,Antolin, I.,Esteban, M. M.,Rodriguez, C. Melatonin prevents apoptosis induced by 6-hydroxydopamine in neuronal cells: implications for Parkinson's disease. *Journal of pineal research*, 1998 24,179-192.

[48] Borah, A.,Mohanakumar, K. P. Melatonin inhibits 6-hydroxydopamine production in the brain to protect against experimental parkinsonism in rodents. *Journal of pineal research*, 2009 47,293-300.

[49] Acuna Castroviejo, D.,Lopez, L. C.,Escames, G.,Lopez, A.,Garcia, J. A.,Reiter, R. J. Melatonin-mitochondria interplay in health and disease. *Current topics in medicinal chemistry*, 11,221-240.

[50] Dowling, G. A.,Mastick, J.,Colling, E.,Carter, J. H.,Singer, C. M.,Aminoff, M. J. Melatonin for sleep disturbances in Parkinson's disease. *Sleep Med.*, 2005 6,459-466.

[51] Medeiros, C. A.,Carvalhedo De Bruin, P. F.,Lopes, L. A.,Magalhaes, M. C.,De Lourdes Seabra, M.,De Bruin, V. M. Effect of exogenous melatonin on sleep and motor dysfunction in Parkinson's disease. A randomized, double blind, placebo-controlled study. *J. Neurol.*, 2007 254,459-464.

[52] Aziz, N. A.,Pijl, H.,Frolich, M.,Schroder-Van Der Elst, J. P.,Van Der Bent, C.,Roelfsema, F.,Roos, R. A. Delayed onset of the diurnal melatonin rise in patients with Huntington's disease. *J. Neurol.,* 2009 256,1961-1965.

[53] Tunez, I.,Montilla, P.,Del Carmen Munoz, M.,Feijoo, M.,Salcedo, M. Protective effect of melatonin on 3-nitropropionic acid-induced oxidative stress in synaptosomes in an animal model of Huntington's disease. *Journal of pineal research*, 2004 37,252-256.

[54] Wang, X.,Sirianni, A.,Pei, Z.,Cormier, K.,Smith, K.,Jiang, J.,Zhou, S.,Wang, H.,Zhao, R.,Yano, H.,Kim, J. E.,Li, W.,Kristal, B. S.,Ferrante, R. J.,Friedlander, R. M. The melatonin MT1 receptor axis modulates mutant Huntingtin-mediated toxicity. *J. Neurosci.*, 31,14496-14507.

[55] Weishaupt, J. H.,Bartels, C.,Polking, E.,Dietrich, J.,Rohde, G.,Poeggeler, B.,Mertens, N.,Sperling, S.,Bohn, M.,Huther, G.,Schneider, A.,Bach, A.,Siren, A. L.,Hardeland, R.,Bahr, M.,Nave, K. A.,Ehrenreich, H. Reduced oxidative damage in ALS by high-dose enteral melatonin treatment. *Journal of pineal research*, 2006 41,313-323.

[56] Mediavilla, M. D.,Sanchez-Barcelo, E. J.,Tan, D. X.,Manchester, L.,Reiter, R. J. Basic mechanisms involved in the anti-cancer effects of melatonin. *Current medicinal chemistry,* 2010 17,4462-4481.

[57] Shirazi, A.,Ghobadi, G.,Ghazi-Khansari, M. A radiobiological review on melatonin: a novel radioprotector. *Journal of radiation research*, 2007 48,263-272.

[58] Sanchez-Barcelo, E. J.,Mediavilla, M. D.,Alonso-Gonzalez, C.,Reiter, R. J. Melatonin uses in oncology: breast cancer prevention and reduction of the side effects of chemotherapy and radiation. *Expert opinion on investigational drugs*, 2012 21,819-831.

[59] Singal, P. K.,Iliskovic, N. Doxorubicin-induced cardiomyopathy. *The New England journal of medicine*, 1998 339,900-905.

[60] Morishima, I.,Matsui, H.,Mukawa, H.,Hayashi, K.,Toki, Y.,Okumura, K.,Ito, T.,Hayakawa, T. Melatonin, a pineal hormone with antioxidant property, protects against adriamycin cardiomyopathy in rats. *Life sciences*, 1998 63,511-521.

[61] Abdel-Wahab, M. H.,Abd-Allah, A. R. Possible protective effect of melatonin and/or desferrioxamine against streptozotocin-induced hyperglycaemia in mice. Pharmacological research : *The official journal of the Italian Pharmacological Society*, 2000 41,533-537.

[62] Granzotto, M.,Rapozzi, V.,Decorti, G.,Giraldi, T. Effects of melatonin on doxorubicin cytotoxicity in sensitive and pleiotropically resistant tumor cells. *Journal of pineal research*, 2001 31,206-213.

[63] Reiter, R. J.,Tan, D. X.,Sainz, R. M.,Mayo, J. C. Melatonin protects the heart against both ischemia/reperfusion injury and chemotherapeutic drugs. *Cardiovascular drugs and therapy* / sponsored by the International Society of Cardiovascular Pharmacotherapy, 2002 16,5-6.

[64] Ravi, R.,Somani, S. M.,Rybak, L. P. Mechanism of cisplatin ototoxicity: antioxidant system. *Pharmacology and toxicology*, 1995 76,386-394.

[65] Rybak, L. P.,Ravi, R.,Somani, S. M. Mechanism of protection by diethyldithiocarbamate against cisplatin ototoxicity: antioxidant system. Fundamental and applied toxicology : *Official journal of the Society of Toxicology*, 1995 26,293-300.

[66] Lopez-Gonzalez, M. A.,Guerrero, J. M.,Rojas, F.,Delgado, F. Ototoxicity caused by cisplatin is ameliorated by melatonin and other antioxidants. *Journal of pineal research*, 2000 28,73-80.

[67] Hara, M.,Yoshida, M.,Nishijima, H.,Yokosuka, M.,Iigo, M.,Ohtani-Kaneko, R.,Shimada, A.,Hasegawa, T.,Akama, Y.,Hirata, K. Melatonin, a pineal secretory product with antioxidant properties, protects against cisplatin-induced nephrotoxicity in rats. *Journal of pineal research*, 2001 30,129-138.

[68] Hassan, M. I.,Ahmed, M. I.,Kassim, S. K.,Rashad, A.,Khalifa, A. Cis-platinum-induced immunosuppression: relationship to melatonin in human peripheral blood mononuclear cells. *Clinical biochemistry*, 1999 32,621-626.

[69] Futagami, M.,Sato, S.,Sakamoto, T.,Yokoyama, Y.,Saito, Y. Effects of melatonin on the proliferation and cis-diamminedichloroplatinum (CDDP) sensitivity of cultured human ovarian cancer cells. *Gynecologic oncology*, 2001 82,544-549.

[70] Arslan, S. O.,Zerin, M.,Vural, H.,Coskun, A. The effect of melatonin on bleomycin-induced pulmonary fibrosis in rats. *Journal of pineal research*, 2002 32,21-25.

[71] Anwar, M. M.,Mahfouz, H. A.,Sayed, A. S. Potential protective effects of melatonin on bone marrow of rats exposed to cytotoxic drugs. Comparative biochemistry and physiology Part A, *Molecular and integrative physiology*, 1998 119,493-501.

[72] Watanabe, M.,Kobayashi, Y.,Takahashi, N.,Kiguchi, K.,Ishizuka, B. Expression of melatonin receptor (MT1) and interaction between melatonin and estrogen in endometrial cancer cell line. *The journal of obstetrics and gynaecology resear*ch, 2008 34,567-573.

[73] Ruiz-Rabelo, J.,Vazquez, R.,Arjona, A.,Perea, D.,Montilla, P.,Tunez, I.,Muntane, J.,Padillo, J. Improvement of capecitabine antitumoral activity by melatonin in pancreatic cancer. *Pancreas*, 2011 40,410-414.

[74] Sanchez-Barcelo, E. J.,Mediavilla, M. D.,Tan, D. X.,Reiter, R. J. Clinical uses of melatonin: evaluation of human trials. *Current medicinal chemistry*, 2010 17,2070-2095.

[75] Raikhlin, N. T.,Kvetnoy, I. M. Melatonin and enterochromaffine cells. *Acta histochemica*, 1976 55,19-24.

[76] Bubenik, G. A. Thirty four years since the discovery of gastrointestinal melatonin. Journal of physiology and pharmacology : *An official journal of the Polish Physiological Society*, 2008 59 Suppl 2,33-51.

[77] Sjoblom, M.,Flemstrom, G. Melatonin in the duodenal lumen is a potent stimulant of mucosal bicarbonate secretion. *Journal of pineal research*, 2003 34,288-293.

[78] Aust, S.,Thalhammer, T.,Humpeler, S.,Jager, W.,Klimpfinger, M.,Tucek, G.,Obrist, P.,Marktl, W.,Penner, E.,Ekmekcioglu, C. The melatonin receptor subtype MT1 is expressed in human gallbladder epithelia. *Journal of pineal research*, 2004 36,43-48.

[79] Mahmud, T.,Scott, D. L.,Bjarnason, I. A unifying hypothesis for the mechanism of NSAID related gastrointestinal toxicity. *Annals of the rheumatic diseases,* 1996 55,211-213.

[80] Alarcon De La Lastra, C.,Motilva, V.,Martin, M. J.,Nieto, A.,Barranco, M. D.,Cabeza, J.,Herrerias, J. M. Protective effect of melatonin on indomethacin-induced gastric injury in rats. *Journal of pineal research*, 1999 26,101-107.

[81] Othman, A. I.,El-Missiry, M. A.,Amer, M. A. The protective action of melatonin on indomethacin-induced gastric and testicular oxidative stress in rats. Redox report : *Communications in free radical research*, 2001 6,173-177.

[82] Brzozowska, I.,Konturek, P. C.,Brzozowski, T.,Konturek, S. J.,Kwiecien, S.,Pajdo, R.,Drozdowicz, D.,Pawlik, M.,Ptak, A.,Hahn, E. G. Role of prostaglandins, nitric oxide, sensory nerves and gastrin in acceleration of ulcer healing by melatonin and its precursor, L-tryptophan. *Journal of pineal research*, 2002 32,149-162.

[83] Konturek, P. C.,Celinski, K.,Slomka, M.,Cichoz-Lach, H.,Burnat, G.,Naegel, A.,Bielanski, W.,Konturek, J. W.,Konturek, S. J. Melatonin and its precursor L-tryptophan prevent acute gastric mucosal damage induced by aspirin in humans. Journal of physiology and pharmacology : *An official journal of the Polish Physiological Society,* 2008 59 Suppl 2,67-75.

[84] Sener-Muratoglu, G.,Paskaloglu, K.,Arbak, S.,Hurdag, C.,Ayanoglu-Dulger, G. Protective effect of famotidine, omeprazole, and melatonin against acetylsalicylic acid-induced gastric damage in rats. *Digestive diseases and sciences*, 2001 46,318-330.

[85] Bandyopadhyay, D.,Biswas, K.,Bandyopadhyay, U.,Reiter, R. J.,Banerjee, R. K. Melatonin protects against stress-induced gastric lesions by scavenging the hydroxyl radical. *Journal of pineal research*, 2000 29,143-151.

[86] Bandyopadhyay, D.,Biswas, K.,Bhattacharyya, M.,Reiter, R. J.,Banerjee, R. K. Gastric toxicity and mucosal ulceration induced by oxygen-derived reactive species: protection by melatonin. *Current molecular medicine*, 2001 1,501-513.

[87] Bandyopadhyay, D.,Bandyopadhyay, A.,Das, P. K.,Reiter, R. J. Melatonin protects against gastric ulceration and increases the efficacy of ranitidine and omeprazole in reducing gastric damage. *Journal of pineal research*, 2002 33,1-7.

[88] Celinski, K.,Konturek, P. C.,Konturek, S. J.,Slomka, M.,Cichoz-Lach, H.,Brzozowski, T.,Bielanski, W. Effects of melatonin and tryptophan on healing of gastric and duodenal ulcers with Helicobacter pylori infection in humans. Journal of physiology

and pharmacology : *An official journal of the Polish Physiological Society*, 2011 62,521-526.

[89] Klupinska, G.,Poplawski, T.,Smigielski, J.,Blasiak, J.,Chojnacki, J. [The effect of melatonin on oxidative DNA damage in gastric mucosa cells of patients with functional dyspepsia]. Polski merkuriusz lekarski : organ Polskiego Towarzystwa Lekarskiego, 2009 26,366-369.

[90] Farrell, R. J.,Peppercorn, M. A. Ulcerative colitis. *Lancet*, 2002 359,331-340.

[91] Terry, P. D.,Villinger, F.,Bubenik, G. A.,Sitaraman, S. V. Melatonin and ulcerative colitis: evidence, biological mechanisms, and future research. *Inflammatory bowel diseases*, 2009 15,134-140.

[92] Mann, S. Melatonin for ulcerative colitis? *The American journal of gastroenterology*, 2003 98,232-233.

[93] Maldonado, M. D.,Calvo, J. R. Melatonin usage in ulcerative colitis: a case report. *Journal of pineal research*, 2008 45,339-340.

[94] Calvo, J. R.,Guerrero, J. M.,Osuna, C.,Molinero, P.,Carrillo-Vico, A. Melatonin triggers Crohn's disease symptoms. *Journal of pineal research*, 2002 32,277-278.

[95] Boden, G.,Ruiz, J.,Urbain, J. L.,Chen, X. Evidence for a circadian rhythm of insulin secretion. *Am. J. Physiol.*, 1996 271,E246-252.

[96] Peschke, E.,Muhlbauer, E. New evidence for a role of melatonin in glucose regulation. *Best Pract. Res. Clin. Endocrinol. Metab.*, 24,829-841.

[97] Paskaloglu, K.,Sener, G.,Ayangolu-Dulger, G. Melatonin treatment protects against diabetes-induced functional and biochemical changes in rat aorta and corpus cavernosum. *Eur. J. Pharmacol.,* 2004 499,345-354.

[98] Negi, G.,Kumar, A.,Kaundal, R. K.,Gulati, A.,Sharma, S. S. Functional and biochemical evidence indicating beneficial effect of Melatonin and Nicotinamide alone and in combination in experimental diabetic neuropathy. *Neuropharmacology*, 58,585-592.

[99] Kadhim, H. M.,Ismail, S. H.,Hussein, K. I.,Bakir, I. H.,Sahib, A. S.,Khalaf, B. H.,Hussain, S. A. Effects of melatonin and zinc on lipid profile and renal function in type 2 diabetic patients poorly controlled with metformin. *J. Pineal. Res.*, 2006 41,189-193.

[100] Tan, D. X.,Manchester, L. C.,Fuentes-Broto, L.,Paredes, S. D.,Reiter, R. J. Significance and application of melatonin in the regulation of brown adipose tissue metabolism: relation to human obesity. *Obes. Rev.,* 12,167-188.

[101] Prunet-Marcassus, B.,Desbazeille, M.,Bros, A.,Louche, K.,Delagrange, P.,Renard, P.,Casteilla, L.,Penicaud, L. Melatonin reduces body weight gain in Sprague Dawley rats with diet-induced obesity. *Endocrinology*, 2003 144,5347-5352.

[102] Rios-Lugo, M. J.,Cano, P.,Jimenez-Ortega, V.,Fernandez-Mateos, M. P.,Scacchi, P. A.,Cardinali, D. P.,Esquifino, A. I. Melatonin effect on plasma adiponectin, leptin, insulin, glucose, triglycerides and cholesterol in normal and high fat-fed rats. *J. Pineal. Res.,* 49,342-348.

[103] Agil, A.,Rosado, I.,Ruiz, R.,Figueroa, A.,Zen, N.,Fernandez-Vazquez, G. Melatonin improves glucose homeostasis in young Zucker diabetic fatty rats. *J. Pineal. Res.*, 52,203-210.

[104] Agil, A.,Navarro-Alarcon, M.,Ruiz, R.,Abuhamadah, S.,El-Mir, M. Y.,Vazquez, G. F. Beneficial effects of melatonin on obesity and lipid profile in young Zucker diabetic fatty rats. *J. Pineal. Res.*, 50,207-212.

[105] Komosinska-Vassev, K.,Olczyk, K.,Kucharz, E. J.,Marcisz, C.,Winsz-Szczotka, K.,Kotulska, A. Free radical activity and antioxidant defense mechanisms in patients with hyperthyroidism due to Graves' disease during therapy. *Clin. Chim. Acta*, 2000 300,107-117.

[106] Venditti, P.,Balestrieri, M.,Di Meo, S.,De Leo, T. Effect of thyroid state on lipid peroxidation, antioxidant defences, and susceptibility to oxidative stress in rat tissues. *J. Endocrinol.,* 1997 155,151-157.

[107] Huang, S. H.,Cao, X. J.,Liu, W.,Shi, X. Y.,Wei, W. Inhibitory effect of melatonin on lung oxidative stress induced by respiratory syncytial virus infection in mice. *J. Pineal. Res.,* 48,109-116.

[108] De Filippis, D.,Iuvone, T.,Esposito, G.,Steardo, L.,Arnold, G. H.,Paul, A. P.,De Man Joris, G.,De Winter Benedicte, Y. Melatonin reverses lipopolysaccharide-induced gastro-intestinal motility disturbances through the inhibition of oxidative stress. *J. Pineal. Res.*, 2008 44,45-51.

[109] Soszynski, P.,Zgliczynski, S.,Pucilowska, J. The circadian rhythm of melatonin in hypothyroidism and hyperthyroidism. *Acta Endocrinol.* (Copenh), 1988 119,240-244.

[110] Mogulkoc, R.,Baltaci, A. K.,Aydin, L.,Oztekin, E.,Tuncer, I. Pinealectomy increases oxidant damage in kidney and testis caused by hyperthyroidism in rats. *Cell Biochem. Funct.*, 2006 24,449-453.

[111] Baydas, B.,Meral, I. Effects of melatonin on lipid peroxidation and anti-oxidant enzyme activity in rats with experimentally induced hyperthyroidism. *Clin. Exp. Pharmacol. Physiol.*, 2005 32,541-544.

[112] Mogulkoc, R.,Baltaci, A. K.,Oztekin, E.,Aydin, L.,Sivrikaya, A. Melatonin prevents oxidant damage in various tissues of rats with hyperthyroidism. *Life Sci.,* 2006 79,311-315.

[113] Blalock, J. E. The syntax of immune-neuroendocrine communication. *Immunology today*, 1994 15,504-511.

[114] Radogna, F.,Diederich, M.,Ghibelli, L. Melatonin: a pleiotropic molecule regulating inflammation. *Biochemical pharmacology*, 2010 80,1844-1852.

[115] Carrillo-Vico, A.,Reiter, R. J.,Lardone, P. J.,Herrera, J. L.,Fernandez-Montesinos, R.,Guerrero, J. M.,Pozo, D. The modulatory role of melatonin on immune responsiveness. *Current opinion in investigational drugs*, 2006 7,423-431.

[116] Wolf, A.,Trendelenburg, C. F.,Diez-Fernandez, C.,Prieto, P.,Houy, S.,Trommer, W. E.,Cordier, A. Cyclosporine A-induced oxidative stress in rat hepatocytes. *The Journal of pharmacology and experimental therapeutics*, 1997 280,1328-1334.

[117] Kumar, K. V.,Naidu, M. U.,Shifow, A. A.,Prayag, A.,Ratnakar, K. S. Melatonin: an antioxidant protects against cyclosporine-induced nephrotoxicity. *Transplantation*, 1999 67,1065-1068.

[118] Kwak, C. S.,Mun, K. C. The beneficial effect of melatonin for cyclosporine hepatotoxicity in rats. *Transplantation proceedings*, 2000 32,2009-2010.

[119] Cagnoni, M. L.,Lombardi, A.,Cerinic, M. C.,Dedola, G. L.,Pignone, A. Melatonin for treatment of chronic refractory sarcoidosis. *Lancet*, 1995 346,1229-1230.

[120] Sutherland, E. R.,Ellison, M. C.,Kraft, M.,Martin, R. J. Elevated serum melatonin is associated with the nocturnal worsening of asthma. *The Journal of allergy and clinical immunology*, 2003 112,513-517.

[121] Hauser, S. L.,Oksenberg, J. R. The neurobiology of multiple sclerosis: genes, inflammation, and neurodegeneration. *Neuron*, 2006 52,61-76.

[122] Sandyk, R.,Awerbuch, G. I. Nocturnal plasma melatonin and alpha-melanocyte stimulating hormone levels during exacerbation of multiple sclerosis. *The International journal of neuroscience*, 1992 67,173-186.

[123] Melamud, L.,Golan, D.,Luboshitzky, R.,Lavi, I.,Miller, A. Melatonin dysregulation, sleep disturbances and fatigue in multiple sclerosis. *Journal of the neurological sciences*, 2012 314,37-40.

[124] Cutolo, M.,Maestroni, G. J. The melatonin-cytokine connection in rheumatoid arthritis. *Annals of the rheumatic diseases,* 2005 64,1109-1111.

[125] Tekbas, O. F.,Ogur, R.,Korkmaz, A.,Kilic, A.,Reiter, R. J. Melatonin as an antibiotic: new insights into the actions of this ubiquitous molecule. *J. Pineal. Res.*, 2008 44,222-226.

[126] Carrillo-Vico, A.,Reiter, R. J.,Lardone, P. J.,Herrera, J. L.,Fernandez-Montesinos, R.,Guerrero, J. M.,Pozo, D. The modulatory role of melatonin on immune responsiveness. *Curr. Opin. Investig. Drugs*, 2006 7,423-431.

[127] Maestroni, G. J.,Conti, A.,Pierpaoli, W. Role of the pineal gland in immunity. Circadian synthesis and release of melatonin modulates the antibody response and antagonizes the immunosuppressive effect of corticosterone. *J. Neuroimmunol.,* 1986 13,19-30.

[128] Guerrero, J. M.,Reiter, R. J. Melatonin-immune system relationships. *Curr. Top Med. Chem.,* 2002 2,167-179.

[129] Nelson, R. J.,Drazen, D. L. Melatonin mediates seasonal changes in immune function. Ann N Y Acad Sci, 2000 917,404-415.

[130] Katila, H.,Cantell, K.,Appelberg, B.,Rimon, R. Is there a seasonal variation in the interferon-producing capacity of healthy subjects? *J. Interferon Res.*, 1993 13,233-234.

[131] Shearer, W. T.,Lee, B. N.,Cron, S. G.,Rosenblatt, H. M.,Smith, E. O.,Lugg, D. J.,Nickolls, P. M.,Sharp, R. M.,Rollings, K.,Reuben, J. M. Suppression of human anti-inflammatory plasma cytokines IL-10 and IL-1RA with elevation of proinflammatory cytokine IFN-gamma during the isolation of the Antarctic winter. *J. Allergy Clin. Immunol.,* 2002 109,854-857.

[132] Guha, M.,Maity, P.,Choubey, V.,Mitra, K.,Reiter, R. J.,Bandyopadhyay, U. Melatonin inhibits free radical-mediated mitochondrial-dependent hepatocyte apoptosis and liver damage induced during malarial infection. *J. Pineal. Res.,* 2007 43,372-381.

[133] Brazao, V.,Del Vecchio Filipin, M.,Santello, F. H.,Caetano, L. C.,Abrahao, A. A.,Toldo, M. P.,Do Prado, J. C., Jr. Melatonin and zinc treatment: distinctive modulation of cytokine production in chronic experimental Trypanosoma cruzi infection. *Cytokine*, 56,627-632.

[134] Gitto, E.,Karbownik, M.,Reiter, R. J.,Tan, D. X.,Cuzzocrea, S.,Chiurazzi, P.,Cordaro, S.,Corona, G.,Trimarchi, G.,Barberi, I. Effects of melatonin treatment in septic newborns. *Pediatr. Res.,* 2001 50,756-760.

[135] Nunes Oda, S.,Pereira Rde, S. Regression of herpes viral infection symptoms using melatonin and SB-73: comparison with Acyclovir. *J. Pineal. Res.*, 2008 44,373-378.

[136] Reiter, R. J.,Tan, D. X.,Korkmaz, A. The circadian melatonin rhythm and its modulation: possible impact on hypertension. *Journal of hypertension Supplement : official journal of the International Society of Hypertension*, 2009 27,S17-20.

[137] Carpizo, R.,Martinez, A.,Mediavilla, D.,Gonzalez, M.,Abad, A.,Sanchez-Barcelo, E. J. Smith-Magenis syndrome: a case report of improved sleep after treatment with beta1-adrenergic antagonists and melatonin. *The Journal of pediatrics,* 2006 149,409-411.

[138] Simko, F.,Paulis, L. Melatonin as a potential antihypertensive treatment. *Journal of pineal research*, 2007 42,319-322.

[139] Zaslavskaia, R. M.,Biiasilov, N. S.,Akhmetov, K.,Teiblium, M. M. [Capozide-50 alone and in combination with melatonin in therapy of hypertension]. *Klinicheskaia meditsina*, 2000 78,39-41.

[140] Zaslavskaia, R. M.,Komarov, F. I.,Shakirova, A. N.,Teiblium, M. M.,Akhmetov, K. [Effect of moxonidine monotherapy and in combination with melatonin on hemodynamic parameters in patients with arterial hypertension*]. Klinicheskaia meditsina*, 2000 78,41-44.

[141] Zaslavskaia, R. M.,Shakirova, A. N.,Komarov, F. I.,Teiblium, M. M.,Akhmetov, K. [Effects of melatonin alone and in combination with aceten on chronostructure of diurnal hemodynamic rhythms in patients with hypertension stage II]. *Terapevticheskii arkhiv*, 1999 71,21-24.

[142] Reiter, R. J.,Tan, D. X. Melatonin: a novel protective agent against oxidative injury of the ischemic/reperfused heart. *Cardiovascular research*, 2003 58,10-19.

[143] Dominguez-Rodriguez, A.,Abreu-Gonzalez, P.,Garcia-Gonzalez, M. J.,Kaski, J. C.,Reiter, R. J.,Jimenez-Sosa, A. A unicenter, randomized, double-blind, parallel-group, placebo-controlled study of Melatonin as an Adjunct in patients with acute myocaRdial Infarction undergoing primary Angioplasty The Melatonin Adjunct in the acute myocaRdial Infarction treated with Angioplasty (MARIA) trial: study design and rationale. *Contemporary clinical trials*, 2007 28,532-539.

[144] Chen, T. Y.,Lee, M. Y.,Chen, H. Y.,Kuo, Y. L.,Lin, S. C.,Wu, T. S.,Lee, E. J. Melatonin attenuates the postischemic increase in blood-brain barrier permeability and decreases hemorrhagic transformation of tissue-plasminogen activator therapy following ischemic stroke in mice. *Journal of pineal research*, 2006 40,242-250.

[145] Barni, S.,Lissoni, P.,Cazzaniga, M.,Ardizzoia, A.,Meregalli, S.,Fossati, V.,Fumagalli, L.,Brivio, F.,Tancini, G. A randomized study of low-dose subcutaneous interleukin-2 plus melatonin versus supportive care alone in metastatic colorectal cancer patients progressing under 5-fluorouracil and folates. *Oncology*, 1995 52,243-245.

[146] Lissoni, P.,Barni, S.,Tancini, G.,Mainini, E.,Piglia, F.,Maestroni, G. J.,Lewinski, A. Immunoendocrine therapy with low-dose subcutaneous interleukin-2 plus melatonin of locally advanced or metastatic endocrine tumors. *Oncology*, 1995 52,163-166.

[147] Lissoni, P.,Barni, S.,Tancini, G.,Ardizzoia, A.,Tisi, E.,Angeli, M.,Rizzi, A. Intracavitary therapy of neoplastic effusions with cytokines: comparison among interferon alpha, beta and interleukin-2. Supportive care in cancer : *Official journal of the Multinational Association of Supportive Care in Cancer*, 1995 3,78-80.

[148] Lissoni, P.,Cazzaniga, M.,Tancini, G.,Scardino, E.,Musci, R.,Barni, S.,Maffezzini, M.,Meroni, T.,Rocco, F.,Conti, A.,Maestroni, G. Reversal of clinical resistance to LHRH analogue in metastatic prostate cancer by the pineal hormone melatonin:

efficacy of LHRH analogue plus melatonin in patients progressing on LHRH analogue alone. *European urology*, 1997 31,178-181.

[149] Lissoni, P.,Paolorossi, F.,Ardizzoia, A.,Barni, S.,Chilelli, M.,Mancuso, M.,Tancini, G.,Conti, A.,Maestroni, G. J. A randomized study of chemotherapy with cisplatin plus etoposide versus chemoendocrine therapy with cisplatin, etoposide and the pineal hormone melatonin as a first-line treatment of advanced non-small cell lung cancer patients in a poor clinical state. *Journal of pineal research*, 1997 23,15-19.

[150] Lissoni, P.,Tancini, G.,Paolorossi, F.,Mandala, M.,Ardizzoia, A.,Malugani, F.,Giani, L.,Barni, S. Chemoneuroendocrine therapy of metastatic breast cancer with persistent thrombocytopenia with weekly low-dose epirubicin plus melatonin: a phase II study. *Journal of pineal research*, 1999 26,169-173.

[151] Lissoni, P.,Barni, S.,Mandala, M.,Ardizzoia, A.,Paolorossi, F.,Vaghi, M.,Longarini, R.,Malugani, F.,Tancini, G. Decreased toxicity and increased efficacy of cancer chemotherapy using the pineal hormone melatonin in metastatic solid tumour patients with poor clinical status. *European journal of cancer*, 1999 35,1688-1692.

[152] Cerea, G.,Vaghi, M.,Ardizzoia, A.,Villa, S.,Bucovec, R.,Mengo, S.,Gardani, G.,Tancini, G.,Lissoni, P. Biomodulation of cancer chemotherapy for metastatic colorectal cancer: a randomized study of weekly low-dose irinotecan alone versus irinotecan plus the oncostatic pineal hormone melatonin in metastatic colorectal cancer patients progressing on 5-fluorouracil-containing combinations. *Anticancer research*, 2003 23,1951-1954.

[153] Lissoni, P. Biochemotherapy with standard chemotherapies plus the pineal hormone melatonin in the treatment of advanced solid neoplasms. *Pathologie-biologie*, 2007 55,201-204.

Declaration of interest: The authors report no conflicts of interest.

Index

A

B

C

D

E

F

G

H

I

J

K

L

M

Q

R

S

T

U

V